Health Education
Creating Strategies for School and Community Health

Glen G. Gilbert

Robin G. Sawyer

Department of Health Education
The University of Maryland
College Park, Maryland

JONES AND BARTLETT PUBLISHERS

BOSTON   LONDON

Editorial, Sales, and Customer Service Offices
Jones and Bartlett Publishers
One Exeter Plaza
Boston, MA 02116
1–800–832–0034
1–617–859–3900

Jones and Bartlett Publishers International
7 Melrose Terrace
London W6 7RL
England

Library of Congress Cataloging-in-Publication Data
Gilbert, Glen G. (Glen Gordon)
   Health education : creating strategies for school and community
health / Glen G. Gilbert, Robin G. Sawyer.
      p.   cm.
   Includes bibliographical references and index.
   ISBN 0–86720–812–0
   1. Health education—United States.   I. Sawyer, Robin G.
   II. Title.
   RA440.5.G48   1995
   613'.071'073—dc20   94–22602
                                                                              CIP

Acquisitions Editor: Joseph E. Burns
Production Editor: Anne Noonan
Manufacturing Buyer: Dana L. Cerrito
Design: Linda Zuk
Editorial Production Service: WordCrafters Editorial Services, Inc.
Typesetting: Sunrise Composition
Cover Design: Beth Santos
Printing and Binding: Book Press, Inc.
Cover Printing: New England Book Components

Quotations by Mohan Singh are from *Cosmic Reflections of Health for All* by Mohan Singh. Ottawa, Ontario: LeCercle des Amis de Mohan Singh, 1983.

Printed in the United States of America

98 97 96 95 94   10 9 8 7 6 5 4 3 2 1

Health Education

086 7208120

We dedicate this book to
Rosemarie, Jessica, Jennifer, and Jeffrey Gilbert
and
Anne Anderson-Sawyer, Katherine, Emily, Meg
and Gillian Sawyer

Contents

Chapter 3   SELECTING AN INTERVENTION/METHOD   47

Chapter 4   METHODS OF INSTRUCTION/INTERVENTION   87

Chapter 8   CONTROVERSIAL TOPICS   247

Appendix A   RESOURCES   279

Appendix B   YEAR 2000 OBJECTIVES   295

SUGGESTIONS FOR FURTHER READING   365

GLOSSARY   367

INDEX   373

Foreword

Having suffered the medieval torture of getting out a book manuscript of this magnitude and complexity, Professors Gilbert and Sawyer warrant the gratitude of the field. But more than size and complexity, the fruits of their labor fill a notable gap in the professional literature between the textbooks on needs assessment on the one side and those on evaluation on the other.

They also strike a balanced middle ground between the fuzzy philosophical precepts of health education and the potentially misplaced precision of prescriptive practice. By placing the question of pedagogy and the selection of instructional methods squarely in a diagnostic planning framework, they avoid the trap of suggesting that some methods are inherently superior to others. The diagnostic-planning approach makes the selection of educational methods context sensitive, culturally relevant, and technologically appropriate to the setting, the population of potential learners, and the resources available.

This book also acknowledges that health education, unlike many other areas of education practiced in schools and most continuing education for adults, must come to grips with behavioral outcomes. It is not enough in health education to be pedagogically correct, entertaining, engaging, and even captivating if nothing happens to improve health-related behavior. Cognitive and affective objectives must be tied very clearly to reducing health-risk behavior or increasing health-enhancing behavior if health education is to fulfill its ultimate mission. The discussion of objectives in this book relates learning objectives not only to behavioral outcomes, but also to the U.S. objectives for the nation in disease prevention and health promotion.

The authors get right down to basics, beginning with the techniques of writing health objectives. Their nuts-and-bolts approach to such topics is spiced with graphics, examples, procedural steps, and even whimsical and ironic aphorisms quoted from that sage of health education, Mohan Singh.

They take the various methods of experts and boil them down to a recommended protocol or worksheet. Their distillation of the myriad ways to express objectives, for example, is presented as a recipe for "self-contained objectives," complete with case studies, lists of suggested verbs, and "common mistakes" made in writing objectives.

They have tied their discussion of down-to-earth procedures to global and national perspectives and standards, such as the competencies expected of health education specialists for certification, the code of ethics of the Society for Public Health Education, and the U.S. objectives for the nation in disease prevention and health promotion.

They give due consideration to the ethical and environmental aspects of the teaching-learning relationship, including the emotional and physical environment in which learning is to occur, and the social and cultural circumstances of special populations.

This book should be expected to endure and grow through many editions with the rapidly expanding array of educational technologies and opportunities for health education in new settings and with new health threats.

Lawrence W. Green
Institute of Health Promotion Research
University of British Columbia
Vancouver, BC, Canada

Preface

The philosophy presented in this text is based in the premise that the core of health education is the *process* of health education. There are many other tools for health educators, such as epidemiology, statistics, and program planning, but what is truly unique about a health educator is the focus on the "doing." To be an effective health educator means that you are skilled in conducting health education. As educators we may have access to the best knowledge available, but unless we are skilled and effective deliverers of this information, the usefulness of our work is clearly compromised.

Health Education is dedicated to the proposition that we must be good at the doing. Further, it is our belief that health educators need a much more systematic approach to the selection of methods of intervention. This text is intended to assist the health educator in reducing the possibility of a poor performance by encouraging the systematic development of sound, effective, and appropriate presentation methods.

This text is designed for any health educator or would-be health educator who wishes to become proficient in conducting health education programs. The authors strongly believe that the skills necessary to plan successfully for, and deliver, effective health education programs are fundamentally the same, regardless of where they are practiced—in a classroom, a workplace, a hospital, or a community setting. The principles of sound methodology remain constant. Therefore, this text is designed for multiple settings. It addresses the needs of the so-called "generic" health educator, and provides the tools for making appropriate programming decisions based on the needs of the clients and the educational settings.

A variety of learning aids are incorporated into the book. Each chapter contains health educator competencies, case studies, objectives, questions, and exercises. Also included are a glossary, a comprehensive resource list, and up-to-date references.

The publisher will make available free to all qualified instructors an adopter's computer disk that contains the instructor's manual, which includes teaching aids, a sample course outline and syllabus, a test bank, a list of Healthy People 2000 objectives, and entry-level health education competencies. The computer disks are available in either Macintosh or IBM format from the publisher.

We know that a good text is a book that fulfills the user's needs. We seek to constantly improve the book and look forward to hearing from students, instructors, and professionals who may have a comment, an idea, or a suggestion regarding the text.

Acknowledgments

The authors wish to give special thanks to:

Carol Jackson and Sandy Walter of the Department of Health Education, University of Maryland, for the graphics used throughout the text.

Jill Black, Springfield College; Loren Bensley, Central Michigan University; Gerald S. Fain, and Karen Liller, University of South Florida; Onie Grosshans, University of Utah; Barbara J. Richards and B. E. Pruitt, Texas A & M University, for reviewing the text.

Marjorie Scaffa, Robert Gold, Lawrence Green, Gail Jacobs, Fran Gover, Bev Monis, Rosemarie Taylor, Jennifer Morrone-Joseph, Susan Karchmer, and Judy Yost.

Our many students over the years at the University of Maryland, University of Virginia, Portland State University, University of North Carolina at Greensboro, South Eugene High School, Colin Kelly Junior High School, Penge High School, London and Calverton School, and the many other schools where we have conducted workshops and classes.

Joe Burns and Anne Noonan of Jones and Bartlett Publishers, and Linda Zuk of WordCrafters Editorial Services.

About the Authors

Glen Gilbert   Glen is currently Professor and Chairperson of the Department of Health Education at the University of Maryland at College Park. He has taught university-level methods of instruction courses for over 10 years and has conducted in-service and consulting programs throughout the United States. He went on leave from his university post for two years to serve as Director of the School Health Initiative for the U.S. Department of Health and Human Services and worked with most states and with most federal agencies. As a former secondary school teacher and community health educator, he can relate to the real-world needs of health educators. He has authored over 70 professional publications and has taught at the University of Maryland, Portland State University, the University of North Carolina at Greensboro, and the Ohio State University. He is a certified health education specialist through examination and has been a health educator for over 20 years.

Robin Sawyer   Robin is currently an Assistant Professor at the University of Maryland at College Park, where he has achieved popular distinction as an outstanding lecturer, teacher, and health educator. A native of Great Britain, Robin has worked in health education for many years on both sides of the Atlantic and has taught at the middle and high school levels in both countries. Known for his innovative instruction, he teaches courses in human sexuality and children's health and also teaches in the professional preparation program. Robin regularly presents on sexuality issues at the national level, and has had great success writing and producing award-winning films in the area of human sexuality.

Chapter 1

Introduction

- Michael is conducting a five-part workshop on health and safety for 45 physical plant employees at a local factory.
- Maria is performing a one-time presentation on the pap and pelvic examination for a group of 15 Hispanic women in a local community center.
- Natalie is conducting an individual birth control session for a sophomore student at a university health center.
- William is teaching a 10-part unit on family life to a class of 25 ninth-grade high school students.
- Tanya is performing a patient education session for two hypertensive middle-aged males at a local hospital.
- Dwayne is lecturing to 500 college students about sexually transmitted diseases and safer sex, as part of a series on contemporary sexual issues.
- Delores is speaking to a congressional panel on the importance of comprehensive health education.

Although these health educators are dealing with very different audiences—from very large groups to individuals, from high school students to elected national officials, from young to old, from the workplace to the school, from the community to the House of Representatives—they all share one crucial factor that will invariably determine success from failure . . . how well they actually educate. The philosophy presented in this text is based in the premise that the core of health education is the *process* of health education. This means that what is most important is how well and effectively we perform the function of educating people about health decisions.

There are many other tools available to health educators, such as epidemiology, statistics, and program planning, but what is truly unique about a health educator is the focus on the "doing." To be a health educator means that you are skilled in conducting health education. As educators we may have access to the best knowledge available, but unless we are skilled and effective deliverers of this information, the usefulness of our work is clearly compromised.

This text is dedicated to the proposition that we must be good at the doing . . . the health education. Our goal is to favorably influence the voluntary decision making of our clients. Further, it is our belief that health educators need a much more systematic approach to the selection of methods of intervention. Anyone who has sat through a poorly prepared, often boring and uninspired presentation/class should question the thought processes that resulted in such a negative experience. This text is intended to assist the health educator in reducing the possibility of a poor performance by encouraging the systematic development of sound, effective, and appropriate presentation methods.

This text is designed for any health educator or would-be health educator who wishes to become proficient in conducting health education programs. The authors of this text strongly believe that the skills necessary to plan successfully for, and deliver, effective health education programs are fundamentally the same, regardless of where they are practiced—in a classroom, a workplace, a hospital, or a community setting. The principles of sound methodology remain constant. Therefore this text is designed for multiple settings. It will address the needs of the so-called "generic" health educator and provide the tools for making appropriate programming decisions based on the needs of the clients and the educational settings.

Case Study   *The government authorizes three million dollars to evaluate a large clinical trial aimed at influencing the health behaviors of Americans. A group of volunteers provides pamphlets and educational counseling at a large shopping mall, and each volunteer spends about an hour with over 5,000 people. The research design for evaluating the program is solid. Proper comparison groups are in place, and the instrumentation for assessing change is of high quality. We know what the behaviors, attitudes, and knowledge were before, during, and after the intervention (treatment), and we are certain threats to internal and external validity of the study have been controlled. The outcome measures are well matched with the objectives of the health education program. According to all measures the intervention does not change anything.*

What Is Wrong?

There are, of course, many possibilities for the no-change results, but there are at least three explanations that we want you to consider.

1. Were the methods selected for the intervention appropriate and properly implemented?
2. Was there adequate time provided for the intervention to successfully achieve the sought objectives?

3. Were the people asked to conduct the intervention properly trained to conduct the intervention? Were they in fact health educators?

- We do not have the objectives before us, but it seems clear that few behavioral objectives could be reached by such an intervention (pamphlets and educational counseling by volunteers).
- An hour is not enough time to change most behaviors unless you have a very highly motivated clientele.
- Volunteers can play important and sometimes powerful roles but do not qualify as health educators.

This only moderately exaggerated example shows why health educators must work to improve the art and science of health education. Becoming a high-quality health educator requires hard work and dedication. A top-quality health educator is always working to develop communication skills, increase current knowledge of the subject matter, and remain a motivator. It is hoped that this text will provide some of the tools needed to accomplish the goals and objectives of health educators.

THE PROCESS OF HEALTH EDUCATION

It is important to remember that health education is, as the name implies, education about health. Health education has its roots in education and public health. It draws on many disciplines including psychology, sociology, education, public health, and epidemiology. It is a unique discipline in many ways. One of the challenges for the health educator is that while the principal tool is education, the sought outcomes are often behavioral. Other disciplines in education focus almost exclusively on knowledge. Health education is called upon to alter people's drug-taking behavior, lower cholesterol, and improve fitness, to name only a few of the many complicated expectations. Other education disciplines are not held to such lofty goals.

Remember always to be grateful for the millions of people everywhere whose despicable habits make health education necessary.
—Mohan Singh

Health educators must learn to set meaningful, appropriate, and achievable goals and objectives. After setting clear, quality objectives the health educator must seek to meet those objectives through appropriate ethical methods.

HISTORY

Health education has been offered in some form since the beginning of time. Humanity has always sought to lead a longer and healthier life. Means' classic text *A History of Health Education in the United States* reviews early health education activities in the United States. It is interesting to note Harvard College required hygiene in 1818 of all seniors (Means, 1962, p. 36). The American Public Health Association was formed in 1872, and the National Education Association started a Department of Child Safety in 1894 (Means, 1962, pp. 46–48). The American School Health Association was formed in 1927 as the then American Association of School Physicians. The Association for the Advancement of Health Education began as part of what is now titled the Alliance for Health, Physical Education, Recreation, and Dance when it began as the American Association for Health and Physical Education in 1937.

Education about health became more common in the 1800s and early 1900s with numerous reports and advocates. Some noted advocates include Horace Mann, Thomas Denison Wood, the American Academy of Medicine, the Metropolitan Life Insurance Company, the U.S. Public Health Service, and the U.S. Office of Education. The first reported academic department of health education was located at Georgia State College for Women around 1917. The first known recipient of a health education degree was Cecile Oertel Humphrey who, after additional course work at Harvard during the summers of his program at Georgia State College, received a bachelor of science in health education. A thesis was required and his was entitled "The Inferiority Complex—Its Relation to Mental Hygiene." No report is available on what has become of Mr. Humphrey (Means, 1962, p. 144). Teachers College, Columbia University, began an undergraduate degree in 1920 and was one of the early granters of graduate degrees in health education.

Health education has functioned as a separate discipline for approximately the last 30 to 60 years. As a relatively new discipline, it has always struggled for a strong sense of identity. One illustration of this is the large number of health education professional organizations, each with overlapping goals. Another example is that health education degrees are sometimes offered at higher-education institutions with few, or in some extreme cases, no health educators on the faculty. Despite these problems, health education continues to evolve into an important discipline with a unique orientation to addressing the health education needs of the world.

Throughout the history of health education, numerous agencies have recognized the potential of health education to address health problems. Federal agencies have supported many studies and projects designed to improve the quality and impact of health education. An important effort was the Role Delineation Project begun in 1978 (funded by the then U.S. Bureau of Health Manpower and carried out by the National Center for Health Education) which examined the role of the entry-level health educator and generated a defined role. This defined role was based on surveys of practicing health educators in 1978. The end product was a defined role for the entry-level health educator. Although obviously in need of updating, the definition of the role was a significant step in the evolution of health education as a discipline. An important finding suggested that the health educator's role was essentially the same regardless of the health education setting. The result was the definition of the *generic health educator.* The generic health educator concept is very important for the training of health educators. It states that health educators should all possess certain common skills. These skills were later more fully defined as Competencies for Entry-Level Health Educators after a panel of experts meeting at Ball State University translated the defined role into competencies for entry-level health educators. Later, these competencies became the basis for the test given to be certified as a health education specialist by the National Commission for Health Education Credentialing. The competencies also used by the National Council for the Accreditation of Teacher Education (NCATE) as part of the teacher-training accreditation review process.

This *generic health educator* concept has important ramifications for the training of health educators because it puts much more emphasis on the acquisition of skills than on health content. It is clear that some skills would be used more in some settings than in others but the basic skills are generic. Health educators need to acquire these basic skills, many of which are the focus of this text. It is ludicrous, for example, for an individual to believe he/she can function well as a health educator without training in educational principles. Health educators practice in a variety of settings often defined as school health education, community health education, worksite health education, or patient health education. The basic skills are now recognized as being the same for all settings, and this text is organized and presented to stimulate the acquisition of many of these basic skills.

GOALS OF THE TEXT

After reading and synthesizing this text, the health educator will be able to:

- plan properly for health education instruction
- develop quality lesson/presentation plans and unit plans
- plan for the special needs of target populations
- select appropriate methods through a systematic approach
- use methods of intervention properly

FORMAT OF THE TEXT

- Each chapter will begin with a listing of the competencies addressed in the chapter.
- Case studies will be used throughout the text.

- Each chapter will begin with a graphic that illustrates the components of proper method selection addressed in the chapter (see Figures 1-1 and 1-2). The method selection representation depicted in Figure 1-1 has been developed by the authors to highlight the key issues in method selection. A graphic resembling Figure 1-2 will be found at the beginning of each chapter and will represent the issues addressed in the chapter.
- Each chapter will be followed by a summary, a series of exercises, and a list of references.
- A glossary can be found at the end of the text.
- Scattered throughout the text can be found health education proverbs from that "not-so-famous" health educator seer (formerly from the east of CDC headquarters) Mohan Singh. We have heard he can sometimes be found roaming the mystic spaces of the Pan American Health Organization in Washington DC. Are his words the mental meanderings of a lunatic or are they pearls of wisdom with deep significance for all health educators? You be the judge.

FIGURE 1-1
Method Selection
in Health Education

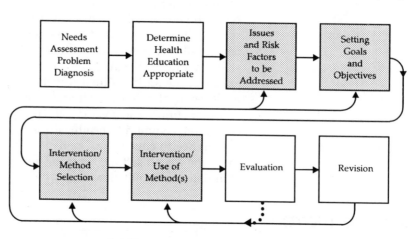

Shaded boxes indicate subjects included in this text.

METHOD SELECTION COMPONENTS

There are many public health and health education texts that deal with program planning and evaluation. This text will deal with the conduct of health education—the pedagogy. Pedagogy is the art or profession of teaching. Pedagogy is what health education practice is about. We are not minimizing the importance of the other components of method selection, but we will address the pedagogy with this text.

1. **Needs assessment and problem diagnosis.** This text begins with the assumption that some type of needs assessment has been done and it has been determined that health education is a viable alternative.

2. **Determination if health education is the appropriate intervention.** This text also begins with the assumption that it has been determined that health education is the appropriate intervention. Health education can be very complicated, expensive, and difficult and therefore this is an important assumption. Often other methods of health promotion may be more appropriate. If we can more effectively alter the environment, for example, it might be better use of our resources. If students are eating unhealthy lunches, for example, it may be easier to ensure they eat lunch at school where they will only be offered healthy choices. This may lead to much better behavior at relatively low cost. However, the long-term behavior may not be altered with only a change in the physical environment.

3. **Issues and risk factors to be addressed.** This text will consider some of the issues to be taken into account when making decisions about what issues and risk factors to address. See Chapters 2, 3, 7, and 8.

4. **Setting goals and objectives.** This is an important component of pedagogy and is addressed in this book. See Chapters 2 and 3.

5. **Intervention/method selection.** This is the major issue addressed in this text. See Chapters 4 through 8 and the Appendix.

6. **Evaluation.** *This is a major issue which simply cannot be sufficiently addressed in this text.* The importance of this area cannot be overestimated. There are entire books and courses dedicated to evaluation, and the authors believe that this text is not the appropriate place to take a piecemeal approach with such important and lengthy material. Therefore, although there are many references to evaluation, this text does not have a chapter dedicated to this issue.

7. **Revision.** Good practical evaluation will lead to revision of any intervention. This is an important tool which should be part of any program. Revision should be based on evaluation and therefore will not be addressed in this text.

Method Selection in Health Education

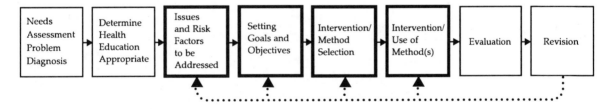

Heavy-bordered boxes indicate subjects addressed in this text; shaded boxes indicate subject(s) of current chapter.

FIGURE 1-2

Each chapter will also begin with a listing of the generic entry-level competencies developed for the National Task Force on the Preparation and Practice of Health Educators, Inc. A complete listing of the competencies can be found in the Appendix.

REFERENCES

U.S. HHS. 1981. National Conference for Institutions Preparing Health Educators: Proceedings, Birmingham, AL, 1981. DHHS Publication 81-50171.

Means, R. K. 1962. *A History of Health Education in the United States.* Philadelphia: Lea and Febiger.

National Task Force on the Preparation and Practice of Health Educators, Inc. 1983. *A Guide for the Development of Competency-Based Curricula for Entry Level Health Educators.* New York.

National Task Force on the Preparation and Practice of Health Educators, Inc. 1985. *A Framework for the Development of Competency-Based Curricula for Entry Level Health Educators.* New York.

_____ Chapter 2 _____

Planning for Instruction

Entry Level Health Educator Competencies Addressed in This Chapter

Responsibility I: Assessing Individual and Community Needs for Health Education
> Competency A: Obtain health-related data about social and cultural environments, growth and development factors, needs, and interests.
> Competency C: Infer needs for health education on the basis of obtained data.

Responsibility II: Planning Effective Health Education Programs
> Competency B: Develop a logical scope and sequence plan for a health education program.
> Competency C: Formulate appropriate and measurable program objectives.

Responsibility III: Implementing Health Education Programs
> Competency A: Exhibit competence in carrying out planned educational programs.
> Competency B: Infer enabling objectives as needed to implement instructional program in specified settings.

Taken from *A Framework for the Development of Competency-Based Curricula for Entry Level Health Educators*, National Task Force on the Preparation and Practice of Health Educators, Inc. 1985. Reprinted by permission.

Method Selection in Health Education

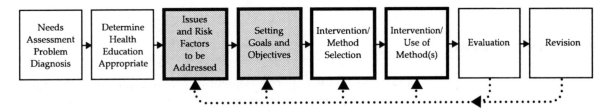

Heavy-bordered boxes indicate subjects addressed in this text; shaded boxes indicate subject(s) of current chapter.

Case Study   *Pat has set the elimination of drug use by all adolescents in her community as her objective for a community-wide drug education program. She plans to work cooperatively with several local agencies including the schools and later to apply for federal funding to support the program. Following two years of this approach, she gets a small local grant to evaluate her program. Preliminary reports show that drugs are used by about 15 percent of adolescents in the community.*

Since Pat's only stated objective was to end drug use, she has failed by her own standards. Pat has not set realistic objectives in measurable terms for her program and because of this mistake the program was virtually certain to fail. Further, Pat has not determined through a needs assessment what the current status of the community is in terms of the prevalence of drug use and its needs and interests. If, for example, Pat had discovered that drugs were being used by 35 percent of adolescents in the community, she could structure her objectives to reflect a modest but realistic behavior or attitude change. Pat has failed to plan carefully for instruction.

After studying the chapter the reader will be able to:

- conduct an appropriate needs assessment for a given community setting
- list the major considerations that should be made before selecting an educational objective
- write behavioral objectives in the cognitive, affective, and psychomotor domains for a given concept or contact area
- list the most common mistakes in objective selection

Key Issues

Program Planning
Conducting a Needs
   Assessment
Relationship of Objectives and
   Evaluation
Selecting Objectives
Objective Domains
Process Objectives

Outcome Objectives
Writing Goals and Objectives
Selecting Verbs
Common Mistakes
Ethics as Part of Planning
Seating Arrangements
The Learning Environment

PROGRAM PLANNING

Method selection is only one element of program planning. Program planning has issues that are beyond the scope of, and therefore not addressed by, this text. We begin with the assumption that the "problem" has been identified and health education has been determined to be part of the needed solution. This is, of course, a major assumption

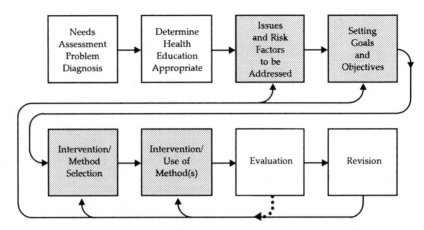

FIGURE 2-1
Method Selection
in Health Education

Shaded boxes indicate subjects included in this text.

but one that is commonly made. There are several quality texts written on program planning for public health programs. We are assuming that the decision to use health education has been made. This assumption is common to school settings where the curriculum framework is usually in place. It is also common for health educators working for a categorical agency that has decided to focus on one or two elements of health education. If the decision has not been made, then the reader should turn to planning models and conduct a thorough diagnosis of the problem before turning to health education and this text.

CONDUCTING A NEEDS ASSESSMENT

Although program goals and objectives are often set for the health educator by some other group, a needs assessment is always appropriate. Outside agencies will often develop excellent objectives, but may still fail to account for special characteristics found at the local level. When goals and objectives are established for us, it reduces the complexity of our needs assessment, but the principles are always important. Generally, we are able to play a significant role in objective establishment either by interpretation or by setting the objectives directly (see Fig. 2-1, step one).

The needs assessment, as the term implies, seeks to determine the needs of the population for whom we are targeting our intervention. We generally call this group the target population. Before we set out to do something, it is important to know where we are and how the target population perceives its needs.[1] Generally, the better we know the

---

[1]Green and Kreuter use the term "diagnosis" to describe this phase of health promotion planning. They describe this phase in detail in their classic text *Health Promotion and Planning An Educational and Environmental Approach*. It is also sometimes referred to as "reconnaissance."

target population, the more we should be able to accomplish. The amount of time and resources we devote to the needs assessment will depend on issues such as the duration, priority, and prior work experience with the group. If we have worked with the group recently, we may need to spend little time, but if this is a new group it may require considerable time and effort. We must review what we know of this target population. A simple sample needs assessment survey is depicted in Figure 2-2.

THE TARGET POPULATION

Demographics
Developmental characteristics
Interest surveys
Knowledge levels
Attitudes held
Health skills
Expert opinion

Statistical Information
National or international trends
Regional
Local

We have many potential sources of information about the needs and interests of our target population. It is important we do what we can to assess this information so that we minimize unneeded work and take into account the desires of the target group. Conducting a needs assessment also puts a group on notice that you recognize its importance and value its opinions. These are necessary ingredients if you hope to be successful.

Prior to a program we should attempt to ascertain what we can about the target population. We may be able to collect demographic information such as age, ethnicity, gender, and other characteristics that may impact objectives and method selection. If we are working with young people, we may turn to information on the developmental characteristics of this age group. Surveys may exist that will tell us something about the knowledge or interests of this age group. If such surveys do not exist, we may be able to conduct such surveys. This data collection, sometimes referred to as baseline data, can provide us information regarding where we are starting. In addition to helping us determine how to conduct our program, such information can provide a basis of comparison. Any major program must include such baseline data since there will always be interest in what benefits have been accrued for the dollars invested.

We should also consider what statistical information may be available. International, national, regional, or local reports can provide vital information on what may be needed. Such reports can also be used to demonstrate the importance of a topic. We must always keep in mind that national or even local reports do not always demonstrate a need for our local target group. Therefore it may be important to conduct our own needs assessment specific to our target population. Collecting such information also demonstrates an interest in tailoring the program to the needs of the local target group and may serve as part of the intervention program by pointing out individual needs. Identification of personal needs often leads to some attempt at behavior change. People who know they are at higher than average risk for some loss of health will sometimes try to reduce that risk. How serious they perceive the risk to be will often determine how they respond. As will be discussed later such information is often very important in selling the program to funding agencies, gathering local support, and encouraging participants to cooperate in the program.

Sources of Data
1. National and regional vital statistics.
2. National health surveys.
3. State reports on health status.

Please answer the following questions as completely and honestly as you can. The information collected will be used in determining the content of the health education workshop.

1. What do you hope to get from this workshop/class?

2. Why are you here?

3. One thing you hope will be covered.

4. One issue that has been covered too much and would be a waste of time for this workshop is?

Other comments?

FIGURE 2-2
Simple Sample Needs Assessment Survey

4. School- or community-based surveys.
5. Self-constructed surveys.

OTHER METHODS FOR PLANNING

Delphi Method   The Delphi method is a technique for "structuring a group communication process so that the process is effective in allowing a group of individuals, as a whole, to deal with a complex problem" (Linstone and Turoff, 1975, p. 3). It originated with a Rand Corporation study sponsored by the U.S. Air Force in the 1950s and was named after the site of an oracle of Apollo, an ancient Greek god (Dalkey and Helmer, 1963). The Rand study was designed to elicit "expert opinion to the selection, from the point of view of a Soviet strategic planner, of an optimal U.S. industrial target system and to the estimation of the number of A-bombs required to reduce the munitions output by a prescribed amount" (Linstone and Turoff, 1975, p. 10).

The Delphi technique has been applied to a number of research issues including technological forecasting, educational and program development, policy decision making, problem solving, and the assessment of planned strategies with respect to their desirability, effectiveness, and feasibility (Linstone and Turoff, 1975). It is a particularly useful approach when accurate, quantitative data are nonexistent or where judgmental, descriptive information is invaluable.

The purpose of the Delphi technique is to create a sort of collective group intelligence regarding a specific issue and to develop an intentionally negotiated group construct of a particular situational reality (Scheele, 1975). This is accomplished through the careful selection of a group of experts in a given topic who respond to a series or rounds of questionnaires that contain controlled feedback (Travis, 1976). In practice, the technique varies in format depending on the nature of the problem, goals and objectives, resources, and characteristics of the researcher (Hentges and Hosokawa, 1980). In order for a Delphi study to be successful, three critical conditions must be met. These include sufficient time, skills in written communication, and motivation among the participants (Hentges and Hosokawa, 1980). The process is a lengthy one and requires sustained effort over a period of time. The written form of the questions, the letters of introduction, and the written feedback between rounds must be clear and concise if the Delphi technique is to produce the desired outcome (Hentges and Hosokawa, 1980).

According to Judd (1972), there are three distinguishing characteristics of the Delphi process. One is anonymity of response, which is accomplished through the use of mailed questionnaires and avoiding face-to-face interactions. A second feature is multiple iterations, that is, the opportunity for respondents to revise their opinions. Lastly, participants are provided with summary feedback of group responses from the previous round of questionnaires. This process facilitates a convergence of the distribution of responses. Typically, this convergence is expressed in terms of descriptive statistics as a statistical group response in the form of a mean/median/mode, standard deviation, and an interquartile range (Judd, 1972; Linstone and Turoff, 1975). An interquartile range is the interval of scores containing the middle 50 percent of the responses and is considered a measure of consensus (Travis, 1976). Consensus, in the Delphi process, generally remains stable after the third round according to Cyphert and Gant (1971). Some researchers have utilized the t-test to compare means of identical items from round to round (Travis, 1976) or to determine differences of opinion among the panel respondents (Jillson, 1975).

Generally, the initial questionnaires are constructed in suggestive, open-ended formats in order not to restrict creative responses. Successive questionnaires, however, attempt to refine and synthesize information gathered in the previous rounds (Scheele, 1975).

One apparent weakness of the Delphi method is that it does not necessarily represent the best judgments of the panelists, but rather a negotiated compromise. As in any attempt to predict the future, the Delphi technique relies on the perceptions, beliefs, and biases of the respondents, not on concrete reality. To the extent that the future is influenced by the images and expectations individuals hold, then the Delphi technique is a useful way to examine present realities and future possibilities (Toohey and Shireffs, 1980).

Case Study   *State legislators have just passed an education bill that requires high school students to complete one mandatory credit of health education in order to graduate. Local county health education coordinators scramble to devise ways to conform with the new law. One far-sighted county administrator decides to employ the Delphi process to achieve this goal. All county middle and high school health education teachers are involved in a lengthy but invaluable process of providing input into the health problems of their students by developing a curriculum, establishing effective teaching methodologies, and identifying quality and useful resources for evaluation and possible adoption. Once this task has been completed, most of the teachers who must implement the new curriculum are extremely satisfied with the outcome. They have been given an active role in the curriculum's development and can take ownership in what has been developed. The teachers continue to show support for the curriculum once the school year begins.*

The county administrator in this example was indeed far sighted! All too often curricula are developed with scant regard for the teachers who will have to implement them. In this example not only did the administrator increase his/her likelihood of support, but because of such a large, cooperative effort by all the county's health education teachers, the chances of developing an innovative, current, and topical curriculum are excellent.

Use of the Delphi Technique in Health-Related Research

Travis (1976) proposed the use of the Delphi technique as a tool for community health educators. The process can identify existing community and/or professional opinion and obtain consensus regarding health problems, needs, and objectives. In a role delineation study of physician's assistants, Travis (1976) identified and rated a number of role statements utilizing the Delphi process. Results indicated that no significant changes in opinion occurred between questionnaires 1 and 3; however, significant differences in opinion regarding the role of the physician's assistant were evident among the professional groups surveyed.

Gilmore (1977) provided a perspective on the use of the Delphi technique by health educators for the purpose of community needs assessment. The emphasis here is not only on the identification of perceived health needs, but also on the prioritizing of these identified needs for the purposes of policy decision making and resource allocation. The Delphi technique has some unique advantages as a needs assessment strategy. It allows the researcher to solicit input from a variety of target group representatives in a wide geographical area. In addition, anonymity of the process allows for consensus to be obtained without the negative influences of group conformity, politics, and power struggles (Gilmore, 1977).

Hentges and Hosokawa (1980) used the technique to involve teachers in the development of a health education curriculum. Teachers provided input into the health problems of students, topics to be covered in the curriculum, teaching methodology, and necessary resources for implementation. The researchers found that the teachers who had participated in the Delphi process felt that they had been well informed and were more likely to support the new curriculum (Hentges and Hosokawa, 1980).

Toohey and Shireffs (1980) attempted to predict the future of the profession and the role of health education in society utilizing the Delphi method. They surveyed 25 national leaders, including chairs of academic departments, former presidents of professional organizations, and directors of governmental and private health education agencies. The experts predicted an expansion of health education services in the health care arena and in corporate workplace settings. In addition, they foresaw, in the near future, the formation of a unified professional association of health educators and the development of a systematic method of dealing with the many variables that impact on health behavior (Toohey and Shireffs, 1980).

A study by Banks (1980) identified the perceptions of health educators regarding the spiritual aspects of health. Three rounds of questionnaires were utilized, each with a different function. The focus of the first questionnaire was on brainstorming, the second, on rating, and the third, on establishing consensus. This research identified and ranked the components of the spiritual dimension of health, delineated important considerations in the teaching of spiritual health, and suggested appropriate methodologies to be used in such a curriculum (Banks, 1980).

He who lives by bread alone
needs sex education.
—Mohan Singh

Simple Multiattribute Rating Technique (SMART)

SMART is one of a variety of approaches classified as Multiattribute utility techniques (MAUTs). Developed as an aid in decision making, MAUT is designed to highlight the utility or value of certain outcomes through the use of "importance weights." An estimate of relevant contribution, standardized weighting allows for ratio comparisons of the relative importance of different outcomes (Clark and Friedman, 1982).

SMART involves the assignment of importance weights on a scale of 0 to 100. Typically, the top-ranked item receives an arbitrary weighting of 100 and other items are assigned weights proportionate to their relative importance (Clark and Friedman, 1982). This means that an item with a weight of 50 is considered half as important as an item weighted 100. This procedure does not preclude the possibility that more than one item may be weighted identically and thus be considered of equal import.

SMART has been used in combination with the Delphi method by Clark and Friedman (1982) to derive a utility function for program effectiveness in mental health. The results of this study indicated that the Delphi technique was appropriate for identifying multiple client outcomes in mental health and the weighting procedure allowed for the transition from generalized statements of client outcomes to specific criteria of overall program effectiveness.

See Chapter 3 for a discussion of models and theories. Health educators need to consider very real and practical motivators for the people they are addressing with their programs.

Case Study

Joe has been asked to make a needs assessment report for a planned health education program targeting the local community. The total budget for the three-month intervention is $2,000 plus 20 to 30 hours of Joe's time. The planned components of the needs assessment include the following:

1. Local health statistics.
2. Planned survey of target audience.
3. Knowledge testing as a pretest.
4. A focus group of neighborhood residents.

The strengths of this plan are that Joe has collected local statistics and is planning to survey the community and hold a focus group. The knowledge testing will provide a baseline, but is knowledge all that is sought as an outcome?

Cost estimates in time and money are not provided, but this program could be too expensive given the total budget. Needs assessment plans need to be realistic.

THE LINK BETWEEN GOALS, OBJECTIVES, AND EVALUATION

Alice "Would you tell me please, which way I ought to walk from here?"
"That depends a good deal on where you want to get to," said the Cat.
"I don't much care where," said Alice.
"Then it doesn't matter which way you walk," said the Cat.
"—so long as I get somewhere," Alice added as an explanation.
"Oh, you're sure to do that," said the Cat, "if you only walk long enough!"
—Lewis Carroll,
Alice in Wonderland and
Through the Looking Glass

You may have heard the statement, "If you do not know where you want to go it is usually impossible to get there." These words of wisdom apply well to all health education endeavors. We often see health educators trying to get somewhere without being clear about where that somewhere might be. Even more interesting, we often see them trying to evaluate what they have done trying to get there. Obviously, this is not a prudent practice. Health educators must state clearly where they want to go. Not only is this vital for evaluation, it is essential for good planning in selecting an intervention. There is clear link between goals, objectives, method/intervention selection, and evaluation.

Let us examine some examples (with discussion) of how inappropriate conclusions can be reached when we have no clear-cut objectives.

1. "My program went well because we distributed 750 pamphlets on drug abuse."
   If the program objective was to distribute pamphlets, then the objective was met but it was a very poor objective. Distribution numbers or numbers of people that visit a booth in a shopping mall are examples of very limited measures that tell us nothing about changes in knowledge attitudes or behaviors.

2. "My program went well because the 40 people attending the lecture on drug abuse seemed very interested and asked many questions."
   Looking interested tells us nothing about what is being learned. It does tell us something about the methods employed (process evaluation). It may indicate that people find the topic or method of presentation interesting, but it tells us nothing about what has been learned.

3. "My program went well because, after the five antidrug television spots were aired, the state drug use numbers went down."
   Although this is a positive trend, it does not tell us if that trend is related to our program. It may have nothing to do with our

activities, and it would be inappropriate for us to assume so without further information.

4. "My program went poorly because, after our intensive intervention with all county high school students, the state drug use numbers went up."

Again, we do not know if this trend had any connection to our program. The number for our students might be much better due to our program, but without clear objectives we cannot adequately measure our outcomes.

5. "My STD prevention program went poorly because, after our intensive intervention throughout the county, our STD statistics showed an increase."

Again, we do not know if this trend had any connection to our program. The statistics for STDs commonly go up for a period of time following an intensive campaign because people seek treatment. If we set objectives to lower incidence rates in a short period of time we would be setting up our program for failure.

It is difficult to evaluate these statements without knowing the objectives, but all suggest that the evaluation measures have not been well thought out.

Case Study

Jerry was extremely enthusiastic about beginning a sexuality education program in his high school. The principal had been skeptical about the potential controversy and had put Jerry off for two years. Finally, the principal gave Jerry the administrative and financial support to begin a program, provided he furnish the principal with a course outline and specific objectives. In his haste to consummate the agreement, Jerry quickly prepared an outline, including objectives that promised a substantial decrease in unintended pregnancy and sexually transmitted disease rates. One year later, with budget reductions looming, Jerry is asked to justify the continued support of his sexuality program. Much to Jerry's chagrin, the principal points to a higher number of pregnancies than last year, and no record whatsoever of any sexually transmitted disease rates.

Through his haste and poorly conceived, unrealistic objectives, Jerry has placed the entire sexuality program in jeopardy. He made the same two fundamental errors in planning as Pat did in an earlier case study. First, Jerry did not conduct a thorough needs assessment before designing program goals and objectives. If Jerry promises a reduction in sexually transmitted diseases, he will need to obtain data as to their existing prevalence in order to make a subsequent comparison. The likelihood of even being allowed to collect such sensitive data in a public school is at best marginal. Second, in constructing his objectives Jerry was extremely unrealistic as to what any single program could accomplish. Constructing program *goals* related to reducing rates of unintended pregnancy and sexually transmitted diseases would be appropriate, but specific behavioral *objectives* which need to be measurable should be much more modest and reasonable in scope. As discussed in Chapter 8, setting such unattainable objectives in a controversial area such as human sexuality can do irreparable and sometimes fatal damage to a program which may be constantly under scrutiny.

WHY USE OBJECTIVES?

Objectives serve many useful functions. They provide the health educator with a clear notion of what is to be accomplished. Therefore it becomes much easier to select methods and to focus all efforts. This focus is vital if we are to develop comprehensive coordinated approaches to influencing health knowledge and behaviors. Therefore it is important to begin with the question, what is the target? (see Figure 2-3). Then we must define the target as specifically as we can. Objectives also make evaluation efforts possible. Without objectives it is impossible to measure the achievement of change—knowledge, attitudes, or behavior. You cannot evaluate any type of change unless you first clearly state exactly what you intend to change . . . and to do that you must construct precise objectives. If we have selected an inappropriate target, it may be impossible to hit the target (see Figure 2-4). Therefore we must select appropriate targets. Objectives moreover make it possible to convey our instructional intent to others. Learners in any setting do better when it is clear what is to be learned. This is true of participants in workshops as well as students in more formal educational settings. Reviewing well-stated objectives allows learners to assess if this program is the correct program for them.

ISSUES TO BE CONSIDERED IN SELECTING OBJECTIVES AND INTERVENTION/METHODS

1. Maturity level of the learner
2. Content to be covered
3. Environment
4. Materials and equipment available
5. Time allotment
6. Group size
7. Time of day

When we set our objectives it is important to make them realistic given our resources. Of course, our objectives are often set by someone

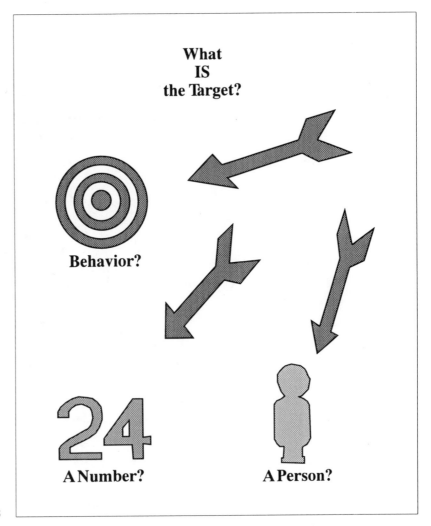

**What
IS
the Target?**

Behavior?

24

A Number?

A Person?

FIGURE 2-3

else, but the principles are the same. What can we accomplish in the time available with the resources at our disposal?

We must take into account the *maturity level of the learner*. Is the information pitched at the correct level for the learner? If it is too high, comprehension will be a problem; too low, boredom and distraction will occur. Are the selected activities sufficiently varied to stimulate audience attention? This is an important concern when working with young people. What type of *content* do you intend to cover? Large amounts of complex, didactic information may need to be broken down into smaller more understandable units, again depending on the level of the learner. Varying strategies might also alleviate the boredom factor and result in more effective learning. What is the physical

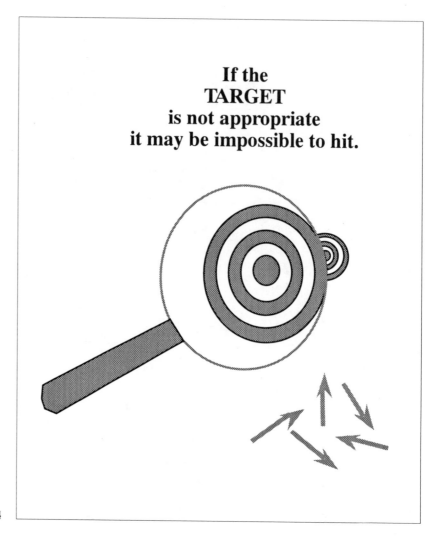

FIGURE 2-4

environment like? Can you, for example, lay out four "Annie" CPR mannequins on the floor of a very confined space to conduct important certification classes? Can you successfully perform group facilitation which might include sensitive issues in a space with little privacy? The available environment cannot be underestimated when considering objectives. Can you obtain the *materials and equipment* you would like to include in a program? For example, is a certain film you would like to use available or affordable? Do you have access to a projector or VCR? Before you include activities in program outlines and strategy selection, check to make sure that the resources are available. How much *time* do you have with specific groups, and how often will you meet? Is it worth spending 20 minutes incorporating an icebreaker exercise with a group that will only meet one time for two hours? The answer to this question depends on the specific objectives that you construct. Should you construct objectives that include behavior change when you will only meet with a group for a total of two hours? You must be realistic about which activities can be utilized and what objectives can be achieved within certain time constraints. *Group size* will certainly drive your method selection. Presenting to a large group of 250 individuals will definitely require a different strategy than group process for a small number of people. Consider what might be the most effective ways to communicate with individuals and groups when considering group size. Anyone who has had early morning classes or dozed during an after-lunch or dinner speech will appreciate the importance of *time of day*. Will you need to wake up the group . . . quiet them down . . . struggle to keep their interest or what? Early morning or postlunch groups might require a wake-up activity, so always consider this issue when developing strategy selection.

Often we must also determine if we can hope to achieve and perhaps measure outcome/impact objectives or if we should focus on process objectives. Time and resources permitting, we should consider both.

PROCESS OBJECTIVES

Some process objectives might include the following:

- Getting people to participate
- Recognition of need
- Quality of workshop presentations
- Needs assessment
- Peer review
- Fidelity
- Self-assessment
- Changes in policy statements
- Quality control standards

Process objectives are concerned with what we hope to do along the path to our outcome objectives. This includes a look at how well we are implementing our methods and whether they are being implemented faithfully. Are we maintaining interest and are we providing high-quality information? Most curriculum packages are not implemented as designed. If we have the time and resources, it is important to measure how faithfully we are implementing our established program. Often programs are evaluated and the outcome of the evaluation is based on the faulty assumption that all users implement the program in the same way. It is most important that if we are successful, partially successful, or unsuccessful we have a clear picture of what was done and not just what we hoped would be done. Often programs are deemed ineffective when in fact the program was not implemented or only a few activities or methods from that program were actually used. This is important to know and it points to the need for training and marketing the total program to the intended user.

OUTCOME/IMPACT OBJECTIVES

Some outcome/impact objectives might include the following:

- Changes in knowledge
- Changes in attitudes
- Changes in skills
- Changes in behavior
- Cost effectiveness

Beware, lest the fragile lotus of health education be trampled by the elephants of reality.
—Mohan Singh

Outcome/impact objectives are concerned with what we are seeking to change in knowledge, attitudes, and behaviors. How will the participants be different as a result of our educational intervention? These outcomes can be assessed after a short-duration program or long-term program. Obviously, what we can expect must be based on the contact time, motivation, and intensity of our program. For a short-term program it may be realistic to expect gains in knowledge, but it may be unrealistic to attempt attitude or behavior change.

STEPS IN WRITING GENERAL GOALS IN HEALTH EDUCATION

Different authors and authorities use a variety of terms and definitions regarding goals and objectives. We will use the term goal to mean a broad statement of direction used to present the overall intent of a program or course. A goal does not need to be stated in measurable terms since it is a broad statement. Objectives will always be stated in measurable terms and will complement and more fully explain the intent of a goal. A goal gives us a general sense of the intent of the program or class.

Some goals might include the following:

1. Participants will be able to prepare healthy meals.
2. The use of non-prescription drugs will be reduced.
3. Participants will develop good parenting skills.
4. Unwanted pregnancies will be reduced.
5. Students will understand the digestion process.
6. Participants will show appreciation for the environment.

Goals from Healthy People

The classic document *Healthy People: The Surgeon General's Report on Health Promotion and Disease Prevention* (1979) contains the following goals:

1. To continue to improve infant health and, by 1990, to reduce infant mortality by at least 35 percent, to fewer than 9 deaths per 1,000 live births.
2. To improve child health, foster optimal childhood development, and, by 1990, reduce deaths among children ages 1 to 14 years by at least 20 percent, to fewer than 34 per 100,000.
3. To improve the health and health habits of adolescents and young adults and, by 1990, to reduce deaths among people ages 15 to 24 by at least 20 percent, to fewer than 93 per 100,000.
4. To improve the health of adults and, by 1990, to reduce deaths among people ages 25 to 64 by at least 25 percent, to fewer than 400 per 100,000.
5. To improve the health and quality of life for older adults and, by 1990, to reduce the average annual number of days of restricted activity due to acute and chronic conditions by 20 percent, to fewer than 39 days per year for people aged 65 and older.

NARROWING YOUR GOALS TO MEASURABLE OBJECTIVES

Goals provide a sense of where we want to go, but they do not provide clear precise statements of our destination. We must break these broad statements into clear measurable objectives. One method for doing this is to use a worksheet to guide us to our objectives. After examining our problem we set general goals. Next we break the problem down as far as we can go. We state our objectives as clearly and precisely as we can. See Figure 2-5 for a sample program planning worksheet.

STEPS IN WRITING SELF-CONTAINED HEALTH EDUCATION OBJECTIVES

Objectives must be much more specific than goals. They must be measurable and clearly indicate what will be different after your health education program. There are many educational experts knowledgeable in the writing of educational objectives. We have taken the components from other systems and have constructed a system called self-contained objectives. That means, of course, that all the elements are contained within the objective statement. The objective can "stand on its own" and make sense. Each objective makes clear what is expected,

SAMPLE PROGRAM PLANNING WORKSHEET

1. What needs to be done? List issue(s) or program(s):

   _____

   _____

   _____

   _____

   _____

2. State the general goal:

   _____

   _____

3. State the objective(s) to be evaluated as clearly as you can:

   _____

   _____

   _____

   _____

   _____

4. Can this objective be broken down further? Break it down to the smallest unit. It must be clear what specifically you hope to see documented or changed–knowledge, attitudes, or a behavior.

   _____

   _____

   _____

   _____

5. Can this objective be evaluated? If not restate it.

FIGURE 2-5

according to what source of information, and is stated in such a way that the achievement is measurable. Objectives need not always be measured but they must be measurable. In the real world there is not always sufficient funds, time, personnel, or the need to measure all objectives, but measurement must be possible or the objective is not clearly stated.

The steps in writing self-contained objectives are as follows.

1. Begin with the phrase: The _____ (student/participant/parent) will be able to . . .
2. Select action verb.
   a. The participant will be able to *list* seven common depressant drugs . . .
   b. The student will be able to *match* drugs with the appropriate classification . . .
   c. The student will be able to *demonstrate* mouth-to-mouth resuscitation . . .
   d. The participant *will show a willingness to take personal action* against drug use in the neighborhood . . .
3. Provide indication of what constitutes evidence of success.
   a. The participant will be able to list seven common depressant drugs *according to the handouts provided.*
   b. The student will be able to match drugs with the appropriate classification *found in the course textbook.*
   c. The student will be able to demonstrate mouth-to-mouth resuscitation *according to the American Red Cross.*
   d. The participant will show a willingness to take personal action against drug use in the neighborhood by *volunteering* to be part of night patrols in the neighborhood or conducting a door-to-door recruitment.
4. Consider if you have selected objectives appropriate to your needs and domains. For example,
   a. Cognitive/knowledge objective requiring recall of information.
   b. Cognitive/knowledge objective requiring some synthesis or recall.
   c. Psychomotor/"doing" objective requiring performance of a skill.
   d. Affective/"attitude" objective seeking willingness to take action.

Sample Objectives

1. Participants will be able to list and describe the four local agencies available to provide child abuse prevention support as presented during the workshop.
2. Participants will report improved self-efficacy in communication with family members according to the guidelines presented during the workshop.

3. Students will show a willingness to take personal action to improve the environment by voluntarily participating in community-organized cleanups or by voluntarily taking personal action to reduce waste in his/her community.

OTHER OBJECTIVE-WRITING FORMATS

There are many styles of writing objectives and the health educator may be forced to adapt to the style adopted by the agency or school. Self-contained objectives are suitable for most purposes and we recommend their use. However, there are advantages to other styles. Some formats make it easier to use objectives over and over again with little change and may be used for different content areas.

1. General instructional objectives (learning outcomes).
   a. Write each objective as an *intended learning outcome.*
   b. Use a verb that is general enough to encompass a domain of student performance. Omit the lead-in phrase, "The student will be able to. . . ." Use verbs such as *knows, understands, applies.*
   c. Include only one learning outcome for each general objective.
   d. Keep these objectives free of subject matter so that they can be used with various units.
   e. State each general objective so that it is definable by a set of specific learning outcomes. (For short units, two to four general objectives will usually suffice.)
2. Specific instructional objectives (learning outcomes).
   a. Place the specific instructional objectives under the general learning objectives. Be certain they are relevant to the general learning outcome under which they are placed.
   b. Use a verb to begin each specific learning outcome. This verb should specify definite, observable student performance. Avoid using verbs such as *sees* and *realizes* which are vague and not observable.
   c. Under each general learning outcome, list a representative sample of specific learning outcomes to describe the performance of those students who have achieved the objective. (It is impossible to list all learning outcomes.)
3. Examples.
   a. Drugs (high school/college level).
      (1) Knows systems of classification.
         (a) Lists various systems of classification.
         (b) Explains the advantages and disadvantages of each system.
         (c) Designs an original system.

    b. Stress control (high school/college level).
      (1) Understands breathing techniques.
        (a) Discusses uses of these.
        (b) Demonstrates them.
        (c) Expresses willingness to use technique.
    c. First aid—choking (junior high/elementary level).
      (1) Knows correct procedures.
        (a) Explains when and when not to use the techniques.
        (b) Recites the steps.
        (c) Performs the procedures.

SUGGESTED GUIDELINES FOR WRITING HEALTH EDUCATION OBJECTIVES

1. Make a rough outline of what you hope to accomplish in this educational setting. Jot down key elements of what you hope to achieve.
2. Ask yourself the following: When they finish with this lesson, workshop, or unit, how will the participants feel or act or what new knowledge or skills will they possess that were not present before this event?
3. Try to state each specific item of information, feeling, and skill as a behavioral objective.
4. Is this something they gained or could gain from your instruction? If the answer is no, it is not a good objective.
5. Check your verb to see that it is specific.
6. Can you measure your objective? Remember you do not have to measure each objective, but it must be possible or it is not a true behavioral objective. Assessment of affective objectives is controversial because many people do not believe they can be measured. Generally, affective assessment is based in a measurable action which a "reasonable person" would assume represents a held attitude or feeling.
7. Pyschomotor objectives represent skills that can be performed (i.e., mouth-to-mouth resuscitation). The focus must be the physical performance. Mouth-to-mouth resuscitation requires cognition but the focus is on the performance of the skill. Visiting an agency is not a psychomotor objective because walking to the agency is not really the focus and because it would generally be an assignment. Assignments are not objectives. Assignments help us to achieve objectives.

After writing your objectives double-check each one with the following questions:

1. Have you avoided "fuzzy" verbs?

2. Can you measure the outcome of your objective?
3. Is the standard by which achievement will be measured clearly stated?
4. Is each objective something that is really worth achieving?
5. Is there a sufficient number of objectives to cover your true intention of instruction?
6. Are you guilty of not stating your true intentions just because you find it difficult?

OBJECTIVE-WRITING EXERCISES

Read the following scenarios, take a few moments to consider strategies for each situation, and then write down what you would consider to be appropriate behavioral objectives. Obviously, you will have to give some consideration to the actual content you would potentially cover in each situation and how you would divide up your time. Remember to consider such basic principles as size of group, setting, time, number of objectives, domain of objectives, and so on.

1. You are a middle school health education teacher. You are about to teach your *first* lesson on heart health to a class of 20 seventh-grade students of mixed academic ability. This particular unit consists of five class periods, and each period is 50 minutes long.
2. You are a community health educator facilitating a program on smoking cessation for 10 middle-aged adults. The program consists of 10 two-hour weekly workshops and you are planning to conduct the *first* workshop.
3. You have been invited to a local high school to deliver a one-hour informational presentation on AIDS to a special assembly consisting of 400 ninth-grade students.
4. You are teaching a two-hour workshop on CPR to 15 Safeway employees in the employee lounge. Your goal is CPR certification of the group.
5. You are a middle school health education teacher beginning the third of five 50-minute class periods on the topic of alcohol. For this period you have decided that the goals should focus on attitudes about the negative aspects of alcohol use. One strategy you have selected is the development of posters by the students depicting alcohol messages. There are 30 students in the class.
6. You are a community health educator who has been asked to facilitate a 90-minute workshop for approximately 25 Hispanic women on the importance of pelvic examinations. Levels of fluency in English are poor.
7. You are a college health educator who has been asked to conduct a one-hour workshop on safer sex for approximately 20 students in a residence hall.

8. Two students in a campus residence hall have recently experienced date rape. As the campus health educator you have been requested by that residence hall's resident assistant (RA) to conduct a one-hour presentation on date rape. The RA expects about 50 students to attend the presentation scheduled to be held in the first-floor lounge.

9. You have been facilitating a weekly six-week course on childbirth. The class meets for 90 minutes and consists of six couples in various stages of pregnancy, from 36 to 41 weeks. This is the last of the six sessions and you are planning objectives that will allow you to wrap up the course.

10. You are a high school health educator teaching in a very progressive and enlightened school district. You are teaching human sexuality and are about to begin a two-day, 50-minute-period unit on homosexuality. You are planning objectives for this first class.

SUGGESTED VERBS FOR HEALTH EDUCATION GOALS AND OBJECTIVES

Goals

Analyze	Apply
Appreciate	Commit
Conceptualize	Create
Demonstrate	Know
Perform	Plan
Synthesize	Use

Objectives

Arrange	Categorize	Choose
Clean	Compute	Conduct
Construct	Define	Describe
Design	Diagram	Discuss
Drink	Eat	Identify
Itemize	Lead	List
Mark	Match	Name
Operate	Perform	Pick
Position	Report	Show a willingness
Sort	Specify	Underline
Volunteer		

Common Mistakes in Objective Selection

1. Selecting an objective that is not achievable.
2. Using verbs that are not specific.
3. Selecting objectives that do not truly represent what you wish to achieve.

4. Selecting objectives that are not realistic given the resources available.
5. Stating an activity and not an objective.

The 1990 Health Objectives

When the 1990 Health Objectives were released, they received little attention outside the Public Health Service. They soon became an important force driving agendas and setting funding priorities for all sectors of government. Having clear specific objectives has forever changed the U.S. Public Health Service. The process in setting the Year 2000 Objectives became much more politicized because public and private groups were aware of their influence. The objectives have become powerful tools in setting government and private policy.

EXAMPLES OF GOAL AND OBJECTIVE SETTING

The National Health Objectives

The U.S. Public Health Service Office of Disease Prevention and Health Promotion was established as a coordinating and policy development unit of the Office of the Assistant Secretary of Health. Since the early days the office has reported to Dr. J. Michael McGinnis, who was charged with coordinating the development of the Surgeon General's reports and the health objectives for the nation. In 1979 the first Surgeon General's report on health promotion was released ("Healthy People: The Surgeon General's Report on Health Promotion and Disease Prevention"), which reviewed the gains made in health promotion. In addition, the report established broad national goals according to life stages and focused on reduction of mortality. During the same period a process was put in place to develop national health objectives. This took over a year, with first drafts developed by 167 invited experts serving on panels centered around 15 subject areas held and sponsored by the Centers for Disease Control in Atlanta. Members were drawn from a variety of backgrounds. The purpose was to develop national, not federal, objectives. It was felt that by establishing clear targets agencies would focus on meeting those objectives—a common practice for business for many years but a new concept for much of government. Available research was used to determine appropriate targets, and the compilation of information pointed to the need for additional data (needs assessment). A major effort was made, but the task became even more complicated when the process was repeated for the year 2000 objectives. By this time people knew that influential people, including virtually all federal funding sources, were paying careful attention to the objectives. As a result, major lobbying efforts became part of the process of setting the objectives. Some of the original drafts of the year 2000 objectives differ significantly from the final product. The Office of Disease Prevention and Health Promotion and the Centers for Disease Control and Prevention are to be commended for pulling together the various factions and completing the target objectives. This is an important example of what needs to be done for any health education program. Clear objectives must be established at the outset if the project is to be successful and to make measurement possible. The national health objectives have resulted in significant changes in the way the U.S. government, and especially the U.S. Public Health Service, does business.

Sample 1990 Objectives

By 1990, every junior and senior high school student in the United States should receive accurate, timely education about sexually transmitted diseases. (Currently, 70 percent of school systems provide some information about sexually transmitted diseases, but the quality and timing of the communication varies greatly.)

By 1990, the proportion of adults who smoke should be reduced to below 25 percent. (In 1979, the proportion of the U.S. population which smoked was 33 percent.)

By 1990, all States should include nutrition education as part of required comprehensive school health education at elementary and secondary levels. (In 1979, only 10 States mandated nutrition as a core content area in school health education.)

By 1990, the proportion of children and adolescents ages 10 to 17 participating regularly in appropriate physical activities, particularly cardiorespiratory fitness programs which can be carried into adulthood, should be greater than 90 percent. (Baseline data unavailable.)

By 1990, the proportion of children and adolescents ages 10 to 17 participating in daily school physical education programs should be greater than 60 percent. (In 1974-75, the share was 33 percent.)

By 1990, the proportion of employees of companies and institutions with more than 500 employees offering employer-sponsored fitness programs should be greater than 25 percent. (In 1979, about 2.5 percent of companies had formally organized fitness programs.)

By 1990, lost workdays due to injuries should be reduced to 55 per 100 workers annually. (In 1978, approximately 62.1 days per 100 workers were lost.)

By 1990, no public elementary or secondary school (and no medical facility) should offer highly carcinogenic foods or snacks in vending machines or in school breakfast or lunch programs.

Sample Year 2000 Objectives

Refer to the Appendix for a complete listing.

4.13 Provide to children in all school districts and private schools primary and secondary educational programs on alcohol and other drugs, preferably as part of quality school health education. (Baseline: 63 percent provided some instruction, 39 percent provided counseling, and 23 percent referred students for clinical assessments in 1987.)

5.4 Reduce the proportion of adolescents who have engaged in sexual intercourse to no more than 15 percent by age 15 and no more than 40 percent by age 17. (Baseline: 27 percent of girls and 33 percent of boys by age 15; 50 percent of girls and 66 percent of boys by age 17; reported in 1988.)

16.3 Reduce breast cancer deaths to no more than 20.6 per 100,000 women. (Age-adjusted baseline: 22.9 per 100,000 in 1987.)

17.13 Increase to at least 30 percent the proportion of people aged 6 and older who engage regularly, preferably daily, in light to moderate physical activity for at least 30 minutes per day. (Baseline: 22 percent of people aged 18 and older were active for at least 30 minutes five or more times per week and 12 percent were active seven or more times per week in 1985.)

18.9 Increase to at least 75 percent the proportion of primary care and mental health care providers who provide age-appropriate counseling on the prevention of HIV and other sexually transmitted diseases. (Baseline: 10 percent of physicians reported that they regularly assessed the sexual behaviors of their patients in 1987.)

19.12 Include instruction in sexually transmitted disease transmission prevention in the curricula of all middle and secondary schools, preferably as part of quality school health education. (Baseline: 95 percent of schools reported offering at least one class on sexually transmitted diseases as part of their standard curricula in 1988.)

Note: Strategies to achieve this objective must be undertaken sensitively to avoid indirectly encouraging or condoning sexual activity among teens who are not yet sexually active.

Sample Community Standards

The Centers for Disease Control are now on their third edition of model standards for communities (Healthy Communities 2000: Model Standards) which formulate model objectives for community adoption. The user simply fills in the blank. Of course, agreement is the more difficult phase but having model objectives that have been formulated by a respected element of the U.S. Public Health Service is very helpful.

By _____ (2000) reduce homicides to no more than (7.2) per 100,000 people. (Age-adjusted baseline: 8.5 per 100,000 in 1987.)

By _____ (2000) reduce weapon-related violent deaths to no more than (12.6) per 100,000 people from major causes. (Age-adjusted baseline: 12.9 per 100,000 by firearms, 1.9 per 100,000 by knives, in 1987.)

By _____ (2000) reduce suicides to no more than (10.5) per 100,000 people. (Age-adjusted baseline: 11.7 per 100,000 in 1987.)

By _____ (2000) increase the high school graduation rate to at least (90) percent, thereby reducing risks for multiple problem behaviors and poor mental and physical health. (Baseline: 79 percent of people aged 20 through 21 had graduated from high school with a regular diploma in 1989.)

By _____ all community prevention programs will have an identifiable strategy for the use of health education including at a minimum:
  a. Specification of population clusters with identifiable health problems or risks
  b. Assessment of behavior related to those problems
  c. Statement of educational objectives
  d. Educational methods to be employed with each target group
  e. Timelines for implementation
  f. Periodic evaluation of educational effectiveness

By _____ programs to promote and distribute condoms including but not limited to television, radio, and print advertising and outreach to those engaged in high-risk behavior should be part of organized community health education.

Reduce the proportion of adolescents who have engaged in sexual intercourse to no more than 15 percent by age 15 and no more than 40 percent by age 17. (Baseline: 27 percent of girls and 33 percent of boys by age 15; 50 percent of girls and 66 percent of boys by age 17; reported in 1988.)

ETHICS AS PART OF PLANNING

There are many ethical issues that are part of health education pedagogy. We are attempting to change people in some way. Will these changes and methods of change be ethical? The answer should be yes, but there are steps that should be taken to ensure that the rights of all are protected. Currently the most widely adopted code of ethics is the SOPHE code (see the Appendix for the complete code). This code is a statement of how a health educator should behave. Influencing people is to be done without coercion and changes of behavior should be voluntary changes. Health educators must always behave in an ethical fashion. A brief version of the SOPHE code is given in Figure 2-6.

When we design programs and select intervention methods, it is important we keep these ethical considerations in mind. For example, if we are conducting any data collection we must go through a formal review process to protect the rights of those involved. These are generally called institutional review boards for the protection of human subjects in research, and they are a requirement for any programs that receive federal funding.

HUMAN SUBJECTS REVIEW

Institutional review boards (IRBs) are established by government, colleges, universities, and other agencies to review ongoing research projects to protect the rights of human subjects. They have formal

To guide professional behaviors of its members toward highest standards, SOPHE adopted a Code of Ethics in 1976 and acknowledged the need for periodic review and improvement of the Code.

- I will accurately represent my capability, education, training, and experience, and will act within the boundaries of my professional competence.

- I will maintain my competence at the highest level through continuing study, training, and research.

- I will report research findings and practice activities honestly and without distortion.

- I will not discriminate because of race, color, national origin, religion, age or socioeconomic status in rendering service, employing, training, or promoting others.

- I value the privacy, dignity, and worth of the individual, and will use skills consistent with these values.

- I will observe the principle of informed consent with respect to individuals and groups served.

- I will support change by choice, not by coercion.

- I will foster an educational environment that nurtures individual growth and development.

- If I become aware of unethical practices, I am accountable for taking appropriate action concerning these practices.

FIGURE 2-6
SOPHE's Code of Ethics (Brief Edition)

guidelines that protect the rights of subjects including the right to know what will happen, the right to privacy, and freedom from harm.

OBLIGATIONS TO EMPLOYER

We are responsible to our employer which means we are obligated to give full effort to our job. If we have been hired to work a 40-hour week, we must ethically devote 40 hours to the work as defined by our employer. It is not ethical for us to define what our work is unless we are self-employed. If we believe our employer is asking us to do something that is unethical, it is our obligation to discuss it with him/her. If it is then clear we are being asked to do something improper, we should report it to the next-higher authority, resign, or do both. If we are asked to teach something we do not believe in due to religious or other conflicts, we are obligated to discuss this with our employer. Perhaps someone else can teach that topic or other accommodation can be made, but it is not ethical for us unilaterally to change the curriculum or lesson to fit our personal beliefs. We must work through channels to either get it changed, teach it, or allow someone else to teach it.

We also have the obligation to keep up to date and to employ the best methods. We often hear of the shortcomings of health education programs. After reading this text you will probably recognize that we do have the tools to be successful, but many practitioners are not applying what we know. This is an ethical issue. Quality health education is not easy and it is not accidental—it takes hard, dedicated work.

Case Study *Nathaniel has been assigned to teach a personal health course at a local community college. The outline calls for two days of coverage of HIV-AIDS issues. Nathaniel is not very conversant in these issues so he substitutes two additional days in the nutrition area which he enjoys. Several students and student reporters go to the dean to urge the dean to be certain AIDS is covered in personal health courses. The dean says that it is part of all personal health courses. Several students have just completed Nathaniel's course and state emphatically that it is not. The dean is very angry when she discovers that Nathaniel has not covered the prescribed material. Can Nathaniel defend his position?*

Nathaniel's actions were poorly thought out and based on selfish motives. If Nathaniel was supposed to teach to an already existing syllabus, then he should have prepared sufficiently to be able to cover all topics. Alternately, Nathaniel could have used a more knowledgeable guest speaker or colleague to cover a particular topic. Nathaniel has certainly not helped himself professionally by angering his dean and his actions would be difficult to defend.

THE LEARNING ENVIRONMENT

The mental/emotional environment can be influenced by the physical environment in which we conduct our classes or workshops. We must do what we can to make the total environment as pleasant as possible. If we have control over the space, we should strive to develop a cheerful positive appearance that is more conducive to learning. It is common sense that a room that is warm and cheerful is important for good learning. Select warm colors and organize the space to be warm and inviting. Adding colorful paper and posters also sets a positive mood. Be certain to change the colors and posters on a regular basis.

Case Study

Susan inherits a classroom that is run down and gloomy in appearance. Many years ago it was painted a battleship gray which has now faded. The bulletin boards are old and worn. She believes that this is contributing to a negative atmosphere and wants to do something about it. She has requested through her principal that it be repaired. She discusses the problem with her students who organize a fund-raising drive which results in $85 for paint and paper. Over the break students volunteer to help scrub and paint the room. The transformation is dramatic. The three days of vacation time spent painting result in a major change in the total environment. Susan notices a significant change in the classroom climate.

Susan has demonstrated an understanding of the effects that the environment can have on learning, and she has shown a great deal of initiative in enhancing her own particular environment. The atmo-

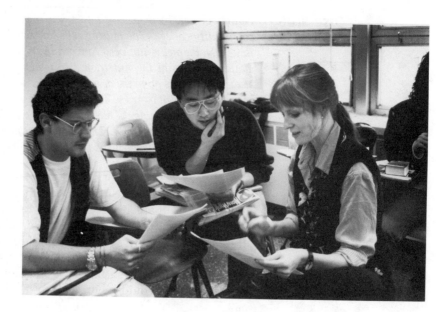

sphere in Susan's classes may not change overnight, but she has optimized the possibility for change. Health educators should not underestimate the effects that the physical environment can have on learning, and in some cases how easily the environment can be improved.

Noise Levels   Noise can be a major distraction in the learning environment. Select a site free of distractions as much as possible. Soft background music can sometimes overcome some noise from the outside. Other noise can come from participants and can also be a distraction or could simply indicate a high degree of interest. Noise must be assessed in terms of what helps achieve learning. Many classrooms are so quiet that learning is unlikely to take place. Students need opportunities to show enthusiasm and ask questions. The reason for the noise is an important consideration. All should have an opportunity to hear and be heard.

Seating Arrangements   The way you organize your seating is very important. Most situations allow for some change. Determine what would be the best seating

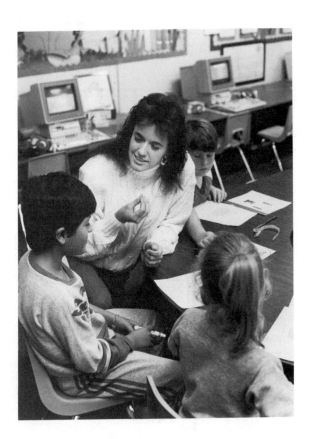

arrangement for the objectives you hope to achieve. If you want inter-action, a circle might be best. If you feel you need most interaction to be between you and the group, a semicircle might be best. If it is a large group, you might consider multiple rows with your position elevated. If you want small group work, you might consider small clusters. Figures 2-7 through 2-12 depict various seating arrangements.

It is important to plan ahead and not let seating happen simply by accident. Arrive early for workshops and plan your environment. Arrange the seating and let people know it is not okay to change it. If you do not want people sitting in the back, then do not place seats in the back. If you are in the classroom, do not let students pick where they sit until you know them well. Certain students should never sit together. Be certain to also consider any special needs students have such as hearing or sight limitations. Putting someone in an incorrect seat can produce a behavioral problem. For example, a student who cannot hear may become very disruptive simply because he cannot participate.

USING THE TOTAL ENVIRONMENT

In the past many health education programs have assumed that the few contact hours of the program could lead to major changes in the target population without giving consideration to the total environ-

FIGURE 2-7
Classroom Seating Objective: Interaction and Small Group Work

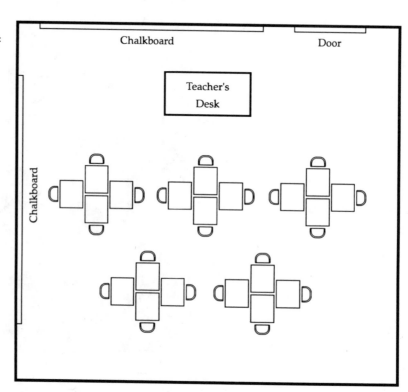

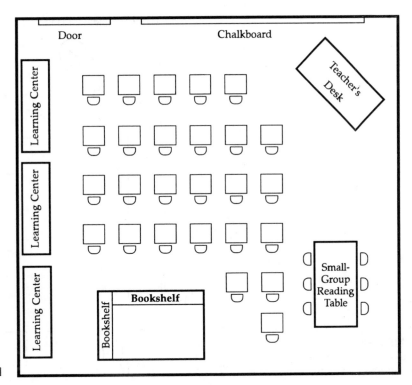

FIGURE 2-8
Classroom Objective:
Flexibility with Control

FIGURE 2-9
Community or School
Objective: Interaction

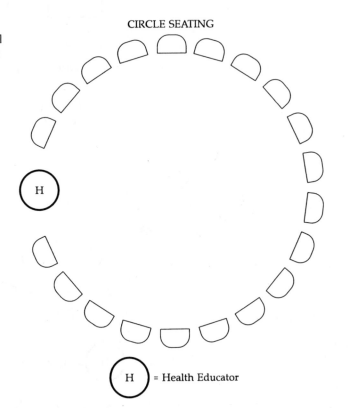

CIRCLE SEATING

$\boxed{H}$ = Health Educator

CLASSROOM U-SEATING

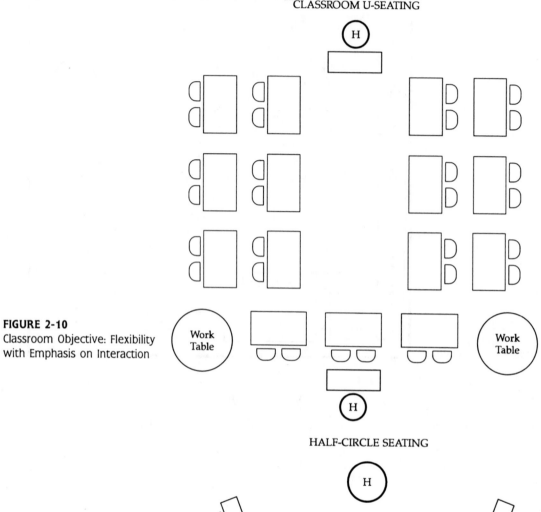

FIGURE 2-10
Classroom Objective: Flexibility
with Emphasis on Interaction

HALF-CIRCLE SEATING

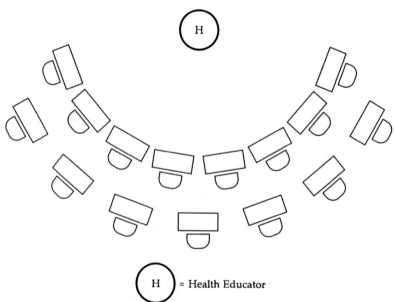

FIGURE 2-11
Classroom or Community
Objective: Controlled
Interaction Health
Educator in
Controlling Position

$\left(\text{H}\right)$ = Health Educator

SEMINAR SEATING

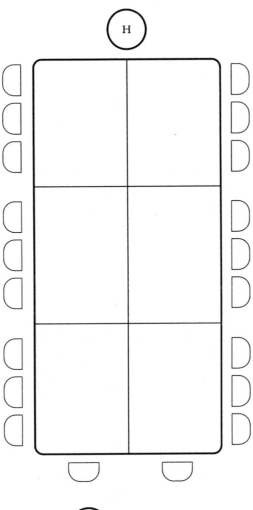

FIGURE 2-12
Community or School
Objective: Controlled
Interaction

(H) = Health Educator

ment in which individual members exist. It is important that we give consideration to the total physical and mental climate in which these people live.

While we may not have the capability to significantly alter this environment, we might provide the knowledge or skills to alter perceptions of the environment. We might overcome feelings of lack of control or helplessness. We might simply provide information on where to get help to change the environment.

Case Study	*Maria has conducted a community workshop on the need for prenatal care. The major objective was to increase knowledge regarding the reasons to seek such care and increase compliance. The workshop was well attended and the information seemed to be received with interest. Post-workshop assessment shows knowledge was significantly increased. However, a six-month follow-up shows no increase in compliance.*

Maria has conducted a useful workshop which obviously provided some needed factual information. However, in preparing for her presentation, Maria failed to consider the total environment of her target population, and just what compliance would necessitate. Maria provided no information on the accessibility of the clinic, how to get there, and failed to emphasize the very low costs involved. She gave no real thought to the total environment of this group or the potential barriers to effecting a positive behavior change.

SUMMARY

Selecting or writing the appropriate educational goals and objectives is important for any health education program.

1. The selection of an objective should always consider the resources available to achieve that objective.
2. A needs assessment is an important step before selecting or writing objectives or selecting methods.
3. Goals may be general but objectives must be specific and measurable.
4. When writing objectives the educational purposes (process or outcome) must be considered.
5. All domains should be considered if adequate time and resources are available.
6. Methods should be selected with proper ethics in mind.
7. The total environment must be considered when planning for instruction.

REFERENCES

Banks, R. 1980. Health and the spiritual dimension: Relationships and implications for professional preparation programs. *Journal of School Health* 50:195–202.

Bloom, B., ed. 1956. *Taxonomy of Educational Objectives The Classification of Educational Goals Handbook I: Cognitive Domain.* New York: David McKay.

Clark, A., and M. J. Friedman. 1982. The relative importance of treatment outcomes: A Delphi group weighting in mental health. *Education Review* 6:79–93.

Cyphert, F. R., and W. L. Gant. 1971. The Delphi technique: A case study. *Phi Delta Kappan* 52:272–273.

Dalkey, N. and Helmer. 1963. An experimental application of the Delphi method to the use of experts. *Management Science* 9:458.

Gilmore, G. D. 1977. Needs assessment processes for community health education. *International Journal of Health Education* 20:164–173.

Green, L. W., and M. W. Kreuter. 1991. *Health Promo-*

tion and Planning An Educational and Environmental Approach. Mountain View: Mayfield.

Green, L.W., D. M. Levine, and S. G. Deeds. 1975. Clinical trials of health education for hypertensive outpatients: Design and baseline data. *Preventive Medicine* 4:417–425.

Green, L. W., D. M. Levine, J. Wolle, and S. G. Deeds. 1979. Development of randomized patient education experiments with urban poor hypertensives. *Patient Counseling and Health Education* 1:106–111.

Hentges, K., and M. C. Hosokawa. 1980. Delphi: Group participation in needs assessment and curriculum development. *Journal of School Health* 50:447–450.

Jillson, I. 1975. The national drug abuse policy Delphi: Progress report and findings to date. The Delphi method: Techniques and applications, edited by H. A. Linstone and M. Turoff. Reading, MA: Addison-Wesley.

Judd, R. C. 1972. Use of Delphi methods in higher education. *Technological Forecasting and Social Change* 4:173–186.

Krathwohl, D., et al. 1956. *Taxonomy of Educational Objectives The Classification of Educational Goals Handbook II: Affective Domain.* New York: David McKay.

Linstone, H. A. and M. Turoff eds. 1975. *The Delphi Method: Techniques and Applications.* Reading, MA: Addison-Wesley.

Morisky, D. E., N. E. DeMuth, M. Field-Fass, et al. 1985. Evaluation of family health education to build social support for long-term control of high blood pressure. *Health Education Quarterly* 12:35–50.

Morisky, D. E., L. Levine, L. W. Green. et al. 1983. Five-year blood pressure control and mortality following health education for hypertensive patients. *American Journal of Public Health* 73:153–162.

Popham, J., and E. Baber. 1970. *Establishing Instructional Goals.* Englewood Cliffs, NJ: Prentice-Hall.

Ross, H. and P. Mico. 1980. *Theory and Practice in Health Education.* Palo Alto: Mayfield.

Scheele, S. 1975. Reality construction as a product of Delphi interaction. In *The Delphi Method: Techniques and Applications,* edited by H. A. Linstone and M. Turoff. Reading, MA: Addison-Wesley.

Taba, H. 1962. *Curriculum Development.* New York: Harcourt, Brace and World.

Toohey, J. V., and J. H. Shireffs. 1980. *Health Education* 11:15–17.

Travis, R. 1976. The Delphi technique: A tool for community health educators. *Health Education* 7:11–13.

U.S. HHS. 1980. *Promoting Health/Preventing Disease: Objectives for the Nation,* U.S. Public Health Service. Washington, DC: Government Printing Office.

U.S. HHS. 1992. *Healthy Communities 2000: Model Standards,* U.S. Public Health Service. Washington, DC: Government Printing Office.

U.S. HHS. 1992. *Healthy People 2000: National Health Promotion Objectives Full Report, With Commentary.* Boston: Jones and Bartlett.

Selecting an Intervention/Method

Entry-Level Health Educator Competencies Addressed in This Chapter

Responsibility I: Assessing Individual and Community Needs for Health Education

Competency A: Obtain health related data about social and cultural environments, growth and development factors, needs, and interests.

Competency C: Infer needs for health education on the basis of obtained data.

Responsibility II: Planning Effective Health Education Programs

Competency B: Develop a logical scope and sequence plan for a health education program.

Responsibility IV: Evaluating Effectiveness of Health Education Programs

Competency A: Develop plans to assess achievement of program objectives.

Responsibility VII: Communicating Health and Health Education Needs, Concerns, and Resources

Competency A: Interpret concepts, purposes, and theories of health education.

Method Selection in Health Education

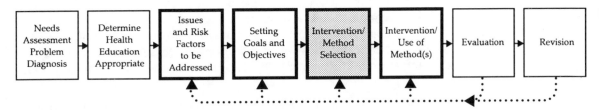

Heavy-bordered boxes indicate subjects addressed in this text; shaded boxes indicate subject(s) of current chapter.

Competency B: Predict the impact of societal value systems on health education programs.

Taken from *A Framework for the Development of Competency Based Curricula for Entry Level Health Educators*, National Task Force on the Preparation and Practice of Health Educators, Inc., 1985. Reprinted by permission.

Case Study

John is offering a workshop for low-income expectant mothers as part of his work for the March of Dimes. He personally likes role playing as a method so he has written up several role plays about life after the delivery. The site for the two-hour workshop is a nice upscale hotel, and he has mailed approximately 100 invitations. This is a very culturally diverse community with many Asians, Salvadorians, and Mexican Americans. John is surprised at the low participant turnout and very indignant when the few mothers-to-be in attendance walk out rather than participate in role plays.

John has much to learn about workshop conduct and method selection. John sent out 100 invitations . . . how many people should he expect to attend? If health educators get a 50 percent attendance rate from invitations, they are usually thrilled! Is it likely that low-income individuals will be willing or even able to travel to an upscale hotel outside their community? John's attendance might have improved had he conducted the workshop at a site in the target community. Because of a personal interest in a strategy, John may have selected an inappropriate method for this population. Did he consult local community leaders about his presentation and discuss the most effective approaches he could utilize? Probably not. When a health educator works with a group that he/she may not be familiar with, it is essential that research and/or consultation of some type be performed in order to optimize effective strategy selection (see also Chapter 7).

Selecting the appropriate educational intervention is vital to achieving your objectives. We use the term intervention to describe the total overall strategy to achieve our objectives. A method refers to one component of the intervention such as an educational game or a health fair. Each is only one of perhaps many methods we may employ to achieve our objectives. The selection of methods to use as part of your intervention should always be based on what you hope to achieve— your objectives. All educators have this process in common, but the health educator must often consider how these strategies might also influence attitudes and behaviors. Further, the health educator must

Special thanks to Marjorie Scaffa for her assistance with this chapter. The section on models and theories is largely from her doctoral dissertation, *The Development of Comprehensive Theory in Health Education: A Feasibility Study,* and is used with permission.

often work with very modest amounts of time and limited resources. Given that we are often asked to modify very complex and deeply held practices, selecting the correct methods is indeed a challenge.

We do have an arsenal of methods and a knowledge base to help us with these decisions. This chapter will review the issues to be considered when selecting an intervention strategy (method).

After studying the chapter the reader will be able to:

- list the major considerations that should be made before selecting an educational intervention/method
- employ appropriate theories and models in method selection
- present a rationale for proper selection of a method
- list the most common mistakes in method selection

Key Issues

Objectives
Educational Principles
Theory and Model Application
Educational Domains
Characteristics of the Learner
  and the Community
Group Size
Contact Time

Budget
Resources/Site/Environment
Characteristics of the
  Educational Provider
Cultural Appropriateness
Using a Variety of Methods
Packaging the Total
  Intervention Strategy

OBJECTIVES

As you have learned, objectives drive the selection of an educational intervention and method. The methods selected must be appropriate for the objectives sought. The previous chapter has described the important components of stating goals and objectives. It is important in the context of selecting appropriate methods that we review our objectives before we select our methods. This is always the first step in selecting any methodology to be applied to our problem. You should always be able to link your selected methods with the objectives they are likely to achieve.

EDUCATIONAL PRINCIPLES

You should also review the basic educational principles. Have you applied as many educational principles as possible such as reinforcement, repetition, and practice? Reviewing these principles will often trigger new ideas about methods to use or not to use.

In order to address health issues through health education, it is important that we draw on the vast knowledge base that education has developed to tell us how to educate learners. The following principles[1] are of enormous importance to health education.

Principles Related to Motivating the Learner

- Learning is more effective when the learner is motivated by goals intrinsic to the experience.
- Individuals tend to repeat behaviors that are rewarded (reinforced).
- Immediate reinforcement is most effective.
- Fear and punishment have uncertain effects upon learning. They may facilitate or hinder learning.
- An individual learns best when he/she believes the learning is important.
- Learners can be helped in the acquisition of a concept, principle, or generalization through varied experiences relating to it and by applying the concept, principle, or generalization to a new situation.

Principles Related to the Needs and Abilities of the Learner

- Behaviors sought should be within the range of possibility for the learner involved.
- Generally, the higher the educational level of any given group, the greater is the reliance on printed words and symbols.
- The lower the educational level, the greater is the reliance on oral or picture media.
- There are marked individual differences in any given group of learners.
- Individuals usually slant persuasive communications to fit their own biases.
- Creative individuals show a preference for the complex and the novel.
- When problems are a common concern, group thinking is an effective approach to learning.

Principles Related to the General Nature of Learning

- In order for learning to occur, repetition is usually required.
- Learning is an active process that involves the dynamic interaction of the learner with that which is to be learned.
- Other things being equal, recent experiences are more vivid than earlier ones.
- According to Gestalt psychology:
  Intellectual processes operate as a whole.
  The whole person tends to respond in a unified way.
  The organism reacts to the total situation.
  We understand the parts by understanding the whole.

---

[1]Adapted from G. G. Gilbert, *Teaching First Aid and Emergency Care.* (Dubuque, IA: Kendall/Hunt, 1981). Used by permission.

- Learning generally proceeds from the general to the specific, then to the general (whole–part–whole).
- Transfer learning is not automatic. We must teach for transfer.
- Behaviors or skills sought must be practiced.
- Learning generally progresses from the known to the unknown, from the concrete to the abstract, and from the simple to the complex.
- Periods of practice interrupted by periods of rest result in more efficient learning than do longer periods of practice with few or no interruptions.
- Time spent recalling what has been read facilitates learning more than does the mere act of rereading.

THEORY AND MODEL APPLICATION

Health educators and researchers from many disciplines have developed numerous theories and models to try to explain human behavior with regard to health practices and ways we might intervene as health educators. These models and theories have important applications in method selection. If we wish to test a model or theory, we should be careful to select a method compatible with that model or theory. If we have theoretical notions we should draw on the available theories and models and related research to improve on our ideas.

How do models and theories such as the health belief model or social learning theory apply to your strategy? How can we utilize these ideas to improve and focus our total intervention and individual methods?

Ideas can be classified in many ways. According to Cornish, they should be classified in two categories: concepts and theories (Cornish, 1980). A concept, he argues, is a generalized notion, a mental map or image of some phenomenon. A theory is a description of two or more concepts and the relationship among them (Cornish, 1980). Thought involves the manipulation of concepts and theories and provides us with models of how the world functions. A model can be defined as a semantic or diagrammatic representation of concepts and their interrelationships which allows for operationalization, experimental assessment, and application of a theory (Parcel, 1984). Not all theories have corresponding models and not all models are founded on specific, well-defined theories.

Current Status of Theory in Health Education

One of the fundamental characteristics of a true profession is that it has a theoretical base underlying its practice within which parameters the profession operates (Shireffs, 1984). As an interdisciplinary field, health education draws its body of knowledge from a variety of sources. Health education relies on the biological sciences for much of its content; the behavioral sciences for its philosophy, program development, and implementation strategies; and education for its methodology (Rubinson and Alles, 1984). Due, in part, to its broad interdisciplinary nature, some argue health education lacks a clearly defined, readily identifiable body of knowledge. We believe that it does but that it is diffuse and hard to identify because of the lack of agreement as to what is the core of health education. As stated earlier, we believe that the core of health education is the process of health education. This means that what is most important is how well and effectively we perform the function of educating people about health decisions. This process of health education is the crucial focus for a health educator. There are many other tools available to health educators, but what is unique about health education as a discipline is that health educators are trained to perform health education. The use of models and theories are among the tools at their disposal.

Typically, in the development of the sciences, theory precedes application. However, health education has been traditionally, and continues to be, very practice oriented. The field has evolved without having a well-developed theoretical base (Creswell, 1984; Dwore and Matarazzo, 1981; Frazer, Kukulka, and Richardson, 1988). A basic premise that has predominated in health education for many years is that knowledge and a positive attitude will lead to health-enhancing behavior change (Shireffs, 1984). This assumption has been demonstrated to be overly simplistic, ill founded, and ineffective, yet much of the field continues to practice health education and conduct research utilizing this principle (Shireffs, 1984; Frazer, Kukulka, and Richardson, 1988).

Neither contemplation of the navel nor the writing of pamphlets can be shown to be cost-effective.
—Mohan Singh

Health education has borrowed and utilized well-defined theoretical frameworks from other disciplines, most notably, social learning theory, problem-behavior theory, theory of reasoned action, communications theory, and social competence theory (Parcel, 1984). Although these models from the behavioral sciences are valuable, it must be recognized that they are not health behavior specific and have been shown to be of limited usefulness in the treatment and prevention of disease and dysfunction (Dwore and Matarazzo, 1981).

A well-developed theoretical base in health education is essential for a variety of reasons. Theory can provide the foundation and context for basic and applied research and program design, implementation, and evaluation. The following is a description of the popular constructs or concepts, theories, and models found in the professional health education literature and a critique of their appropriateness for health education practice and research. This is not meant to be an exhaustive account of relevant theoretical approaches, but rather a sampling in order to illustrate the current state of theory in health education.

Constructs Of all of the social-psychological variables that may impact on health-related behavior, three appear to receive the most attention in health education literature. These are: locus of control, self-efficacy, and behavioral intent. These constructs can aid us in method selection or evaluation. Depending on our goals and objectives, they can be useful tools.

Health Locus The health locus of control construct was first described by Wallston et
of Control al. (1976). It was developed as a health-specific adaptation of the internal-external locus of control concept postulated by Rotter in 1954 as one component of social learning theory. Locus of control was considered a means of predicting behavior based on an individual's expectations of reinforcement. Reinforcement was believed to be either under the control of the individual (internal locus) or under the control of outside forces (external locus). Externality has been associated with feelings of powerlessness, and internality with self-motivated behaviors (Wallston and Wallston, 1978).

Health locus of control, it was suggested, could be used to predict a variety of health behaviors, including information seeking, compliance with medication regimens, smoking cessation, and appointment

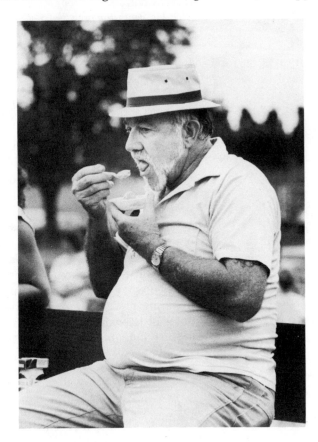

keeping (Wallston and Wallston, 1978). Levenson (1974) expanded the health locus of control construct to include two dimensions of externality: belief that reinforcement is due to fate or chance and belief in control by powerful others. If an individual perceives that an event is contingent upon his/her own actions, then the person is considered to have an internal locus of control. If, on the other hand, an individual perceives that an event is contingent upon the actions of powerful others or due to luck or chance, then he/she is considered to have an external locus of control (Parcel, Nader, and Rogers, 1980).

Currently, several health-specific locus of control scales exist. These include the original health locus of control scale by Wallston et al. (1976), the multidimensional health locus of control scale by Wallston, Wallston, and DeVillis (1978), and the children's health locus of control scale by Parcel and Meyer (1978).

Case Study

Marcel is working with a community group on a series of workshops designed to improve general levels of health, particularly related to nutrition and heart health. As he begins his introductory statements on the benefits of good food, Marcel notices several cynical looks and some careless whispering. Putting aside his carefully prepared notes, Marcel stops the workshop to query the participants' reactions. After several minutes of discussion what becomes clear to Marcel is that many of the participants feel that they cannot influence their own health behavior. Instead of continuing on with the planned presentation, Marcel decides to employ a health locus of control instrument and finds over 50 percent of the group feel external forces control their health status. Marcel then decides to modify his programming by designing an intervention that not only includes factual information related to heart health, but also strategies to address the issue of locus of control.

Marcel deserves a good deal of credit for being intuitive about the concerns of the group. It takes courage to realize that the presentation is not going as planned and then making the conscious decision to stop and reorganize the material. It is probably unrealistic to expect Marcel to whip out a health locus of control instrument that he conveniently had in his back pocket! However, the important point being made is that health theory plays an important role in determining the most effective ways of delivering health messages and information. When preparing presentations such theories should be considered and elements of relevant models utilized to increase the effectiveness of the intervention. If nothing else, this approach forces the presenter to consider the very specific intent of the presentation and facilitates the development of behavioral objectives.

Self-Efficacy

Self-efficacy is defined as the individual's perception that he/she will be able to perform a specific behavior successfully (Bandura, 1977). A belief in one's own competence to execute a task is required to produce a desired outcome. Self-efficacy expectations are derived from several sources of information: previous performance accomplishments, vicarious experiences (modeling), verbal persuasion, and emotional arousal (Bandura, 1977).

Successful performance increases expectations of mastery, while repeated failures diminish them. The effects of failure, however, are partially dependent on the timing and the pattern of the negative experiences. Watching others who are similar to oneself, overcoming obstacles by determined effort increases self-efficacy. Diversified modeling by a variety of individuals is more effective than repeated modeling by a single individual. Self-efficacy is increased if the modeled behavior has clear and observable outcomes. Verbal persuasion is an effective adjunct to performance accomplishments and modeling, but rarely increases self-efficacy when used in isolation. Certain physiological and emotional states are perceived to be indicators of stress. High levels of arousal usually interfere with performance and lower efficacy expectations. Behavioral control of arousal levels and cognitive reappraisal of these physiological and emotional states can increase self-efficacy (Bandura, 1977).

It is hypothesized that these efficacy expectations influence what behaviors will be initiated, the degree of effort expended, and the

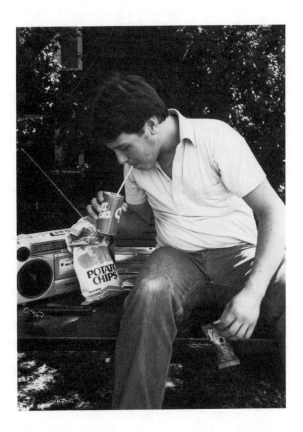

persistence of the behavior over time. Perceived self-efficacy has a direct influence on an individual's choice of activities and settings (Bandura, 1977). Expectation of successful performance alone will not produce the desired behavior; necessary skill capabilities and incentives are also required.

Efficacy expectations change over time and vary on several dimensions, including magnitude, generality, and strength (Bandura, 1977). Magnitude refers to the level of difficulty with which an individual experiences a sense of competence. Generality refers to an ability to extend one's sense of efficacy beyond a circumscribed situation. Strength refers to the degree to which the expectation can be extinguished by disconfirming experiences. Weak expectations are easily abandoned, whereas strong expectations persist in spite of some negative experiences (Bandura, 1977).

Case Study

Nancy is working with a group of senior smokers. Although Nancy is an ex-smoker herself, the group, being much older, does not see her as a role model. Instead of simply moving ahead and ignoring this issue, Nancy decides to bring in a panel of older ex-smokers to review the skills needed to stop smoking. The individuals on the panel discuss in depth their experiences with stopping smoking and the group seems to relate well to the session. Nancy finds a pronounced difference in group response following this panel. Self-efficacy has clearly improved. Nancy is pleased that she was able to incorporate a strategy that seemed to facilitate learning, but is somewhat angry at herself for not anticipating this problem before it arose.

Like Marcel in the previous case study, Nancy should feel very positive about recognizing a problem and then confronting the issue with the intent to make a program more effective. In some instances the easiest way to deal with a problem is to ignore it . . . ultimately ignoring the fact that an intervention might have become totally ineffective. Nancy identified a problem and devised a strategy to alleviate her difficulties. Health educators working in the area of addictions should be aware that there exists in the field of prevention and treatment a belief by some that only individuals who have experienced addiction themselves can fully relate to the problem. Although this philosophy is not necessarily held by the majority, this issue needs to be considered by health educators when planning interventions of this nature. Nancy's experience is not an unusual one.

Behavioral Intent

Behavioral intent, according to Ajzen and Fishbein (1973), is the immediate antecedent of overt behavior. It is an individual's resolution to perform a specific act with respect to a given stimulus in a given situation. It is the attitude about a specific behavior that is relevant, not attitudes toward objects, people, or situations.

Behavioral intent is a function of two basic factors. One is personal in nature and the other is reflective of social influences. The personal factor is the individual's attitude, positive or negative, toward performing a specific behavior and whether he/she is in favor or against engaging in this behavior. The social factor is the individual's perception of the social pressures to act or not to act in a specific manner. This is often referred to as the subjective norm. These two factors in isolation are not sufficient to determine behavioral intent. Ajzen and Fishbein (1973) state that the person's motivation to comply with the subjective norm is also necessary.

Behavioral intent can be an excellent evaluation method before and after intervention. Such needs assessment and evaluation tools can be very helpful. Measuring this trait is particularly useful when efforts to evaluate actual behavior change may be too costly or time consuming to be practical. We must, of course, have realistic expectations for our health education program.

Case Study

John is involved in teaching CPR to a group of metal shop employees. He has little time or resources to carry out an extensive evaluation but is concerned that in previous training workshops participants appeared to have little confidence and seemed unlikely to use the skills covered. John considers his options and decides to utilize simulation mannequins, which will help participants gauge their skills, and use a pretest/posttest questionnaire to measure any changes in levels of behavioral intent. He employs questions regarding self-assessed skill level and the likelihood of using CPR if faced with a real situation. He is elated to see a marked increase in scores after his 10-hour inservice.

John did a good job of taking into account the important elements of self-efficacy and behavioral intent when considering the impact of his workshop. It would have been much easier to simply go through the mechanics of teaching CPR and at the conclusion of the workshop make the assumption that most individuals were sufficiently trained. Utilizing a simulation helped participants gauge their individual skill levels and the pretest/posttest questionnaires allowed John to evaluate an often-ignored element of CPR training: Are people likely to use their training in a real-life situation?

Many theories have been referred to in the health education literature, but two are cited more frequently than others: social learning theory and theory of reasoned action. Again, theories can provide a basis for method selection. Much needs to be done to test these theories and to link theories to appropriate health education interventions.

Social Learning Theory

In Social Learning and Clinical Psychology, Rotter (1954) established the foundation for social learning theory which has recently been renamed social cognitive theory (Bandura, 1986). He postulated that it was an individual's expectations of the consequences of a particular action that determined whether or not that behavior was performed.

Bandura (1977) expanded on Rotter's work and developed the concept of self-efficacy as an integral component of social learning theory. Self-efficacy is defined as the individual's perception that he/she will be able to successfully perform a specific behavior (Bandura, 1977). It is the belief in one's own competence to execute an action that will achieve the desired outcome. The most basic postulate of social learning theory is that individuals perform behaviors that result in certain outcomes. However, both the behaviors and the outcomes are mediated by expectancies. An expectancy is the value an individual places on a particular outcome (Bandura, 1977).

Efficacy expectations, whether or not an individual believes in his/her ability to perform a given behavior, are derived from personal performance attainments, vicarious experience, verbal persuasion, and emotional arousal. Successful accomplishment of a behavior enhances one's expectation for future endeavors. The more similar the current task to ones performed successfully in the past, the greater are the efficacy expectations. Observation of others, who are perceived as being similar to oneself, engaging in activities and achieving the desired outcome can also increase one's expectations for accomplishment. Verbal encouragement and permission to try a specific behavior and a perceived physiological and emotional state conducive to successful execution of the task will also enhance an individual's confidence and self-efficacy relative to that behavior, according to the theory.

Outcome expectations are the individual's belief that a given behavior will lead to specific outcomes (Bandura, 1977). The locus of control construct is considered an element of outcome expectations by Bandura (1977) and others (Rosenstock, Strecher, and Becker, 1988; Wodarski, 1987; DiBlasio, 1986; Eiser, 1985). The interaction of the constructs of self-efficacy and locus of control forms the foundation for social learning theory and is the basis on which behavior can be predicted (Bandura, 1977). It is expected, according to the theory, that individuals who have high levels of self-efficacy and an internal locus of control will be more likely to attempt to execute a particular behavior. These individuals would have a high level of confidence in their ability to successfully accomplish the task and tend to believe that performance of the behavior would directly affect the outcome (Rosenstock, Strecher, and Becker, 1988). Individuals with low levels of self-efficacy and an external locus of control would be least likely to attempt a given behavior, as they have low levels of confidence in their ability to perform the behavior and believe that their actions would not produce the desired outcome anyway (Rosenstock, Strecher, and Becker, 1988).

Behavior change, in the social learning theory paradigm, can be achieved directly by reinforcement of particular behaviors; indirectly, through social modeling or observing someone else being reinforced for the behavior; and thirdly, through self-management or by having the individual monitor and self-reward (Parcel and Baranowski, 1981). According to Rosenstock, Strecher, and Becker (1988), lifestyle changes will occur if the individual believes:

1. The current behaviors pose a threat to a personally valued outcome, for example, health or appearance (environmental cue).
2. The specific behavior change will be likely to reduce these threats (outcome efficacy).
3. He/she is personally competent to perform the desired behavior (efficacy expectation).

Applications of Social Learning Theory in Health Education

Several studies have utilized the social learning theory (SLT) approach in examining health behaviors. DiBlasio (1986) investigated the drinking and driving behavior of students in grades 10 through 12. Five SLT constructs were operationalized and measured through self-report. These constructs included exposure to and identification with various groups; modeling; differential reinforcement; personal attitudes and beliefs; and positive or negative social rewards or consequences. The theory was supported, as all of the constructs significantly contributed to the adolescents' decisions to drive under the influence or ride with someone who was intoxicated. The greatest predictor of all of the constructs was exposure to or identification with specific groups. Di-

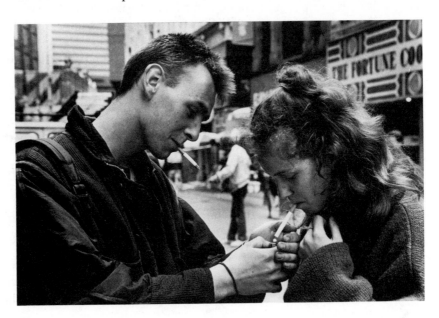

Blasio's (1986) recommendation, based on these results, was to include parents and peers in the planning of prevention programs for driving under the influence. Such findings are very important for method selection.

Wodarski (1987) evaluated the usefulness of SLT in the development and implementation of an educational intervention for adolescents on drinking and driving. A teams/games/tournament approach was designed to enhance self-efficacy and to provide positive social outcomes for the desired behaviors. The results indicated that, when compared to a control group, the intervention students demonstrated a significant decrease in self-reported alcohol consumption and a significant increase in knowledge and self-efficacy related to drinking behavior.

Parcel and Baranowski (1981) described the application of SLT as it relates to phases in the behavior change process. They concluded that the various constructs of SLT were relevant at different stages in the process of behavior change. Baranowski's four phases of behavior change include the pretraining, training, initial self-testing, and continued performance stages. In the pretraining phase expectancies are the key constructs. What a person believes about a given health problem, what anxieties are associated with these beliefs, and the perception of changeability are all relevant issues during this phase.

In the training phase the focus is on developing the capability to perform the desired behaviors and on learning to cope with problems associated with the change process itself. The construct of behavioral capability states that if an individual is to engage in a specific behavior, he/she must have *knowledge* of the parameters of the behavior and the *skill* to carry it out successfully. According to SLT, behavioral capability can be acquired through the observation of others engaged in the behavior or social modeling, as well as direct skill training (Parcel and Baranowski, 1981).

In the self-testing phase the construct of self-efficacy appears to be the most influential. Confidence in one's ability is essential if the skills learned in the training phase are to be implemented. The technique of successive approximations is particularly useful in the development of self-efficacy.

In the final phase, continued performance, the construct of self-control is the most salient. In order for a behavior to be maintained over time, an individual must be able to resist the temptation to discontinue the behavior and to delay gratification. Contracting and self-monitoring are methods of enhancing self-control (Parcel and Baranowski, 1981).

In general, social learning theory provides a unique perspective for health education practice. The constructs of self-efficacy, outcome expectancy, behavioral capability, modeling, reciprocal determinism, and self control appear to be particularly relevant for the development of health education interventions.

Case Study   *Jessica is working with a group of young people at the YMCA with the hope of increasing their resistance skills to offers of drugs. After reading about various models and theories of health behavior, Jessica plans to cover ways of saying "no thanks." She makes a determined effort to have each person practice saying "no" in a role play in front of the other group members. Each session is critiqued by the other members, and other suggestions for strategies are fully discussed. Even though this is a time-consuming methodology, each person has three such sessions of saying "no." The self-confidence of the group members regarding the possession of needed skills and the feeling that they can and will use the skills is greatly enhanced.*

Jessica's approach is one that is based on health education theory and is an approach that has become commonplace in drug education today. The emphasis, particularly in schools, is to spend less time on didactic, factual learning and more time on developing practical skills to avoid becoming involved in drug use/abuse. Elements of health education models such as self-efficacy, locus of control, and behavioral intent are all utilized in an attempt to equip the individual to combat risky health behavior. Jessica's method selection allows participants to experience and develop their own skills on a personal level rather than simply hearing facts about drugs in an impersonal, abstract manner.

Theory of Reasoned Action

Attitude theory serves as the basis for the work of Fishbein and Ajzen and the theory of reasoned action. This theory postulates that an individual's attitude toward an object is a function of his/her beliefs about the object. Attitudes are defined as learned predispositions to consistently respond to objects in favorable or unfavorable ways (Fishbein, 1973).

The theory of reasoned action is based on several assumptions. One assumption is that human beings are usually very rational and make systematic decisions based on available information. It dismisses the notion that unconscious motives can influence behavior and insists that individuals carefully consider the implications of their behavior before engaging in specific activities (Ajzen and Fishbein, 1980).

A second assumption is that most behavior is under volitional control and that in a specific situation an individual forms an intent to act which subsequently influences overt behavior (Ajzen and Fishbein, 1973). This behavioral intent is viewed as the most immediately relevant predictor of behavior. According to the theory, behavioral intent is determined by the individual's attitude toward the behavior, normative beliefs regarding the behavior, and motivation to comply with the norms (Ajzen and Fishbein, 1973).

Attitude toward the behavior, in this context, is defined as the individual's positive or negative evaluation of performing the behavior. Normative belief, or subjective norm, refers to the individual's perception of the social pressures to perform or not to perform the behavior in question. Conflict between an individual's attitude toward the behavior and the subjective norm is not uncommon. Assigning relative weights to these two determinants greatly enhances the predictive value of the behavioral intent construct and the explanatory value of the theory (Ajzen and Fishbein, 1980).

According to Ajzen and Fishbein (1973), the central equation of the theory is that behavior is determined by behavioral intent which is equal to the individual's attitude toward the act (multiplied by an empirically determined weight) plus the individual's normative belief multiplied by his/her motivation to comply with the norm (multiplied by an empirically determined weight).

The theory of reasoned action has several limitations. Although it makes reference to attitudes toward behavior, it does not include attitudes toward objects, people, or institutions. These attitudes may also have an impact on behavioral intent. In addition, other factors that may influence behavior, such as personality variables and demographic characteristics, are not considered. Ajzen and Fishbein (1980) contend that it is unnecessary to attempt to link these external variables to behavioral phenomenon, as the intervening factors, that is, behavioral intent, can account for these effects.

Another limitation is the degree of specificity necessary for the theory to accurately predict behavior. The relationship between attitude, behavioral intent, and behavior is not consistently supported in the literature. Behavioral intent appears to be a relatively good predictor under specific conditions. The more abstract or generalized the measure of intention, the less is its predictive capability. A measure of behavioral intent such as "I intend to exercise" is much less predictive than the statement "I intend to walk two miles, three times a week for the next three months." The longer the time interval between the measure of intent and the observation of the behavior, the less likely the behavior is to occur. Behavioral intent appears to be unstable and variable over time which limits its usefulness as a predictor of behavior.

Other Selected Theories Relevant to Health Education

Several other theories applicable to health education will be described briefly. These include problem-behavior theory, communications theory, and behavioral theory.

Jessor and Jessor (1977) developed problem-behavior theory which has its conceptual roots in social psychology. It is an attempt to develop a profile of vulnerability or predisposition toward health-threatening behaviors, such as alcohol consumption, drug use, smoking, and risky sexual behavior. This theoretical framework is based on the interrelationships and interactions among three major explanatory concepts: personality, perceived environment, and behavior. Each concept has specific variables that have implications for the incidence of problem behaviors. A major contribution of this theory is its application in the explanation of risk-taking behavior of adolescents in the normal developmental process.

Communications theory is not a single theory but rather many approaches designed to change people's attitudes and behavior through persuasive techniques (Parcel, 1984). One eclectic approach is known as the information-processing paradigm (McGuire, 1981). In this model the communication-persuasion process occurs in six phases and consists of five components. The components of communication are described as source, message, channel, receiver, and destination. The phases, or behavioral steps, in the process of persuasion are presentation, attention, comprehension, yielding, retention, and overt behavior (McGuire, 1981). Communications theory has been used effectively in health education in the design and conduct of a public health campaign (McGuire, 1981). It may also be useful in an attempt to inoculate children against persuasion in the media and peer pressure (Parcel, 1984).

Behavioral theories are multiple and are variations derived from Watson and Skinner's notions of behaviorism. Behavior modification is a technique, based on behavioral theory, designed to develop new behaviors or alter existing behaviors (Stainbrook and Green, 1982). Basically, the presupposition of behavioral theory is that behavior is a function of reinforcement conditions. If a behavior is reinforced, then it will increase in frequency. Reinforcement may be positive, as in the administration of some pleasurable consequence, or negative, as in the removal of some pleasant condition.

In its most radical form, behaviorism focuses on the study and control of external environmental variables. Internal constructs such as attitudes and mental processes are dismissed as unimportant at best, and irrelevant at worst (Stainbrook and Green, 1982). Behavioral strategies have proven effective in the treatment of habit disorders, behavior or conduct problems, and in skill acquisition and development.

MODELS

Clearly, two models relevant to health education are very popular in the literature. One, the health belief model, is a model of the precursors of health behavior; the other, the PRECEDE-PROCEED model, is a program planning and evaluation tool. A third lesser known model, the activated health education model, is also described.

Health Belief Model

The health belief model (HBM) is one of many models of health-related behavior. Cummings, Becker, and Maile (1980), in a review of 14 models used in health education research, concluded that there is considerable overlap in the constructs or variables that make up these frameworks. Cummings, Becker, and Maile (1980) attempted to develop a unified framework for explaining health behavior by involving the authors of the various models in categorizing over 100 variables derived from the models. Six factors emerged from the multidimensional scaling analysis: (1) access to health care services; (2) attitudes toward health care; (3) perception of threat of illness; (4) characteristics of the social network, interactions, norms, and structure; (5) knowledge about disease; and (6) demographic characteristics (Cummings, Becker, and Maile, 1980).

Of all of the models studied by Cummings, Becker, and Maile (1980), the health belief model is, by far, the most extensively utilized. The health belief model was originally developed by Hochbaum, Kegeles, Leventhal, and Rosenstock to explain preventive health behaviors, but was quickly adapted to study sick role and illness behavior (Becker, 1974; Kirscht, 1974). The model is based on theories from social psychology, most notably, Lewin's aspiration theory (Maiman and Becker, 1974). Two underlying premises of the model, borrowed from Lewinian tradition, are the phenomenological orientation and the historical perspective. The phenomenological orientation states that it is the individual's perceptions that determine behavior, not the envi-

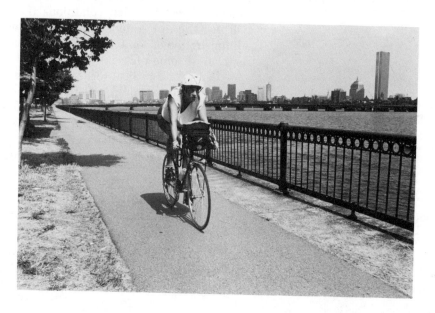

ronment. A historical perspective mandates a focus on the current dynamics affecting an individual's behavior, not on past history or prior experiences (Rosenstock, 1974).

The health belief model describes the relationships between people's beliefs about health and their health-specific behaviors. The beliefs that mediate health behavior are, according to the model, perceived susceptibility, severity, benefits, and barriers (Figure 3-1). In addition to the previously mentioned beliefs, cues to action are viewed as necessary triggers of behavior. Perceived susceptibility is the individual's subjective impression of the risk of contracting a disease or illness. Perceived severity refers to the convictions a person holds regarding the degree of seriousness of a given health problem. Perceived benefits are the beliefs a person has regarding the availability and effectiveness of a variety of possible actions in reducing the threat of illness. Perceived barriers are those costs or negative aspects associated with engaging in a specific health behavior. Cues to action are defined as instigating events that stimulate the initiation of behavior. These cues may be internal, such as perceptions of pain, or external, such as feedback from a health care provider (Rosenstock, 1974).

According to the model, in order for a person to take action

FIGURE 3-1
The Health Belief Model
Source: M. Becker (ed.), *The Health Belief Model and Personal Health Behavior* (NJ: Slack, 1974), p. 7. Reprinted with permission.

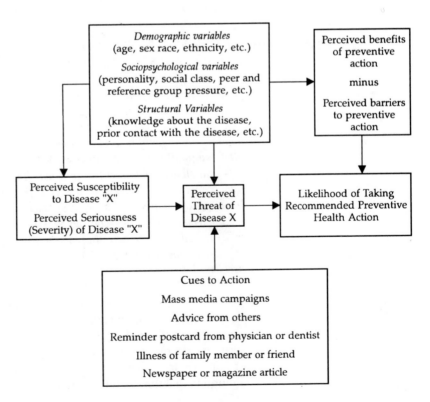

The lotus, like health education, floats upon still waters; alas, while many admire their perfection, neither hath visible means of support.
—Mohan Singh

to avoid illness, the positive forces would need to outweigh the negative forces. If an individual believes that

    (a) (s)he is personally susceptible to the disease or illness;

    (b) the occurrence of the health problem is severe enough to negatively impact his/her life;

    (c) taking specific actions would have beneficial effects; and

    (d) the barriers to such action do not overwhelm the benefits, and the individual is exposed to cues for action, then it is likely that the health behavior will occur. (Rosenstock, 1974)

The health belief model has been applied to a variety of populations and a diversity of health issues, including alcoholism (Bardsley and Beckman, 1988); compliance with a diabetes regimen (Becker and Janz, 1985); breast self-examination (Champion, 1985); contraceptive behavior (Herold, 1983; Hester and Macrina, 1985); and medication compliance among psychiatric outpatients (Kelly, Mamon, and Scott, 1987). Although it is true that the majority of studies are retrospective in nature and the predictive value of the model is still in doubt (Kegeles and Lund, 1982), recent studies have used the model to make some predictions (Stein et al., 1992; Harrison, 1992).

Case Study

Bill is teaching a unit on AIDS to ninth-grade classes in a local high school. He is dismayed to find that his students are bored and restless, despite this being a topic which is related to sex. After class, Bill questions several students about their attitudes and discovers that although the students consider AIDS to be a serious disease, they feel that because they are heterosexual and do not use drugs the problem has little relevance to their lives. Bill ponders the issue of how to increase the students' perceived susceptibility to HIV and finally develops a strategy. With permission from school administrators, Bill shows his students a film which dramatically depicts the story of a high school student who contracts HIV from heterosexual sex. In addition, a local speakers bureau provides a speaker for Bill's classes. The speaker is a young woman who has contracted HIV through heterosexual intercourse while in college. Both activities have a sobering effect on Bill's students, and, at least in the short term, they no longer view AIDS as "someone else's problem."

Bill is another good health educator who is aware enough to realize when his approach might need an adjustment to make a program more effective. In theoretical terms his students were demonstrating extremely low perceived susceptibility to HIV/AIDS. This lack of concern is endemic among adolescents, and Bill was perceptive enough to feel that he needed to change his plans. Bill's strategy was to show a dramatic film about AIDS and bring in a speaker who was HIV positive. Both methods had two key elements in common . . . the major character in the film and the guest speaker were very close in age to Bill's students and both had contracted HIV through heterosexual sex—something Bill's students had failed to take seriously before exposure to these strategies. Bill had successfully applied his knowledge of health education theory to enhance his program delivery.

PRECEDE-PROCEED Model

The PRECEDE model was developed by Green, et al. (1980) (Figure 3-2) with financial support from the National Institutes of Health. It is a planning model for health education based on principles, both theoretical and applied, from epidemiology, education, administration, and the social/behavioral sciences. The acronym PRECEDE stands for predisposing, reinforcing, and enabling causes in educational diagnosis

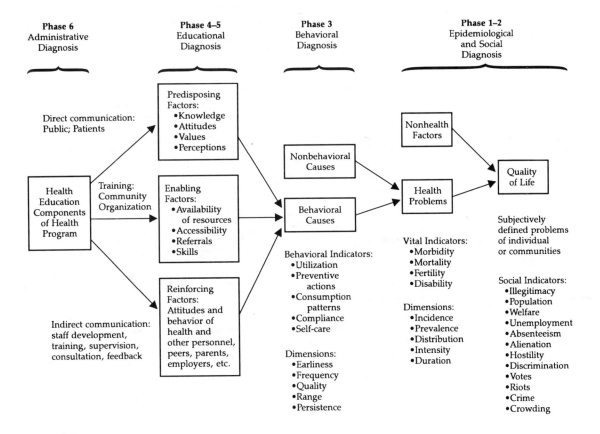

FIGURE 3-2

The PRECEDE Model

Source: L. W. Green, M. W. Kreuter, S. G. Deeds, and K. B. Partridge. *Health Promotion Planning: An Educational and Environmental Approach* (Mountain View, CA: Mayfield, 1980), pp. 14–15. Reprinted by permission.

and evaluation (Green et al., 1980). Between 1980 and 1991, the model was revised in an effort to accommodate the evolving nature and broader perspective of health promotion. The addition of a new set of steps called PROCEED (policy, regulatory, and organizational constructions in educational and environmental development) has been superimposed on the original model (Green and Kreuter, 1991) (Figure 3-3).

The PRECEDE model was designed to be acceptable to health educators with various philosophical and theoretical orientations and to be readily applicable across a variety of settings. It is intended to give structure and organization to health education program planning and evaluation. Application of this approach occurs in several phases and involves the diagnoses of variables in five domains: social, epidemiological, behavioral, educational, and administrative (Green et al., 1980). It is unique in that it begins with active engagement of the target population in defining the desired final outcome and works backward asking what are the factors that must precede that result.

Phase 1 of the model is social diagnosis. An analysis of the social problems that exist in a community is a necessary prerequisite in

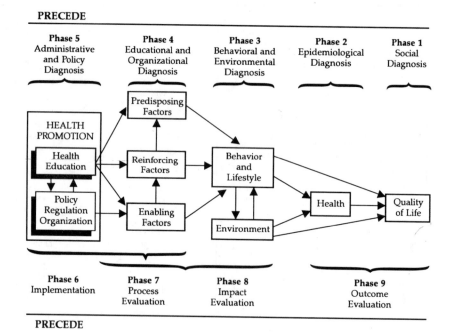

FIGURE 3-3

The PRECEDE-PROCEED Model

Source: L. W. Green and M. W. Kreuter, *Health Promotion Planning: An Educational and Environmental Approach* (Mountain View, CA: Mayfield, 1991), p. 14. Reprinted by permission.

assessing the quality of life of the target population. The purpose of this phase is to obtain maximum feasible participation in ascertaining the relationship between a given health problem and the social problems of the population. Phase 2, epidemiological diagnosis, is an evaluation of the health problems associated with the community's quality of life. Morbidity, mortality, fertility, and disability are the primary indicators of the health of a population (Green et al., 1980).

Behavioral diagnosis, the third phase, attempts to identify the health-related behaviors that impact on the health problems isolated in the epidemiological diagnosis. It is important at this stage to also acknowledge the nonbehavioral factors, such as age, gender, and environment, that may contribute to the health problem of interest. Behavioral factors are then rated on a scale of importance and changeability. In the PRECEDE-PROCEED model (Green and Kreuter, 1990, 1991), equal weight is given to an environmental diagnosis at this stage in the diagnostic process. Factors rated high in importance and changeability are usually selected as the targets for intervention (Green et al., 1980).

In the fourth phase, educational diagnosis, the theories described previously are used to identify factors influencing the health behaviors stated in the behavioral diagnosis. These are differentiated by three categories of influence: predisposing, enabling, and reinforcing factors. Predisposing factors provide the motivation or rationale for the behavior, for example, knowledge, attitudes, values, and beliefs. Enabling factors include personal skills and assets and community resources. Predisposing and enabling factors are antecedent to the health behavior and allow for the behavior to occur. Reinforcing factors supply the reward, incentive, or punishment of a behavior which contribute to its maintenance or extinction. Similar procedures are applied to an organizational diagnosis of factors influencing the environment in the combined PRECEDE-PROCEED model. Each group of factors is analyzed in terms of importance and changeability, and priorities are established for the intervention. Based on the nature of the targets for intervention, educational methodologies are selected (Green et al., 1980).

The final phase of the process (phase five), administrative diagnosis, assesses budgetary implications, identifies and allocates resources, defines the nature of any cooperative agreements, and sets a realistic timetable for the intervention. Neglect of this important step can doom an otherwise viable intervention to failure. The PROCEED modifications (Green and Kreuter, 1991), at this point in the model, include an assessment of policies, regulations, and organizational factors that impact on the resourcing and implementation of health promotion programs and the development of strategies to effectively manage these influences. In addition, the revised PRECEDE-PROCEED model includes a discussion of implementation issues as well as process, outcome, and impact evaluation.

The PRECEDE model has been used in a variety of settings with a number of different populations, including planning an adolescent school-based sexuality program (Rubinson and Baillie, 1981); analysis of school health education programs (Green and Iverson, 1982); and educational interventions for hypertension control (Green, Levine and Deeds, 1975, 1979; Levine, 1979).

Activated Health Education Model

This eclectic model has as its focus active participation in the assessment of one's health, awareness of health values, and individual responsibility for health behavior (Dennison, 1984). Activated health education was developed through a review of the health education literature and was based on the components of successful interventions. These interventions were examined for commonalities in procedures and strategies and these were subsequently classified into clusters of principles (Dennison, 1977).

The three fundamental premises of the model are active involvement, awareness, and responsibility. Active involvement is viewed as a necessary prerequisite, if health education is to have a behavioral impact. Awareness of the various positive and negative influences on health and acceptance of personal responsibility for health also impact significantly on health behavior. Standardized procedures have been developed by the author to impact on these three areas which correspond to the three phases of intervention in the model (Dennison, 1984). Each phase of intervention has its own set of objectives. In the experiential phase participants are expected to record/measure their health status; chart/plot normative data related to specific health behaviors; participate in modeling, role playing, and demonstration activities; and practice skill development in the behavior of interest. In the awareness phase participants assess influences on their health; evaluate their individual susceptibility; and examine the basic empirical, physiological, and behavioral information available regarding the health topic of concern. The third phase, responsibility, has as its objectives the identification and clarification of health-related values; the recognition of barriers that interfere with the establishment of healthy behavior; and the establishment of personal goals and self-management strategies to improve the target behaviors (Dennison, 1984).

Various intervention strategies are suitable at different phases of the process. In the experiential phase the methodology is usually instructor centered, formal, and activity oriented with massive reinforcement. In the awareness phase the strategies are more cognitive, interactive, and attempt to create dissonance between what is and what should be relative to health behavior. Finally, in the responsibility phase the intervention is more participant centered, informal, facilitative, and dissonance reducing (Dennison, 1984).

The activated health education model draws its foundation from social learning theory, operant conditioning, self-management theories, and the health belief model. According to its creator, the model is most appropriate for target health behaviors that have a physiological base. This approach has been used successfully for a variety of health concerns including cardiovascular health (Wolfgang and Dennison, 1981), nutrition (Dennison, Frauenheim, and Isu, 1983); and alcohol education (Dennison, Prevet, and Affleck, 1980). It has been used primarily with high school and college student populations. Mental and emotional health issues are less amenable to this approach (Dennison, 1984).

Limitations and Future Directions

Among health education professionals and in the health education literature, there is much confusion over the terms theory, model, and paradigm (Parcel, 1984). Many of the "theories" described in professional journals are not theories at all, but rather constructs or models. In addition, those theories that do satisfy the criteria described by Strauss and Corbin (1990) are not specific to health concerns. Theories currently in vogue often fall short in their ability to accurately predict or explain much of the variance in health behavior. In addition, these theoretical frameworks fail to address the complexity of human health behavior, typically lack a description of the relationships among the variables in the theory, and do not account for interaction effects or synergism among the constructs. Poorly operationalized variables and constructs and a lack of valid measures are also limitations of existing theories. Someone planning an intervention must sort out as much as possible the constructs to be employed before selecting the methods.

It has been suggested that the essence of the health education discipline is to understand and identify methods of managing the

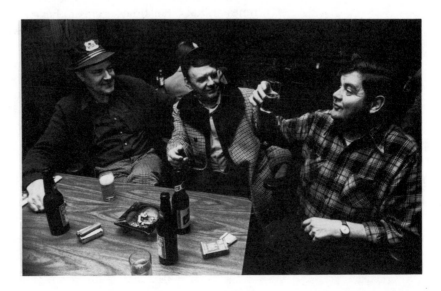

influence of multiple variables on health behavior, whether this behavior be health destructive or health generating (Toohey and Shireffs, 1980). We can contribute to the scientific basis of health education by utilizing and testing theories and models as appropriate. These theories and models can be important tools in method selection as they potentially can lead us to more effective health education interventions.

Programs would be much stronger if they utilized what we know of models and theories. In selecting methods/strategies for interventions, it is important to take these issues into consideration.

There are many other issues to consider in method selection. One important consideration is the educational domain.

EDUCATIONAL DOMAINS

An important consideration is the domain in which we are working. Most health education programs work in more than one domain as defined in the classic, *Taxonomy of Educational Objectives*. The three major domains are cognitive, affective, and psychomotor. Cognitive refers to the recall and synthesis of information. Affective refers to the change of an attitude. Psychomotor refers to the performance of a physical skill. Sometimes skills are also included as a domain. Skill refers to the development and application of a skill. Examples include refusal skills or the ability to analyze the unscientific nature of appeals used in health advertising.

There is disagreement as to the relationship of these domains and health behavior. Knowledge, attitudes, physical performance, and skills all have important relationships, but they act in different ways at different times and with different people. Knowledge can change behavior at times and at other times seems to have no relationship. Most people if they know their partner is HIV positive will take extra precautions or avoid sexual contact all together. However, although most of us know the relationship of diet to heart disease and cancer, we will still elect to eat high-fat, low-fiber foods on occasion. Several highly respected health educators, for example, are overweight. What motivates one person may not motivate another. A model or theory may never explain the behavior of some individuals. Therefore it is important we use a variety of methods addressing as many domains as practical.

CHARACTERISTICS OF THE LEARNER AND THE COMMUNITY

We must always consider the characteristics of the individuals and groups we are working with. Such elements as age, gender, reading ability, language skills, biases, and readiness to learn are examples of important considerations. This is what application of the previously mentioned theories and models seeks to do. Motivation is also an important consideration. If this is a court-ordered alcohol education program, you may have good attendance in terms of the number of bodies, but it is usually a great challenge to get their minds interested and in attendance. Most community workshops mix ability groups, making it a further challenge to maintain interest levels.

Some of the Characteristics of the Learner to Be Considered:

Age

Gender

Reading ability

Language skills

Biases

Readiness to learn

Group Size   The size of the group will play an important role in method selection. Large groups, say over 100, make individual interaction difficult and often frustrating. Methods must be selected keeping in mind the size of the group. Lecture is a way to share a considerable amount of cognitive information in a short time but usually is not effective for reaching affective or psychomotor objectives. Small groups offer flexibility in many ways but also put more pressure on the individual to participate.

Contact Time   The time you have to spend with a group will play a major role in the selection of appropriate methods. Certain methods simply cannot be used in a short period of time. Many activities require a certain amount of trust to be successful. This often involves icebreaking activities which usually require time in order to develop openness among the participants. Short workshops do not lend themselves to these activities.

Case Study   *James is conducting a two-hour workshop on alcohol abuse with 20 individuals who have been referred to this mandatory workshop for drinking and driving offenders. James has not worked with this type of group before and decides to use an icebreaker exercise which is designed to reveal personal details of the participants. The group members immediately become hostile and barrage poor James with comments like, "I don't want to be here anyway," "This information is no one's business but mine," "Just get on with the facts and let's all get out of here!" James cuts short the icebreaker and concludes the workshop as quickly as possible with a less than successful lecture on the dangers of alcohol abuse and driving.*

James obviously had not made a good match between his strategy selection and learner characteristics. In addition, using a revealing icebreaker exercise in a short, once-only workshop where trust could never be established was an error and not a good use of limited contact time. This example points to the necessity of thoroughly examining all the elements of learner characteristics and presentation conditions (group size, contact time) before proceeding with an intervention. Too many health educators have had to learn the hard way . . . through painful experience.

Budget   Quality health education need not be expensive, but it does require an appropriate budget. To compete successfully with the often unhealthy media messages and long-held unhealthy habits, we need and deserve a chance through a reasonable budget. Do you have enough money to use the best methods for the health educational program? If you have limited resources, can you still achieve your objectives or would you be

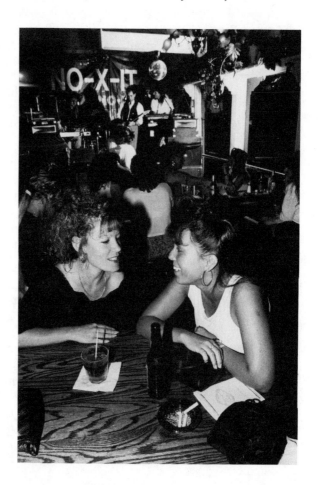

better off limiting the number of programs but improving the quality of the programs offered?

Quality health educators should receive quality salaries for their time and that requires an appropriate budget. Photocopies, videotapes, computer software, and other tools of the health educator all cost money.

Resources/Site/ Environment

You must consider all the resources you have at your disposal. Do you have good facilities to break out into small groups? If you have access to a microcomputer lab, it opens up totally new possibilities. Will you have a quiet space for presentations? What about parking or transportation? If you have access to well-appointed teaching facilities, it opens up the use of many methods. This is especially true of those methods that include technology. Of course, many quality health education programs have been offered without any facilities by reaching into homes or utilizing community settings. You work with what is available, and often the local setting is much better for achieving your objectives.

Characteristics of the Educational Provider

If you are the primary provider what are your strengths as a health educator? What methods are you uncomfortable using? Although you should be willing to take some chances if you are to be successful, it is important you not set yourself up for disaster by selecting a method that will make you so uncomfortable that you cannot do a credible job. If certain methods seem central to achieving your objectives, it may be vital to employ them. Therefore you may need to practice the method so you can be effective in using it or bring in an outsider to conduct the method. Using such guests can often increase your comfort with a method while providing a needed activity for your target population. Again, the important principle is to use the correct method given your objectives.

SALLY FORTH HOWARD & MACINTOSH

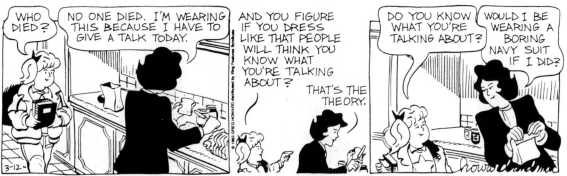

Reprinted with special permission of North America Syndicate. © 1993.

Cultural Appropriateness

It is most important that you consider the cultural characteristics of the group you are targeting. Many programs have failed because of this issue. The best protection is to establish an advisory group from the group being targeted. This small group can review your methods and give you some idea of what response to expect from the participants. Another less formal way to get some idea is to sit down with a few participants prior to the event and ask them if they think the method would work and be appropriate.

Using a Variety of Methods

Why Use a Variety of Methods?

1. It makes it more likely you will achieve your objectives.
2. It may prevent disruptive behavior.
3. It may maintain participant interest.
4. It is more fun for the presenter.
5. Not all learners respond positively to the same methods.

Using a variety of educational methods is important for a number of reasons. First, we all get tired of the same presentation method. Remember, in health education we are often working with hard-to-reach groups. Always do what you can to make it interesting and you will have a better chance of achieving your objectives. By keeping people interested we also minimize disruptive behavior. In the classroom this is shown by lack of attention or outright hostility. During community workshops it might be demonstrated by participants walking out. The first time you have a large number of people walking out on your presentation you will be very upset and it may simply be due to your lack of variety or poor method selection. The final reason for variety is that it is more fun for you. You too will lose interest if you do things the same way each time. Try new methods and you will find it much more enjoyable.

Some Comments on Method Choice

At the elementary and secondary levels, straight lecture or textbook methods are *considered nonfunctional.* (Fodor and Dalis, 1974, p. 53)

Each instructor must develop his/her own technique of facilitating. Learning is greatly increased if students are motivated and interested in what they are doing. One of the major criticisms of health education programs is that they are dull. Developing a caring, humanistic approach toward students should help health teachers make their classes more exciting and challenging for the students. The learning process can and should be made enjoyable and interesting. (NEA-AMA, 1966)

Any teaching technique or procedure must actively involve the learner if it is to be effective. Active participation can be either direct or vicarious. Direct participation exists where the student is himself physically involved in the activity; vicarious, where he is a viewer of an activity that is going on in another place or another time. Either way, the individual must be affected positively and provided perceptions and experiences contributing to the attainment of desirable long-range cognitive, affective, and action goals. (Kime, Schlaadt, and Tritsch, 1977, p. 96)

Different learning opportunities should not be used for the sake of variety alone. A variety of learning may be of value since variety tends to break the monotony for the teacher as well as for the student. There are, however, more important reasons for using different learning opportunities: (1) to meet a variety of objectives, (2) to meet a variety of student needs and interests, and (3) to stimulate a variety of senses. (Oberteuffer, et al., 1972, pp. 138–139)

One of the most important generalizations that emerges from systematic comparisons of programs and experiments with positive results and those with negative findings (no effect) is that the greater the variety in educational methods used, the more likely the program or experiment will show positive results. This generalization applies both with individuals and with populations. At the individual level, variety in education methods apparently helps to surround the learner with communications appealing to different senses and modes of learning which are mutually supportive. (Green, 1976, p. iv)

Cohen believes that learning is related to the method selected. The more active and involved the learner becomes the more likely he/she will learn. This is represented by the pyramid below.

FIGURE 3-4

Adapted from M. Cohen, A comprehensive approach to effective staff development: Essential components, Presented at Education Development Center sponsored capacity-building meeting for Comprehensive School Health Education Training Centers (Cambridge, MA: March 1991).

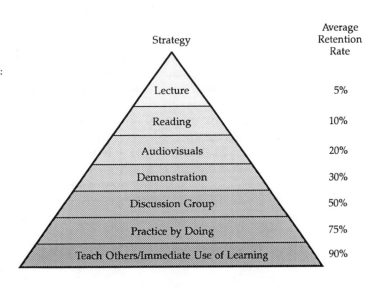

Strategy	Average Retention Rate
Lecture	5%
Reading	10%
Audiovisuals	20%
Demonstration	30%
Discussion Group	50%
Practice by Doing	75%
Teach Others/Immediate Use of Learning	90%

PACKAGING THE TOTAL INTERVENTION STRATEGY

How your methods fit together to form your intervention package is important in achieving your objectives. Are the methods complementary and reinforcing? Do the methods break up the time together so that you hold the attention of your intended audience? Have you appealed to different styles of learning? Have you applied as many educational principles as possible such as reinforcement, repetition, and practice?

Common Mistakes in Method Selection

1. Selecting a method that you personally like but that is not the best method for achieving your stated objectives.

2. Underestimating the time required to conduct a method properly.

3. Overestimating the time required to conduct a method properly.

4. Selecting an inappropriate method for the characteristics of the group.

5. Not reinforcing key points.

USING A SYSTEMS APPROACH TO METHOD SELECTION

A systems approach is a predictable and orderly series of events or steps applied to decision making. In method selection this is a very appropriate approach to ensure we are giving appropriate consideration to the options that are available. We can apply these principles without technology although the use of such technology should allow for a much more comprehensive review.

There are efforts underway to apply expert system technology to health education which has very interesting potential. Robert Gold, Lawrence Green, Marshall Kreuter, James Ross, and others are developing an expert system called EMPOWER (expert methods for planning and organization within everyone's reach), which is a computer program that takes the user through a decision matrix designed around the PRECEDE-PROCEED model. It is a user-friendly application of the model which will allow the user to call upon top expertise to make decisions about program planning, implementation, and evaluation. The following is a summary of this project provided by Robert Gold.

Application of Technology to Disease Prevention and Health Promotion

A group of health educators (Bob Gold, Larry Green, Marshall Kreuter and Jim Ross) are in the midst of a project designed to develop and test an extension of existing technology to help decision makers design cancer prevention and control programs. It is their hope that these efforts will contribute to the planning and implementation of community-based programs that are on target with the health education needs of communities with diverse minority and other high-risk populations.

A three-phase effort has been used in the development of an expert system called EMPOWER: needs assessment and design specification; product prototype development and testing; and final development and preparation for dissemination. The following technical objectives guided the development of EMPOWER:

1. To evaluate the health education science base in terms of level and quantity of expertise, and the needs of health programmers to assess the feasibility of encapsulation of such expertise for use in an expert system format.
2. To identify the best mechanisms for serving the intended audiences, assess pertinent content to include in the system, and select the most appropriate modes of delivery.
3. To investigate the needs of health professionals for an expert system to provide technical assistance in the planning, implementation, and management of community-based cancer prevention programs for minority and other high-risk populations.
4. To develop a preliminary design for a software product to provide technical assistance and management support to health professionals in the planning, implementation, management, and evaluation of community-based cancer prevention and control programs.
5. To prepare a design strategy for this application with complete specifications.

Significance

The timeliness and significance of EMPOWER stem from two converging developments:

- The technology related to artificial intelligence and expert systems now provides an opportunity to extend expertise to meet unmet needs in much the same way that a group of human experts would be consulted if they were accessible.
- A growing body of literature concerning program planning for health promotion interventions now calls for professional training and experience, or access to technical assistance from experts, or both.

Project Objectives

The feasibility phase suggested the following specific objectives of this effort:

1. To develop a fully functional expert system that will provide technical assistance to community-based health promotion program planners with a special emphasis on planning community-based cancer prevention interventions for minority and other high-risk populations.
2. To evaluate the expert system for reliability, validity, utility, and acceptability to potential users.

Design

The PRECEDE-PROCEED model developed by Green and Kreuter provides a framework around which to provide technical guidance and assistance to those involved in the complex process of planning and implementing community-based cancer prevention interventions. It is this model that forms the core of the program planning and evaluation system which we tentatively call EMPOWER.

Structure

EMPOWER is an expert system designed around the PRECEDE-PROCEED planning model. There are seven separate subsystems and several external databases linked dynamically to provide guidance to program managers and directors. Six of the seven subsystems are outgrowths of the PRECEDE-PROCEED model, and the seventh is designed to link any of these subsystems to global, national, or provincial goals, policies, or standards for evaluation, such as the Health for All 2000 goals of the World Health Organization and the Year 2000 Health Objectives and Community Model Standards of the United States. The project has linked these seven subsystems to census data, appropriate morbidity and mortality data, and other specific databases that may assist the potential user in the development of synthetic estimates useful for planning at the local level when actual data are unavailable and too costly to generate.

Purpose

EMPOWER will provide expert guidance and technical assistance to its users in any component of the program planning and evaluation of community-based cancer prevention and control interventions. It will do this by prompting the user through a series of algorithms based on the PRECEDE-PROCEED framework while at the same time providing the capacity for the user to make inquiries regarding the reasoning and rule processes used during the consultation.

Tasks EMPOWER Will Help the User Accomplish

Examples of specific steps in the planning and community organizing process that will be addressed by EMPOWER are:

1. Data-gathering procedures essential to the planning, conduct, or evaluation of community-based cancer prevention programming.
2. Organizing the involvement of community residents or representatives in the planning process.
3. Setting priorities and setting initial and long-term objectives.
4. Preparing full program and evaluation plans.
5. Organizing coalitions or other interagency and intersectoral collaboration arrangements.
6. Assessing the plausibility of the intended outcomes in light of the nature of the proposed activities, the level and manner of implementation of the program, and the gap between required resources and available resources.
7. Assessing policies and developing proposals and strategies for policy changes.
8. Identifying elements of the plans that are working at odds with each other and that reduce the plausibility of achieving the intended program outcomes.
9. Assessing organizational and regulatory constraints and strategies for reorganization and regulations.
10. Assessing whether the program has succeeded in attracting the target population for which it was designed and in the expected numbers.
11. Assessing the impact of cancer prevention programming on community awareness, interest, motivation, attitudes, beliefs, perceptions, behaviors and environmental changes.
12. Recommending evaluation designs and methods to address the needs of the program and the interest of stakeholders.

Specific Nature of the Projected Users of the EMPOWER

1. Program managers and health promotion directors and staff of provincial, state, and local health departments.
2. Program managers, directors, and staff of Canadian or American Cancer Society units and divisions.
3. Program managers and directors of other community-based cancer prevention programs.
4. Directors of worksite health promotion programs.
5. Health directors or coordinators of SEAs, LEAs, and school districts.
6. Community organizers with little or no health science background.

TABLE 3-1
Methods Selection Matrix

	Method	Cognitive Objectives	Affective Objectives	Skill Objectives	Psychomotor Objectives	Time Required Minutes	Ages/Years	Size/Suggested Max	Budget	Community Setting	School Setting	Comments
1	Getting acquainted activities	X	P		P	15+	All	None	Low	X	X	
2	Audiotapes	X	P	P	P	15+	All	None	Low	X	X	Equipment required
3	Audiovisual materials	X	P	P	P	15+	All	None	Mod	X	X	Equipment required
4	Brainstorming	X				20+	All	20	Low	X	X	
5	Cartoons/ humor	P	P			5+	All	None	Low	X	X	Equipment helps
6	Computer-assisted instruction	X	P	P		30+	10+	Ratio	High		X	Equipment required
7	Cooperative learning	P	P	P	P	30+	All	20	Low	X	X	
8	Debates	P	P			30+	All	30	Low	X	X	
9	Displays/ bulletin boards	X			P	30+	All	None	Low	X	X	Special materials required
10	Educational games	X				20+	All	30	Low	X	X	
11	Experiments and demonstrations	X		X	X	30+	All	Ratio	Mod+		X	Equipment required
12	Field trips		P	P		60+	All	Ratio	Mod	X	X	
13	Guest speakers	X	P			30+	All	None	Low+	X	X	
14	Guided imagery		X	X	P	30+	All	None	Mod	X	X	Equipment required
15	Lecture	X		P		5+	All	None	Low	X	X	
16	Mass media	X				5+	All	None		X	X	Access required
17	Models	X		P	P	5+	All	None	Low+	X	X	Equipment required

X = Yes common use.
P = Possible.
Blank = uncommon.

TABLE 3-1
Continued

	Method	Cognitive Objectives	Affective Objectives	Skill Objectives	Psychomotor Objectives	Time Required Minutes	Ages/Years	Size/Suggested Max	Budget	Community Setting	School Setting	Comments
18	Music	P	X			5+	All	None	Low	X	X	Equipment required
19	Newsletters	X				120+	All readers	None	Mod	X	X	Equipment and duplication required
20	Panels	P	X			30+	All	None	Low	X	X	
21	Peer education	P	X	X		120+	All	Ratio	Mod	X	X	Special training needed
22	Personal improvement projects		X		P	600+	10+	None	Low+	X	X	Requires adequate time
23	Problem solving	P	P	P		30+	All	25	Low	X	X	
24	Puppets	X	X			30+	All	25	Low+	X	X	Equipment required
25	Role plays		X	P	P	30+	10+	25	Low	X	X	
26	Self-appraisals		X			15+	10+	None	Low	X	X	Handout or computer required
27	Simulations	X	X	X	X	30+	10+	25	Mod+	X	X	Special materials required
28	Value clarification		X	P		30+	14+	30	Low	X	X	
29	Word games and puzzles	X				10+	10+ readers	None	Low	X	X	Handout required

X = Yes common use.
P = Possible.
Blank = uncommon.

SIMPLE SYSTEMS APPROACH

Table 3-1 is an example of a simple systems approach. When considering the selection of a method, the user reviews the objectives to be achieved and then considers how each of the listed methods might be employed (all listed methods are covered in detail in Chapter 4). A cost-benefit analysis is done to determine if the method will become part of the program. At any time the user can return to the table to reconsider. This simple chart can be a powerful tool to improve method selection.

Read Chapter 4 which describes each method in more detail and then return to this table.

EXERCISES

1. Select one of the theories/models or elements of a theory/model described in this chapter and apply it (them) to a specific health intervention. For example, consider HIV education for a community youth group. You could apply the HBM as a whole, elements of the HBM, or maybe you want to focus on self-efficacy of condom use. State the health issue on which you will focus, select the theory/model/element, and then briefly outline an intervention describing the methods that will operationalize the theory.

2. One of the educational principles related to motivating the learner states: *Fear and punishment have uncertain effects upon learning. They may facilitate or hinder learning.* You are conducting a workshop for middle-aged women on preventing cervical cancer.

Briefly describe how this educational principle could have an impact on your workshop.

3. One of the educational principles related to the needs and abilities of the learner states: *The lower the educational level, the greater is reliance on oral or picture media.* You are conducting a workshop for 10-year-old children on safety in the home. Briefly describe how this educational principle could have an impact on your presentation and give concrete examples of how you would incorporate this principle.

4. You are planning to conduct a series of community workshops on weight control. List four *characteristics of the learner* which you feel should be considered in planning and briefly describe why each is important.

SUMMARY

Selecting the appropriate educational intervention is vital to achieving your objectives.

1. The selection of a method should always take into account the objectives to be achieved.

2. Some of the other important considerations include:
   Educational Principles
   Theory and Model Application
   Educational Domain
   Characteristics of the Learner

   Group size
   Contact time
   Budget
   Resources/site/environment
   Characteristics of the educational provider
   Cultural appropriateness
   Using a variety of methods
   Packaging the total intervention strategy

REFERENCES

Ajzen, I. and M. Fishbein. 1973. Attitudinal and normative variables as predictors of specific behaviors. *Journal of Personality and Social Psychology* 27:41–57.

Ajzen, I. and M. Fishbein. 1980. *Understanding Attitudes and Predicting Social Behavior.* Englewood Cliffs, NJ: Prentice-Hall.

Bandura, A. 1977. Self-efficacy: Toward a unifying theory of behavioral change. *Psychological Review* 84:191.

Bandura, A. 1977. *Social Learning Theory.* Englewood Cliffs, NJ: Prentice-Hall.

Bandura, A. 1986. The explanatory and predictive scope of self-efficacy theory. *Journal of Social and Clinical Psychology* 4:359-373.

Bardsley, P. and L. Beckman. 1988. The health belief model and entry into alcoholism treatment. *International Journal of the Addictions* 23:19-28.

Becker, M., ed. 1974. *The Health Belief Model and Personal Health Behavior.* Thoroughfare, NJ: Slack.

Becker, M. and N. Janz. 1985. The health belief model applied to understanding diabetes regimen compliance. *Diabetes Educator* 11:41-47.

Champion, V. 1985. Use of the health belief model in determining frequency of breast self-examination. *Research in Nursing and Health* 8:373-379.

Cornish, E. 1980. Toward a philosophy of futurism. *Health Education* 11:10-12.

Creswell, W. H. 1984. Health education issues. In *Health Education: Foundations for the Future,* edited by L. Rubinson and W. F. Alles. St. Louis: Times Mirror/Mosby.

Cummings, K. M., M. H. Becker, and M. C. Maile. 1980. Bringing the models together: An empirical approach to combining variables used to explain health outcomes. *Journal of Behavioral Medicine* 3:123-145.

Dalkey, N. and O. Helmer. 1963. An experimental application of the Delphi method to the use of experts. *Management Science* 9:458.

Dennison, D. 1977. Activated health education. *Health Education* 8:24-25.

Dennison, D. 1984. Activated health education: The development and refinement of an intervention model. *Health Values* 8:18-24.

Dennison, D., K. A. Frauenheim, and L. Isu. 1983. The DINE microcomputer program: An innovative curricular approach. *Health Education* 14.

Dennison, D., T. Prevet, and M. Affleck. 1980. *Alcohol and Behavior: An Activated Health Education Approach.* St. Louis: C. V. Mosby.

DiBlasio, F. A. 1986. Drinking adolescents on the roads. *Journal of Youth and Adolescence* 15:173-189.

Dwore, R. B. and J. D. Matarazzo. 1981. The behavioral sciences and health education. *Health Education* 12:4-8.

Eiser, J. R. 1985. Smoking: The social learning of addiction. *Journal of Social and Clinical Psychology* 3:357-446.

Fishbein, M., ed. 1967. *Readings in Attitude Theory and Measurement.* New York: Wiley.

Fodor, J. and G. Dalis. *Health Instruction: Theory Application.* Philadelphia: Lea and Febiger.

Frazer, G. H., G. G. Kukulka, and C. E. Richardson. 1988. An assessment of professional opinion concerning critical research issues in health education. In *Advances in Health Education: Current Research,* vol 1, edited by J. H. Humphrey. New York: AMS Press.

Gilbert, G. G. 1981. *Teaching First Aid and Emergency Care.* Dubuque, IA: Kendall/Hunt.

Green, L. 1976. Determining the impact and effectiveness of health education as it relates to federal policy. Prepared for the office of the Deputy Assistant Secretary for Planning and Evaluation/Health, HEW.

Green, L. W. and D. Iverson. 1982. School health education. *Annual Review of Public Health* 3: 321-328.

Green, L. W. and M. W. Kreuter, 1991. *Health Promotion Planning: An Educational and Environmental Approach.* Mountain View, CA: Mayfield.

Green, L. W., M. W. Kreuter, S. G. Deeds, and K. B. Partridge. 1980. *Health Education Planning: A Diagnostic Approach.* Palo Alto, CA: Mayfield.

Green, L. W., D. M. Levine, and S. G. Deeds. 1975. Clinical trials of health education for hypertensive outpatients: Design and baseline data. *Preventive Medicine* 4:417-425.

Herold, E. 1983. The health belief model: Can it help us understand contraceptive use among adolescents? *Journal of School Health* 53:19-21.

Hester, N. and D. Macrina. 1985. The health belief model and the contraceptive behavior of college women: Implications for health education. *Journal of American College Health* 33:245-252.

Jessor, R., and S. Jessor. 1977. *Problem Behavior and Psychosocial Development: A Longitudinal Study of Youth.* New York: Academic.

Jillson, I. A. 1975. The national drug abuse policy delphi: Progress report and findings to date. In *The Delphi Method: Techniques and Applications,* edited by Linstone and Turoff. Reading, MA: Addison-Wesley.

Kelly, G., J. Mamon, and J. Scott. 1987. Utility of the health belief model in examining medication compliance among psychiatric outpatients. *Social Science Medicine* 25:1205-1211.

Kerlinger, F. N. 1973. *Foundations of Behavioral Research.* New York: Holt, Rinehart, and Winston.

Kime, R., R. Schlaadt, and L. Tritsch. 1977. *Health Instruction: An Action Approach.* Englewood Cliffs, NJ: Prentice-Hall.

Kirscht, J. 1974. The health belief model and illness behavior. In *The Health Belief Model and Personal Health Behavior,* edited by M. Becker. Thoroughfare, NJ: Slack.

Kuhn, T. S. 1970. *The Structure of Scientific Revolutions.* Chicago: University of Chicago Press.

Levenson, H. 1974. Activism and powerful others: Distinction within the concept of internal-external control. *Journal of Personality Assessment* 38: 377–383.

Levine, D. M. 1979. Health education for hypertensive parents, *Journal of American Medical Association* 241:1700–1703.

Levine, D. M., D. E. Morisky, L. R. Bone, C. Lewis, K. B. Ward, and L. W. Green. 1982. Data-based planning for educational interventions through hypertension control programs for urban and rural populations in Maryland. *Public Health Reports* 97:107–112.

Maiman, L. and M. Becker. 1974. The health belief model: Origins and correlates in psychological theory. In *The Health Belief Model and Personal Health Behavior.* edited by M. Becker. Thoroughfare, NJ: Slack.

McGuire, W. 1981. Behavioral medicine, public health and communication theories. *Health Education* 12:8–13.

Mullen, P. D. and D. Iverson. 1982. Qualitative methods for evaluative research in health education programs. *Health Education* 13:11–18.

Oberteuffer, D., et al. 1972. *School Health Education.* New York: Harper and Row.

Parcel, G. & T. Baranowski, 1981. Social learning theory and health education. *Health Education,* 12:14-18.

Parcel, G. S. 1984. Theoretical models for application in school health education research. Special combined issue of *Journal of School Health* 54:39–49 and *Health Education* 15:39–49.

Parcel, G., and M. P. Meyer. 1978. Development of an instrument to measure children's health locus of control. *Health Education Monographs* 6:149–159.

Parcel, G., P. R. Nader, and P. J. Rogers. 1980. Health locus of control and health values: Implications for school health education. *Health Values* 4:32–37.

Rosenstock, I. 1974. Historical origins of the health belief model. In *The Health Belief Model and Personal Health Behavior,* edited by M. Becker. Thoroughfare, NJ: Slack.

Rosenstock, I. M., V. J. Strecher, and M. Becker. 1988. Social Learning Theory and The Health Belief Model. *Health Education Quarterly* 15:175–183.

Rotter, J. B. 1954. *Social Learning and Clinical Psychology.* Englewood Cliffs, NJ: Prentice-Hall.

Rubinson, L. and W. F. Alles, eds. 1984. *Health Education: Foundations for the Future.* St. Louis: Times Mirror/Mosby.

Rubinson, L., and L. Baillie. 1981. Planning school based sexuality programs utilizing the PRECEDE model. *Journal of School Health* 51:282–287.

Scaffa, M. 1992. The development of a comprehensive theory in health education: A feasibility study. Unpublished Doctoral Dissertation. University of Maryland.

Shireffs, J. A. 1984. The nature and meaning of health education. In *Health Education: Foundations for the Future.* edited by L. Rubinson and W. F. Alles. St. Louis: Times Mirror/Mosby.

Stainbrook, G., and L. W. Green. 1982. Behavior and behaviorism in health education. *Health Education* 13:14–19.

Strauss, A., and J. Corbin. 1990. *Basics of Qualitative Research: Grounded Theory Procedures and Techniques.* London: Sage.

Suggested School Health Policies, 5th ed. 1966. NEA-AMA Committee.

Tarabokia, J. R. 1985. Forecasts by selected professional health educators and their implications for health education: A delphi application. Doctoral Dissertation. Brigham Young University. Dissertation Abstracts International, #8526331.

Toohey, J. V. and J. H. Shireffs. 1980. Future trends in health education. *Health Education* 11:15–17.

Travis, R. 1976. The delphi technique: A tool for community health educators. *Health Education* 7: 11–13.

Wallston, K. A., and B. S. Wallston. 1978. Preface to health locus of control. *Health Education Monographs* 6:101–105.

Wallston, K. A., B. S. Wallston, and R. DeVillis. 1978. Development of the multidimensional health locus of control scales. *Health Education Monographs* 6:160–170.

Wallston, K. A., B. S. Wallston, G. D. Kaplan, and S. A. Maides. 1976. Development and validation of the health locus of control scale. *Journal of Consulting and Clinical Psychology* 44:580–585.

Wodarski, J. 1987. Evaluating a social learning approach to teaching adolescents about alcohol and driving: A multiple variable evaluation. *Journal of Social Science Research* 10:121–144.

Wolfgang, J. and D. Dennison. 1981. The effects of a heart health education workshop. *Journal of School Health* 51:356–359.

Chapter 4

Methods of Instruction/Intervention

Entry Level Health Educator Competencies Addressed in This Chapter

Responsibility III: Implementing Health Education Programs

Competency A: Exhibit competence in carrying out planned educational programs.

Competency C: Select methods and media best suited to implement program plans for specific learners.

Competency D: Monitor educational programs, adjusting objectives and activities as necessary.

Taken from *A Framework for the Development of Competency-Based Curricula for Entry Level Health Educators*, National Task Force on the Preparation and Practice of Health Educators, Inc. 1985. Reprinted by permission.

Method Selection in Health Education

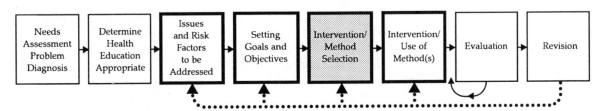

Heavy-bordered boxes indicate subjects addressed in this text; shaded boxes indicate subjects(s) of current chapter.

Case Study

Pam has been asked to develop a health education program for the local community. During her years in college the only teaching method she experienced was lecture. She therefore develops an intellectual lecture presentation on the evils of drugs for the five parents of adolescents who are believed to have drug problems. When the parents seem disinterested in her approach, she is disappointed. One of the parents suggests she just sit down and talk with them. Another parent who is a physician says they are all aware of the evils of drugs but need help in relating to their children.

Pam needs help in her method selection. She needs to review her objectives and select more appropriate methods. She has selected an inappropriate method for the target population and has failed to take advantage of an excellent opportunity for small-group techniques.

There is an arsenal of methods available to us in health education. It is important we consider the objectives first and then focus on the methods to meet those objectives within the context of the resources we have at our disposal. This chapter will focus on the many methods available to the health educator.

After studying the chapter the reader will be able to:

- describe the major advantages and disadvantages of using each method
- describe how to use each method
- provide a rationale for using each method
- match methods with objectives

Key Issues

Method Description	Advantages
When to Use	Disadvantages
How to Use	Examples

Following is a list of the methods discussed in this chapter.

1. Getting acquainted activities
2. Audiotapes
3. Audiovisual materials
4. Brainstorming
5. Cartoons/humor
6. Computer-assisted instruction
7. Cooperative learning
8. Debates
9. Displays/bulletin boards
10. Educational games
11. Experiments and demonstrations
12. Field trips
13. Guest speakers
14. Guided imagery
15. Lecture
16. Mass media
17. Models
18. Music
19. Newsletters
20. Panels
21. Peer education
22. Personal improvement projects
23. Problem solving
24. Puppets
25. Role plays
26. Self-appraisals
27. Simulations
28. Value clarification
29. Word games and puzzles

CONSIDERING YOUR OPTIONS AND USING METHODS AS A FRAMEWORK

Each method should be considered a "framework." Every possible method should be considered for each objective to be achieved. An important step in making the decision is to use the preceding list of activities/methods and consider how each one might conceivably be employed to meet your objectives. This will force you to consider the many options available for achieving your objectives and make it less likely you will pick a method for inappropriate reasons.

This chapter will present a variety of methods and one or more examples of the application of the method. The reader should remember that the methods presented can be converted to other subject matter with relative ease. Each method is a framework that can and should be adapted to meet your needs. Always think of how each method might be applied to meet your objectives. Health educators often "crash" into a method without thinking through what is the best method to achieve the desired outcome.

Of all the beasts in the jungle, we most often resemble the crashing boar.
—Mohan Singh

METHOD/INTERVENTION 1: GETTING-ACQUAINTED ACTIVITIES

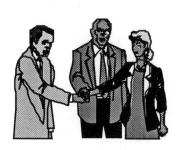

Getting-acquainted activities are used to set the tone for a workshop or class. These activities are generally easy to follow and fun. They range from introducing yourself to more complex activities designed to show what will be covered or why the lesson is being presented.

Advantages

1. Can serve to create an atmosphere of mutual trust and respect.
2. Can help the facilitator learn the names of participants.
3. Set the ground rules for participant interaction.

Disadvantages

1. Can be time consuming.
2. May make participants unnecessarily uncomfortable.

Example 1: Getting-Acquainted Activity: The Name Game

1. Sit in a circle so that all faces can be seen.
2. After reviewing all rules, begin.
   You cannot write names down.
   All will participate.
   Associate names with faces since we will change places later.
3. First person says his/her own name (generally only first name).
4. Second person says first person's name and then his/her own.
5. Procedure is repeated until final person says all names plus his/her own.
6. Reverse directions and have first person say all names in reverse order.
7. After several persons have completed game in reverse, change places and pick several people to say names.
8. Repeat until all are comfortable saying all names.

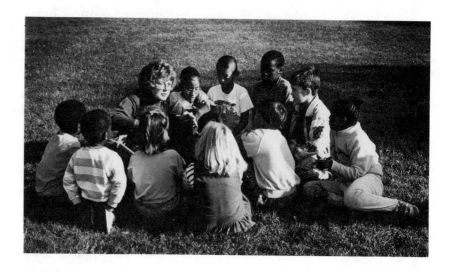

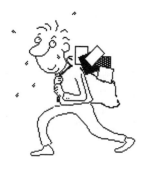

Example 2: Get It Off My Back

Purpose

1. To introduce a new area of instruction.
2. To get a group better acquainted.
3. To review.

Background

The facilitator must do background work on the topic to be covered and identify key vocabulary words. Examples include drug names, nutrients, diseases, and pollutants.

Player Objective

To identify the word on your back.

Materials

Three-by-five-inch cards and masking tape.

Rules of Play

1. After reviewing all rules, a three-by-five-inch card with a word on it is placed on the back of each participant. It is important that no one sees the card placed on his/her back.
2. You can ask only yes-and-no questions.
3. You can ask each person only one question. If you have asked a question of all participants, you may repeat the process.
4. You must get at least three yes answers to your questions before you can guess the word on your back.
5. The first person to guess correctly is the winner. Continue the game until at least half of the group has been successful.

6. Instruct participants to answer "I don't know or I am not certain" if appropriate. It is important that they not guess as this will ruin the game. If no one is certain of the correct answer, direct them to the facilitator.
7. Repeat the game if there is time.
8. Debrief by discussing the logic followed in getting to the answer.

Example 3:
Special Name Tags

Construct special name tags to include information that will open up common ground.

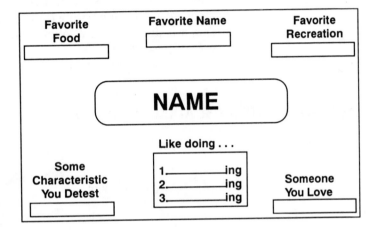

After completing the answers to the questions posed on the name tag, each person pairs up with another and asks clarifying questions. Participants can decline to answer any question but generally find these questions nonthreatening. This is a good beginning activity and promotes some safe self-disclosure which generally contributes to a positive atmosphere.

METHOD/INTERVENTION 2: AUDIOTAPES

Audiotapes can be used as a method or to assist with another method. You can use audiotapes in many ways.

Advantages

1. Low cost.
2. Provide a structured experience.
3. Easy to use.
4. Can provide excellent feedback.

Disadvantages

1. Appeal to only one sense.
2. Require equipment.
3. Require special equipment for large groups.
4. Material can be boring.

Example 1   Interviews with experts played back for group.

Example 2   Interaction with self. Have a conversation with yourself. The tape asks questions and you provide the answers. One example would be to have a conversation with a crystal ball. Control the on-and-off button and ask the crystal ball about your future if you behave in certain unhealthy ways.

See also Chapter 5.

METHOD/INTERVENTION 3: AUDIOVISUAL MATERIALS

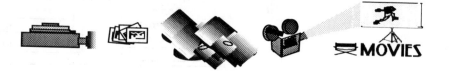

Audiovisual materials include videotapes, films, overhead transparencies, videodiscs, and filmstrips. The use of audiovisual equipment will be discussed in detail in Chapter 5. Therefore it will not be discussed extensively here.

Advantages

1. Provide potential for variety.
2. Attention-getter.
3. Blank videotapes are relatively cheap and easy to use.
4. Tapes can be made as a class or individual project.
5. Overhead transparencies are inexpensive.

Disadvantages

1. Outcome may be unpredictable.
2. Require equipment.
3. Some equipment is expensive.
4. Interactive videodiscs are still expensive but prices are coming down.

5. Some may be unwilling to participate and allow others to do all the work.

See also Chapter 8.

Examples

1. As a supplement to lecture.
2. Group-made tapes (audio or video).
3. Videotapes of community problems. Can be done like an investigative reporter.
4. Using videotapes to monitor behaviors such as drug transactions.

METHOD/INTERVENTION 4: BRAINSTORMING

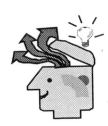

Brainstorming is a method of eliciting ideas and information from a group. It can be used to define a problem or to consider possible solutions to a problem. It can be very effective in developing a positive group attitude since it recognizes the importance of each group member. It often provides a sense of group empowerment. Basically, it is a free-thinking forum with the facilitator working to elicit as many possible solutions to a problem as possible. This is followed by grouping and reorganizing ideas until they are well understood and all are considered.

Rules

1. There are no bad ideas. Do not make negative remarks about ideas as this will stifle creativity.
2. All ideas/solutions will be considered (listed).
3. Go around the group in a circle and list ideas that are possible solutions to the problem or issue at hand. If possible, use large sheets of paper and hang them on the walls. If not available, use a chalkboard or transparencies.
4. Individuals can pass on their turn if they feel they have no new idea to contribute.
5. Continue the process until people run low on new ideas. Make certain not to stop before all new ideas are presented.
6. The process can end here or can move to a second step.
7. The second step is to consolidate common themes and ideas. This must be done with the full consent of the group. It may be possible to consolidate the list to a more manageable list without losing the essence of the ideas presented.
8. The third step is to prioritize the ideas. This step may not be necessary but if needed it should be done with ample time for discussion. If consensus cannot be reached, some form of voting

may be necessary. Consider the group dynamics before deciding on an oral or secret ballot.

Advantages

1. Provides an opportunity for all to be important contributors.
2. Requires little equipment.
3. Builds a cooperative environment.

Disadvantages

1. Outcome may be unpredictable.
2. Some individuals may be uncomfortable and feel forced to contribute.
3. Can be time consuming if taken through all steps.
4. Some may not be willing to participate.

Examples

1. A health problem of concern to the group such as school littering, access to local services, or using a condom.
2. Approaches to intervening with an identified problem such as teenage pregnancy, poor food selection, or drugs sales in the neighborhood.

Sample Operational Procedures Using Brainstorming for Objective Setting

1. Brainstorm objectives—use large wall charts.

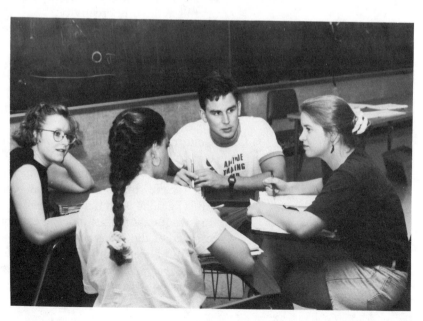

2. After creating an exhaustive list, quickly review the intentions/wording of each stated objective.
3. Establish priority objectives.
4. Assign suggested implementation responsibility.

Assumptions

1. All contributions are welcomed and should be considered.
2. All suggested objectives will be reported unless withdrawn by the person making the suggestion.
3. It is permissible, in fact encouraged, to overlap with other groups.
4. Rotation input will be used but anyone can decline to make suggestions.

METHOD/INTERVENTION 5: CARTOONS/HUMOR

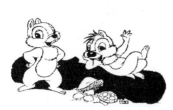

Cartoons can be used as interesting attractions or reinforcing activities. Common usage is to make copies on an overhead transparency, have students collect cartoons of interest, or ask students to make up their own cartoons and/or messages. Political cartoons are often excellent sources. Humor is an important tool for health educators. It can liven up a meeting and help to establish rapport with an audience. It is important to note that not all people view humor in the same way. Be certain to avoid humor that may offend.

Advantages

1. Provide an element of fun.
2. Easy to acquire.
3. Provide variety.
4. Can address affective information or issues in a palatable format.

Disadvantages

1. Outcome may be unpredictable since everyone has a different sense of humor.
2. Require special setup.
3. May require permission to use.

Examples

1. Ask group to design cartoons that would influence a target group.
2. Use cartoons with text removed and ask group to write new text that would influence target population.
3. Ask group to write humorous health sayings.
4. Photocopy cartoons or humorous health sayings and make transparencies to spice up presentation.

Bumper Sticker: "Support Mental Health or I Will Kill You"
Funny to many but upsetting to others.

How in the Health Are You?" May still offend some.

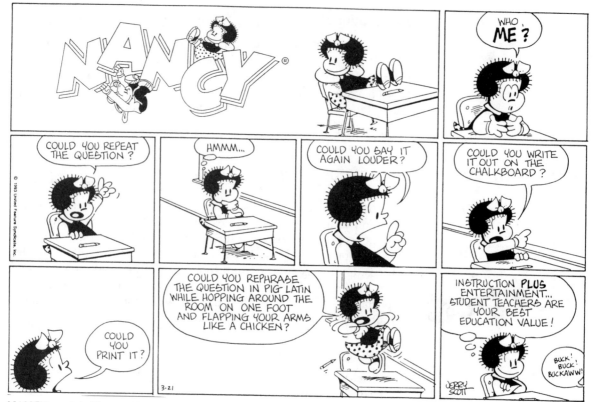

NANCY reprinted by permission of UFS, Inc.

METHOD/INTERVENTION 6: COMPUTER-ASSISTED INSTRUCTION

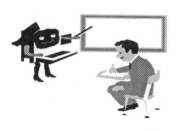

Computer-assisted instruction is not really a teaching method by itself. Rather, it is a tool that is capable of employing other teaching techniques. It allows the combining of audiovisual materials with sound and graphics. The main issue is to find appropriate software that meets your objectives and a setting that has the hardware and software to implement the program. The possibilities are very exciting but the costs can still be very high. The use of such technology is currently much more common in school settings but could be used in community settings. Many people have computer access at home and if the program could be distributed this could be a major way to reach large numbers of people. Apple Macintosh and IBM and compatibles dominate the market and software would need to be compatible to support a large audience. Health education software has been slow to develop because it is often difficult to make a profit on software that can be very high in developmental costs. The market is often small and unfortunately much of the software has been shared through software pirating.

Other possible approaches to gain access to adequate hardware are to use local community colleges or to purchase portable machines. Libraries generally have computers for public use and often lend public domain software. Public domain software can also be obtained over networks and public systems via a modem. The future will make such applications even more feasible for community and school projects.

Portable projection systems are now available making use of a large screen. This means one computer can be used to reach a large audience. Changes can be made on the spot and new technology permits on-screen movement and sound. Custom lessons can be developed which are very professional attention-getters.

Advantages

1. Can provide an element of fun.
2. Considered innovative.
3. Provides variety.
4. Can involve participants actively in the process.
5. Almost immediate feedback.
6. Self-pacing exercises possible.
7. Some applications such as simulations require higher-level thinking.
8. Can provide individualized programs.
9. Can be used to reinforce other lessons.

Disadvantages

1. Can be expensive.
2. Requires special equipment.
3. Requires special software.
4. Requires special training in computer use.
5. Can be frightening to someone new to computers.

Examples

1. Dietary analysis programs.
2. Health risk appraisals.
3. Health games.
4. Monitoring compliance such as medications.
5. Simulations.

6. Expert system applications.
7. Using computers to plot trends such as birth rates or violent acts.
8. Automatically sending reminder notices using computer database.

See also Chapter 5.

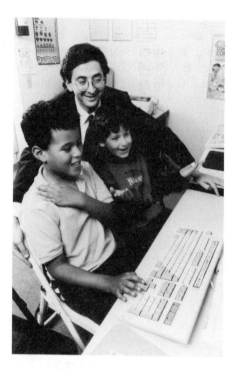

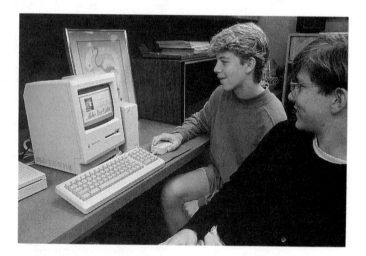

METHOD/INTERVENTION 7: COOPERATIVE LEARNING

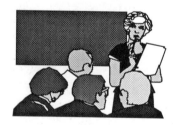

Cooperative learning is a broad category of learning experiences which centers on learning from fellow participants. Generally participants are working toward a common goal. It includes group work such as brainstorming but can be as straightforward as permission to share personal experiences. It has the potential to enhance group spirit and can be very important in group situations.

When to Use

Working in small groups can be an effective strategy in both the school and community settings. The health educator must first establish some very clear behavioral objectives before deciding whether or not small group work is even appropriate. There are many reasons for incorporating group work into the learning process. Group work can facilitate cooperative learning, problem solving, the sharing of ideas, brainstorming, or be nothing more than a device to allow the members of the group to get to know one another. The ability to use group work may be driven by the overall number of participants, their willingness to participate, facilities that allow for small group setup, and the health educator's aptitude for running small group exercises.

Advantages

1. Can provide an element of fun.
2. Potentially creates an atmosphere of cooperation.
3. Utilizes multiple thinkers and therefore can create high-quality innovative answers.
4. Allows participants to learn in a more active and involved manner, therefore decreasing the potential for boredom.
5. Encourages cooperation and collaboration that a large group setting might inhibit.
6. Stimulates innovation in thought, which again might not be encouraged in a large group.
7. Allows participants to quickly become acquainted with each other. This is particularly useful in making people feel at ease in a new situation.
8. Exposes individuals to a variety of viewpoints and ideas that might not surface in a large group setting.
9. Can foster an acceptance of differences in heritage, socioeconomics, or disabilities, for example.

Disadvantages

1. Sometimes difficult to predict outcomes.
2. In the school setting this type of activity has the potential for being very disruptive. School health educators must be very clear about their expectations regarding behavior and noise levels and be prepared to end an activity prematurely should the students get out of control.
3. In both school and community settings, small groups can sometimes be dominated by overassertive individuals. Facilitators need to circulate among the groups to minimize the effects of such behavior. In the school setting, if there are tasks to be performed within groups (such as recorder or reporter), the health educator should appoint these individuals before the groups begin work to avoid disruptive arguments.
4. Small groups, particularly in the school setting, have the potential to wander off the track of their activity. Again, the health educator can minimize this problem by regularly checking in with individual groups and bringing them back on task.

Examples

1. Brainstorming how to prevent drug sales on certain street corners.
2. Sharing of personal experiences.

3. Individual presentations—instructor assigns group work and presentation. Instructor reviews format prior to presentation and ensures quality experience will be provided.
4. Planning an environmental day such as earth day.
5. Designing an antismoking ad poster or 30-second videotape.
6. Forming dyads or triads for problem-solving tasks.
7. Preparing and practicing delivery of a report (small group practice and critique).

METHOD/INTERVENTION 8: DEBATES

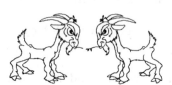

Debates are the organized discussion of differing points of view. By providing structure we hope to achieve better understanding of multiple points of view and perhaps some wisdom. Debates also can potentially develop skills in oral persuasion.

Advantages

1. Can provide an element of fun.
2. Can develop many skills.
3. Provide variety.
4. Can expose group to many diverse opinions.

Disadvantages

1. Require careful controls.
2. May reinforce current positions.
3. May develop into controversy.
4. Some people may not feel comfortable and may refuse to participate.

Debates can be inspirational events or the dull sharing of opinions. What happens is a result of organization and planning. First, you must review your objectives and determine if a debate will be helpful in achieving them. Do you wish to bring in outside debaters, use a debate team, or plan a notable debate and invite the community? What would be useful? If you wish to use your group or class, it is important to structure the debate so you can be certain to achieve your objectives. Since you are not teaching debate, remember that debate skills are an important secondary benefit but not the primary objective. The primary objective is usually the knowledge gained from preparation and observation of the debate or considering an issue from an alternative viewpoint.

Case Study *Pat Thomas, a school health educator, decides to have a debate on the issue of abortion. She asks for volunteers for the debate from the class. They select their position, and the debate follows in one week. The students provide excellent arguments on both sides of the issue. Pat feels good about the experience until she notices hostility among the students following the debate. Upon questioning the class she learns almost no one changed his/her position in any way and many feel upset that others will not change their position given the righteousness of their cause.*

Questions for discussion

What happened?
What could improve the chances that learning will take place and students will consider all sides?

Common debate characteristics

1. Not knowing which side—pro or con—you will present until the last minute. This forces preparing both sides of an issue. Also forces considering both sides.
2. Structured time frame set in advance. For example, 5 minutes opening arguments followed by 3 minutes rebuttal and 3 minutes closing.
3. Order drawn at random.
4. Consider ascertaining the participants' position on an issue and assign them to debate the opposite side.

Examples of Debate Issues in Health Education

1. Mandatory helmet laws.

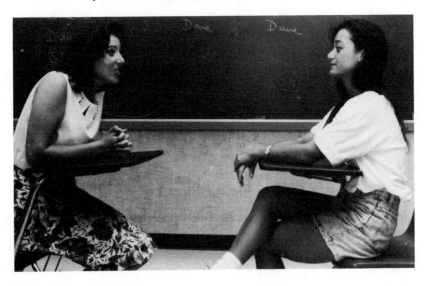

2. Providing condoms to minors on demand.
3. Parental notification for all medical procedures (STD treatment, abortion etc.).
4. Abortion.
5. Free needles and sterilization kit handouts.
6. Who is responsible for a problem—pollution, violence, poverty.

METHOD/INTERVENTION 9: DISPLAYS/BULLETIN BOARDS

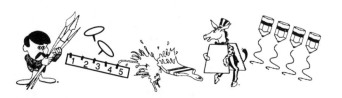

Displays and bulletin boards are graphics and text combined in formats to attract attention. They can provide a positive educational environment and reinforce important points. They can also reach groups not attending any formal presentation or course.

Advantages

1. Set a positive environment.
2. Can be an ongoing educational tool.
3. Can reach special populations such as "walk-bys."
4. Provide variety.

Disadvantages

1. Can be expensive.
2. Require special materials.
3. Can be very time consuming.
4. Issue of vandalism can be a concern.

Good bulletin board planning begins by analyzing its various elements: the title materials to be used, their arrangement, lettering, and color choices. Interest will be aroused by attention-getters such as puns, riddles, exaggeration, associations, comic strip figures, and other familiar figures.

Elements to be used should be considered in terms of the following variables:

1. *Topic selection.* Focus attention on single theme or subject. Message should be short and to the point.
2. *Materials (background).* Those that are to be best used will vary with theme or subject. Once you have a rough sketch, take time to

decide which materials will create the desired effect. You can use construction paper, white newspaper print, burlap, wall paper, newspaper, gift-wrapping paper, and/or corrugated paper.

3. *Display materials.* Use actual objects and three-dimensional objects whenever possible. You can also use drawings, next best to real objects, cartoon and stick figures, pictures, or cotton roving (this can be used to tie the board together, indicate direction, or add decorative touch).

4. *Arrangement.* Can be formal with two sides balanced—all items quickly seen. May tend to be boring because it is best suited for complicated arrangements. An informal or unbalanced arrangement is more interesting and eye catching. Key elements dominate. With either arrangement use captions employing left-to-right principle. Place these at the bottom only when bulletin board is at eye level. Frames give appearance of completeness. Can use construction paper corners or paper strip corners for final touch.

5. *Lettering.* Must balance yet not overshadow the rest of the board. Bold even stroke of about ⅙ of letter found to be most legible. Capital letters, manuscript letters, fancy, or textured. Can use felt pens, rope, paint, cutouts, ribbon or yarn, spray paint, stencils, twigs, popsicle sticks, and so on.

6. *Color.* Attention, force, and meaning are obtained through skillful contrasting of color. Choose colors that catch attention and not those that blend into the background. Can pick for shock effect. Red, green, and blue are good at all times, but dark and light tones add dramatic and pleasing effect.

Contrast makes the difference!

METHOD/INTERVENTION 10: EDUCATIONAL GAMES

Educational games are activities that utilize an element of competition. They differ from other games in that the educational objectives are clear and are the main focus of the activity. Games are generally competitive activities, and the user should consider the effects on all participants of using such a format.

Advantages

1. Provide an element of fun.
2. Competition can be motivating.
3. Gaming provides variety.
4. Can provide opportunities for repetition of important information.
5. Can be excellent introduction activities or good reviews.
6. Can encourage and enhance teamwork.

Disadvantages

1. Tend to focus on cognitive information for the most part.
2. Some games can be embarrassing for individuals who know little of the topic.
3. Can place too much emphasis on competition.
4. Enthusiasm can get out of control and become disruptive.
5. Winning sometimes becomes more important than learning.

Often participants can design their own games and rules. Utilizing existing frame games is a good way to develop interest. Use the format followed in current popular TV game shows.

**Example 1:
Football Game**

(Can be adapted to baseball, basketball, etc.)

Purpose

1. To review (could be used as a means of oral evaluation).
2. To start a card file collection of good testing items for future tests, reviews, and oral evaluations.

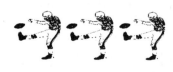

Background

Facilitator must make up a large number of appropriate questions.

Rules of Play

1. Divide into two teams.
2. Flip a coin to see which team will be on offense first.
3. First offense begins from the team's own 40-yard line.
4. Questions are asked in rotating order. If the answer is correct, the team advances 10 yards.
5. If the first person fails to answer the question, the next member is permitted to answer the question but a down is lost. If the first question was a true-false question, a new one is asked.
6. If the question is missed by the fourth person, the ball is lost on downs.
7. Questions are asked from pile 1 down to the 30-yard line.
8. Questions are asked from pile 2 between the 30-yard line and the 10-yard line.
9. Pile 3 contains the touchdown questions when the team reaches the 10-yard line.
10. Pile 4 contains the point after touchdown conversion.
11. From the 20- or 10-yard lines, a field goal may be attempted from pile 5.
12. After a touchdown and conversion attempt, the team scored on starts a new offensive from its own 40-yard line.
13. If a field goal attempt is successful, the team that kicked starts a new offensive from its own 40-yard line. If unsuccessful, the defense takes over on its own 20-yard line.

14. A five-minute halftime is taken in the middle of the period for consultation with team members and references on questions missed during the first half. Change possession of ball for second half.
15. In case of a tie score, the team with the most first downs (in this case the most correct answers) shall be the winner.

Materials Needed

1. A series of questions on three-by-five-inch cards or cards that look like footballs, separated into piles.
2. Place cards showing numbers of piles.
3. Football field could be a model or magnetic board or you could draw one on a blackboard, showing line divisions.
4. Prepare a place on blackboard or scoreboard for showing the team scores and first downs.
5. Progress of ball:
   a. By marking the blackboard with chalk (use colored chalk if you have it).
   b. If using a model, by moving a small indicator of some kind back and forth on top of it.
   c. Using a magnetic board.

Example 2: Baseball Game

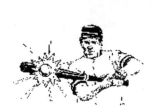

Rules of Play

1. Three outs to a side (three misses).
2. Limit singles to a maximum of three per inning. This will keep one team from dominating time.
3. Score by force-in only. This will prevent arguments. Be certain to explain.
4. Play as many innings as time permits (not more than nine).
5. If question correctly answered, runner advances the corresponding bases.
6. Singles are easy questions, doubles harder, and so on.
7. If game ends in a tie, decide winner by total number of correct answers.

Alternate Rules of Play

1. Divide into two teams.
2. Make up series of questions: true-false for singles, easy questions for doubles, harder questions for triples and home runs.
3. Runner must be forced in to score.
4. Limit of three singles and three doubles per inning.
5. Talking by team at bat results in an out; talking by team on defense results in an out for the next inning.
6. Winner scores most runs.
7. May add third-inning stretch for study.
8. Missed questions may be used again later.

**Example 3:
Hollywood Squares**

Basic Rules

Introduction

Hollywood squares is a cognitive (knowledge) oriented game. It is especially suitable as an introductory game or as a review activity. The basic design (frame) is taken from the television game of the same name, and questions may be based on any desired content area. The instructor can make up questions or have students develop them as an assignment. Consider using another more current TV game show format.

Setting

1. Select nine people to act as celebrities and ask them to leave the room. They might be selected earlier and come prepared.
2. Arrange chairs in the front of the class.
   a. Three chairs in a straight row facing away from the blackboard toward the rest of the class. Allow room for three persons to stand behind and three to sit on the floor in front.
   b. Put lectern at back of class as shown, with two captains.

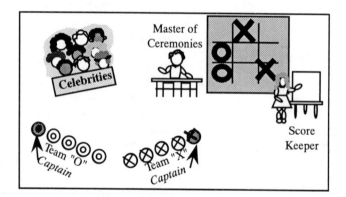

3. Prepare a scoreboard to one side of the blackboard in case there is time for more than one game.
4. Divide remainder of class in half alternately.
   a. Advise (name: _____) that she is captain of team X and seat her.
   b. Advise (name: _____) that he is captain of team O and seat him.
   c. Be sure to seat X on right of lectern, O on left.

Celebrities Briefing

Celebrities wear tags and take on the role of famous people or they can just be themselves.

1. Questions will be directed to you; answer independently.

2. If you do not have a good answer, alibi or bluff—but make up your mind quickly because there will be a time limit.
3. When you come back into the room, situate yourselves in the front of the room as I direct you.
4. Please, no conversation, except to answer or bluff.
5. Do not be afraid to ask for a question to be repeated.
6. Any questions?

Return to Class

1. Celebrities seated.
2. Check to see that teams are situated.
3. Brief class on the game.
   a. The object of the game is to get three squares in a row either up and down, across, or diagonally. To do this, the team must decide whether or not a celebrity is giving the right answer or making one up.
   b. Each completed game is worth 250 points. The team with the most points at the end of class will win a fabulous prize. The winning team will be given some prize, perhaps be allowed to leave early. If used with a community group, provide gold stars or prizes.
   c. Since we are deviating from the original format of "Hollywood Squares" in as much as teams will compete instead of single contestants, it is necessary to set a time limit of 30 seconds on deliberation between captain and team. Final decisions on how to answer each question will be left to the captain of each team. Please answer as quickly as possible.
   d. The facilitator will be the final judge of whether an answer is correct.
4. Are there any questions?

Begin

1. X, you start by choosing a square.
2. Question 1.

Questions

Questions should be based on important concepts and stated objectives. They should also be asked in such way that they lend themselves to bluffing.

Materials Needed

Nine large cards with "X" on one side and "O" on the other side. Two cards to designate teams; one "O" card and one "X" card.

Example 4:
Health Bingo

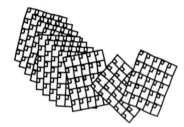

Purpose

1. To review information.
2. To introduce information.
3. To evaluate workshop or class.

Background

Facilitator must make up a list of questions suitable for the game. Each round requires 24 questions.

Player Objective

To achieve "bingo" by getting five correct answers in a row/column or diagonal.

Materials

Bingo cards and pencils.

Rules of Play

1. Each person randomly assigns numbers (1–24) to the small corner boxes of their Bingo cards.

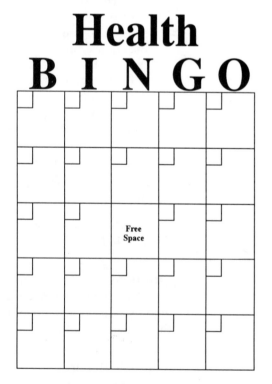

Health BINGO Cards

2. Facilitator begins game by drawing or otherwise randomly selecting the first number and reads a question.
3. Players locate square and write the correct answer (if they know it).
4. The process is repeated until someone calls "bingo."
5. The facilitator then checks the card to ensure there are five correct answers. If one or more is incorrect, play resumes; otherwise the person is named the winner.
6. At this point the facilitator reviews the questions and answers.

Example 5: Educational Relay

Purpose

1. To introduce a new area of instruction.
2. To get people up and active.
3. To review material.

Background

The facilitator must prepare a set of cards for each team (usually there are three teams with 15 to 20 cards each). Each set of cards should be the same except for a mark identifying each team. Three different-colored sets of cards could be used, for example. Cards each have a word appropriate to the topic being covered. Each container is labeled with the name of the category. An example would be containers labeled with food groups and cards with names of foods.

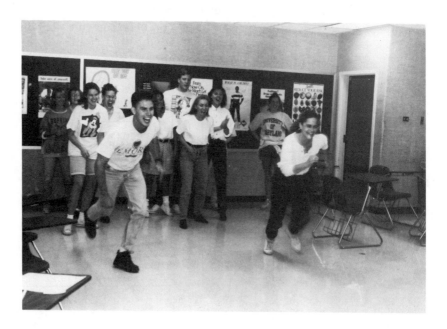

Player Objective

To get the cards in the correct container, and also to complete the task first.

Materials

1. Three sets of three-by-five-inch cards.
2. Three containers (large brown bags work fine).

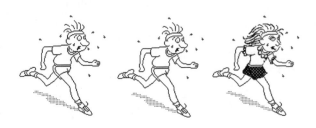

Rules of Play

1. Teams are selected and the room is cleared to allow running a relay.
2. Each member must start behind a line, pick up a card, run and place it in the correct container, and return to tag the next person in line. The next person repeats until all cards are used.
3. The winning team (first team to deposit all cards) receives 5 points for best speed; the second team receives 3 points; the third team receives 1 point.
4. The facilitator moves to the containers and removes the cards, checking with the group for correct answers. Each *correct* answer is worth 1 point.

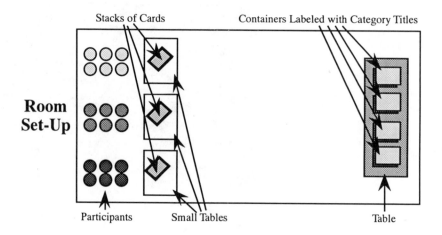

Room Set-Up

Stacks of Cards

Containers Labeled with Category Titles

Participants   Small Tables   Table

5. The team with the highest point total is the winner.
6. Be extra careful with safety. Make certain the room is safe for a relay. Encourage people to walk if appropriate.

METHOD/INTERVENTION 11: EXPERIMENTS AND DEMONSTRATIONS

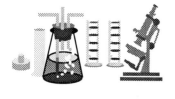

Experiments and demonstrations can serve as important tools for the health educator. Providing a factual demonstration is important for presenting information, reinforcing information, and enhancing recall. They can be used in community settings with careful planning. Such demonstrations are often remembered for a long time.

Advantages

1. Visual and often hands on.
2. Can serve to teach the scientific method.
3. Usually high interest level.
4. Reinforce theoretical aspects of a topic.

Disadvantages

What I hear, I forget.
What I see, I remember.
What I do, I learn.
—Chinese proverb,
author unknown

1. Can be costly.
2. Time-consuming setup.
3. Require special equipment.
4. Outcomes can be unpredictable.

Example 1: The Fish Tank Ecology Demonstration

Materials Required

1. Fish.
2. Fish tank.
3. Small fishnet.
4. Litter, assorted sizes.
5. Appropriate story.
6. Clearance of agency or school to conduct activity (human subjects clearance may be required).

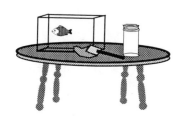

Description

One medium-sized fish tank is set up in plain view of the audience. Inside the tank is a goldfish. Next to this tank is a smaller tank or large jar with clean water. A fishnet is evident and in plain view.

Procedures

1. The facilitator sets up the demonstration without explanation but makes certain the audience sees all components, especially the fishnet.

2. The facilitator introduces someone to present a story. An excellent choice would be the Dr. Seuss story, *The Lorax*. The story is then read to the group.

3. Every so often the facilitator adds a piece of litter to the fish tank. This is done in full view of the audience. Hold up the litter item and examine the label before placing it in the tank.

4. As the story goes on, the litter becomes increasingly toxic. Progress from solid objects such as cans to soap products and oil.

Discovery is learning.
—Francis Bacon

5. If someone says to stop littering, ignore that person, but if someone takes action, allow that person to put the fish in the clean tank.

6. The activity ends when the story is over and the tank is thoroughly polluted or someone saves the fish.

7. The story reader usually leaves after reading the story.

8. Debrief the group as follows:

> *Question:* What happened?
>
> The usual response is, "You killed the fish."
>
> *Question:* Who killed the fish?
>
> *Response:* You all the killed the fish. You all knew what was happening but did nothing to save the fish. That is exactly what is happening to our environment. We talk a lot but do nothing. Everyone of you could have saved this fish but made excuses and did nothing.
>
> If someone saves the fish, present the fish to that person and commend him/her for taking action.
>
> *Caution:* This activity requires clearance and may evoke emotional responses. You must be prepared to deal with these issues from animal rights groups and others. Be certain this is appropriate for the age group involved.

Example 2:
Smoking Experiment
Accumulation of
Tar 1[1]

A. Purpose
   To show the accumulation of tar in water by change of color and smell.

B. Appropriate Age Group
   Middle through secondary school.

C. Equipment
   1. Gallon jar with a two-holed stopper.
   2. Cigarettes and matches.
   3. Delivery tubes (glass, plastic, or rubber hose).
   4. Cigarette holder.
   5. Hand squeeze pump or vacuum pump.

---

[1]From G. G. Gilbert and M. Ziady, *Science and Health Experiments and Demonstrations in Smoking Education* (U.S. Public Health Service, 1986). Also available from the American School Health Association.

D. Procedure
1. Assemble cigarette tar separating apparatus as shown in the diagram.
2. Fill the gallon jar half full with water.
3. Place cigarette in intake and light.
4. Using vacuum pump, draw smoke from cigarette into gallon jar and water.
5. Pump until cigarette is burned completely. Replace with additional cigarettes until tars can be seen in water.
6. Examine color and smell of water.

E. Key Points for Discussion
1. What happens to your lungs when you smoke?
2. What are the similarities between this experiment and what happens to your lungs?
3. What chemicals are in the water?
4. Where can we find out more about the effects of smoking?
5. How does your body rid itself of these tars?

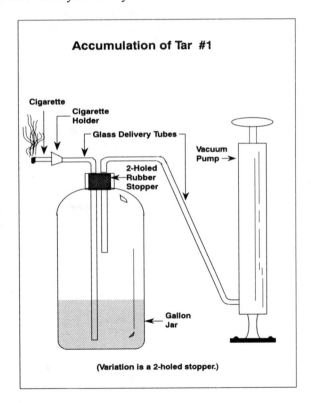

Accumulation of Tar #1

Cigarette

Cigarette Holder

Glass Delivery Tubes

Vacuum Pump →

2-Holed Rubber Stopper

Gallon Jar

(Variation is a 2-holed stopper.)

**Example 3:
Smoking Experiment
Accumulation of
Tar 2[2]**

A. Purpose
To show the accumulation of tar in cotton balls.

[2]From G. G. Gilbert and M. Ziady, *Science and Health Experiments and Demonstrations in Smoking Education* (U.S. Public Health Service, 1986). Also available from the American School Health Association.

B. Appropriate Age Group
   Primary school.
C. Equipment
   1. Plastic window cleaner container or other empty plastic container, transparent if possible.
   2. Ball point pen barrel or other tubing approximately the size of a cigarette.
   3. Cotton.
   4. Cigarettes and matches.
   5. Ash tray or other item to catch ashes.
D. Procedure
   You may wish to conduct experiment outside or with the windows open to avoid side-stream smoke.
   1. Rinse the container thoroughly.
   2. Make an opening in the cap of the container to fit the tubing into the cap.
   3. Place the tubing in the opening and seal tight with cement or clay if needed.
   4. Insert loosely packed cotton ball into tubing.
   5. Insert cigarette into open end of tubing.
   6. Press firmly on the plastic container to force air out, light the cigarette, and then proceed with slow and regular pumping action.

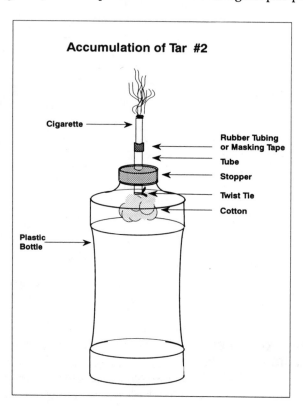

Accumulation of Tar #2

Cigarette

Rubber Tubing
or Masking Tape

Tube

Stopper

Twist Tie

Cotton

Plastic
Bottle

7. Withdraw cotton from tubing to show accumulation of tar.
8. Pass container around for individuals to smell and to observe that smoke continues to be expelled for a period of time.

Variation

1. Divide into groups and conduct several experiments, keeping a close watch for safety.
2. Try same experiment with filter cigarette.
3. Compare filter and nonfilter cigarettes.

E. Key Points for Discussion
1. What happens to your lungs when you smoke?
2. Is this experiment similar to what happens to your lungs?
3. Consider this effect multiplied by 20 or 30 times per day for 5, 10, or 20 years.

Other Examples of Experiments

1. Putting powder on doorknob that is only visible under a black light. Follow-up using black light to discuss transmission of disease.
2. Testing local streams for contaminates.
3. Testing wall paints for the presence of lead.

METHOD/INTERVENTION 12: FIELD TRIPS

Field trips are visits with individuals, to sites of interest, or both. Such visits provide special opportunities to put people or activities in the context of the environment. Such activities are common in many schools but should also be considered in community health programs. If you expect individuals to use services, for example, it would be a good idea to visit the site and get acquainted with the personnel. Chances are much greater that these services will be utilized.

When to Use

It is appropriate to use field trips when you believe the trip will actually help meet your objectives. Being on site affords special opportunities not found elsewhere and visiting a site can often have a demystifying effect. If you want to ensure that your group is more comfortable in using a facility, for example, a field trip would be a good idea. Knowing how to get there can be an important issue. Which bus to take or where to park can be important considerations. This has been shown time and again to be a major barrier for action.

You may gain access to special expertise or equipment that is important to reaching your objectives only through field trips. Prior planning is most important if you want to ensure a successful trip. You should always personally visit the site first before taking a group. Only

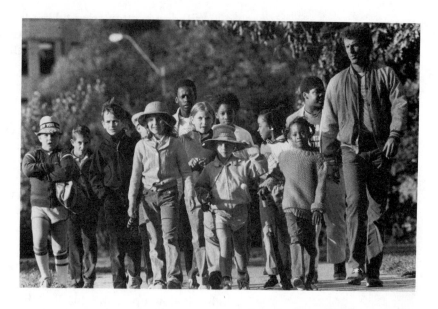

take a group that you are certain you can handle. This is especially important with any group that will be in a potentially dangerous area. One method often used is to establish a list of questions to be answered by each visitor and collect the responses following the trip. Always conduct a debriefing session after the visit.

Case Study *Meshah took a group of high school students to a comprehensive community health clinic to meet with the staff. The agenda was so full the students had little opportunity to ask questions. On the bus home Meshah engaged the students in discussion about the football season. Unknown to Meshah, the students still had many questions about privacy issues, access to care, and the qualifications and training of staff. Many students went away with incorrect assumptions due to the lack of follow-up.*

Health Museums or Health Education Centers

There are several centers around the country that specialize in health education activities. These are very exciting places that have a wealth of materials on display. Most are hands on places that schedule group visits. Generally, they have specially trained staff who will lead tailor-made sessions.

Examples of such centers include:

1. The Center for Health Education in Indianapolis.
2. The Poe Center for Health Education in Raleigh, North Carolina.
3. The National Health Museum at Walter Reed Hospital in Washington, DC.

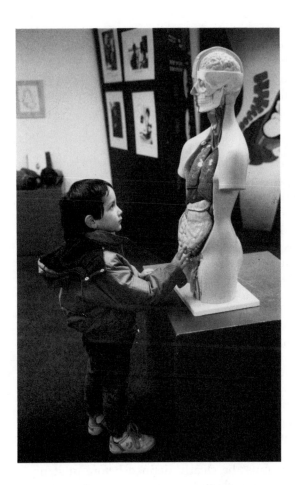 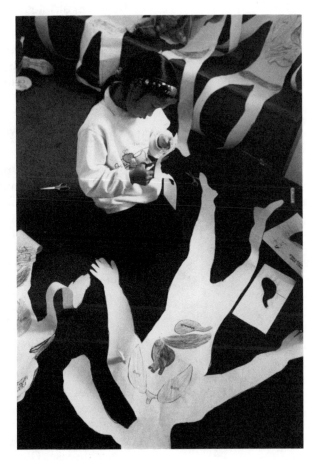

4. The Denver Museum of Natural History: Hall of Life Health Education Center.

Advantages

1. Can be structured to address difficult objectives.
2. Often very entertaining and enjoyable.
3. Put people in the context of their environment.
4. Often have models and materials not available elsewhere.

Disadvantages

1. Transportation is usually required and can be costly.
2. Can be very time consuming.
3. Outcome can sometimes be unpredictable due to uncertainty of interaction.
4. Liability coverage often an issue.

Other Examples

1. Visit to an emergency room.
2. Visit a public health clinic and take on the role of a client.
3. Ride with a police officer for an evening.
4. Interview individuals who have experienced a health problem of special interest.

METHOD/INTERVENTION 13: GUEST SPEAKERS

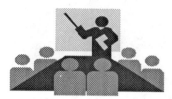

Guest speakers can potentially be a tremendous resource in both the school and community settings. Many individuals have qualifications or experiences that make them uniquely qualified to add a great deal to health-related topics. Individuals who have experienced or are experiencing health problems can help bring alive and personalize what might be viewed as dull, unimaginative, and all too irrelevant health information. Other speakers might be experts in a field who can bring up-to-date information about topical health issues. One caution must be made, however. Health educators must think carefully about what they are trying to achieve before using guest speakers (see the information on constructing behavioral objectives in Chapter 2). For example, all too often school and college health educators, in an attempt to increase the students' awareness of their own susceptibility to HIV, will bring in a guest speaker who is HIV positive. The speaker is a middle-aged man who discusses how he contracted the virus through homosexual sex. The students usually feel moved by the tragedy of the situation and the courage of the individual, but leave the presentation with their stereotypical view strongly reinforced, that HIV is still really a gay disease. Objectives must be clearly defined before utilizing a speaker, and the health educator should avoid the trap of using someone simply because "it seemed like the right thing to do!"

Advantages

1. Allow groups access to experts in the field and the opportunity to obtain up-to-the-minute information.
2. Enable participants to personalize or put a face to a health issue that up to this point might have seemed very abstract.
3. Can help to give the participants a "break" from the regular presenter or teacher.
4. Allow participants to meet individuals who might be influential at the local, state, or even national levels. This opportunity can facilitate networking.

Disadvantages

1. The individual might be a poor speaker. Many individuals may have some good information to share, but because their speaking skills are so poor, their presentations become dull, boring, and

ultimately ineffectual. Every effort should be made to hear the speaker present *before* extending an invitation.

2. The single guest speaker tends to bring one viewpoint to an educational setting, which, of course, is not always a bad thing. However, care must be taken to at least consider this factor, and, when discussing controversial issues in particular, perhaps some type of effort should be made to provide a balanced viewpoint.

3. When working in a school setting, notification and permission from the administration to use any guest speaker should be obtained. This is of particular importance when considering "sensitive" issues such as human sexuality or drug education.

4. In the community setting will the participants be able to relate to the speaker? Issues such as the speaker's race, gender, age, and national origin are all important factors to consider when bringing in a guest speaker to a community. Close consultation with community leaders is an effective way to facilitate the choice of speaker.

5. Although many speakers will not charge any type of fee, those individuals who have a particular expertise, who are regular speakers, and who have a good reputation will invariably charge a speaking fee. This can range from a few hundred to a thousand or more dollars per engagement. Always be sure to ask about a fee before arranging a presentation!

Example

You have been asked to teach a small unit on eating disorders to college students. You have covered the "theory" of the issue, but it is clear to you that despite the statistics you have given related to the prevalence of this problem, the students are having a difficult time understanding how individuals become involved with eating disorders. After a little research on your part, you discover that the campus has an eating disorder support group which provides students who are willing to share their stories with other students. A student from the group attends your class, and suddenly eating disorders has a face and a personality . . . and because the face and personality probably look very similar to those of the regular class members, the effects of using such a guest speaker can be profound.

METHOD/INTERVENTION 14: GUIDED IMAGERY

Guided imagery as a method involves experiencing through a guided sensory journey some health-enhancing behavior. It generally involves closing of the eyes and being guided through some experience. It is commonly used in stress management or sports psychology.

When to Use

It is appropriate to use guided imagery when you believe the experience will actually help meet your objectives.

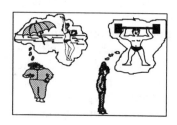

Advantages

1. Can positively influence attitudes and values such as efficacy.
2. Can be entertaining and enjoyable.
3. Low cost.
4. Can be motivational.

Disadvantages

1. Requires some training and practice.
2. Can be time consuming.

Example: A Basic Experience for Pain Control[3]

Now relax, close your eyes, take a deep breath, and repeat mentally to yourself each sentence after I say it:

My arms and legs are heavy and warm. (six times)

My heartbeat is calm and regular. (six times)

My body breathes itself. (six times)

My abdomen is warm. (six times)

My forehead is cool. (six times)

My mind is quiet and still. (three times)

My mind is quiet and happy. (three times)

I am at peace.

I feel my feet expanding lightly and pleasantly by 1 inch. (two times)

My feet are now expanding lightly and pleasantly by 12 inches. (two times)

The pleasant 12-inch expansion is spreading throughout all the parts of my legs. (two times)

My abdomen, buttocks, and back are expanding 12 inches lightly and pleasantly. (two times)

My chest is expanding 12 inches pleasantly and lightly. (two times)

My arms are expanding 12 inches lightly and pleasantly. (two times)

My neck and head are joining in the 12 inches of expansion. (two times)

My entire body is relaxed, expanded, and comfortable. (six times)

My mind is quiet and happy. (two times)

I withdraw my mind from my physical surroundings. (two times)

I am free of pain and all other sensations. (two times)

My body is safe and comfortable. (six times)

My mind is quiet and happy. (two times)

I am that I am. (pause two minutes)

Each time I practice this exercise my body becomes more and more comfortable. And I carry this comfort with me to my normal awareness. As I prepare to return to my normal awareness, I will bring with me the ideal comfort which I have created in my focused concentration. As I open my eyes, I take a deep comfortable breath and a big comfortable stretch.

Other Examples
1. Stress reduction—soft music such as sea sounds accompanied by directions to experience a walk on the beach.
2. Imagine yourself at your ideal weight and how well it feels and looks.

METHOD/INTERVENTION 15: LECTURE

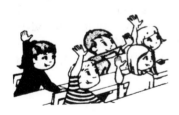

Lecturing is a primary tool of the health educator. It is often maligned as a method, but in fact it is the most common tool in health education. It is often poorly utilized and requires practice and organization. Most of us will not become world-class orators, but we can become competent speakers. We strongly urge you to read some books on public speaking, take a course, or join a toastmasters club to improve your skills. You will constantly be called upon to make presentations as a health educator. Whether you are in school or community health education, you must develop skills in making presentations. Your presentations may be to small or large groups, but the basic principles are the same.

Any time you must lecture for over 20 minutes, utilize some of the other methods or prepare a truly stirring presentation. It is unlikely that you can keep the attention of your audience much beyond this time frame unless audience members are personally highly motivated (i.e., graduate students or victims of the disease you are discussing and you clearly have information they want) or you are charismatic. Preparation is the key to a successful presentation.

See also chapter 6.

Advantages

1. Able to cover large amounts of information in a short time.
2. Can be used with very large groups.
3. Requires little equipment although a microphone is important for large groups.

Disadvantages

1. Can be difficult to hold the attention of an audience.
2. Requires very high level of expertise on the topic to do well without other aids.
3. Difficult to attract audience unless speaker is well known and respected.

Prepresentation Tasks

1. Select or write objectives (see Chapter 2).
2. Analyze audience—needs assessment (see Chapter 2).
3. Develop appropriate content for lecture. Be careful not to cover too much material at one time. Consider providing a handout to reinforce important points.
4. Develop lecture notes as part of your lesson plan (see Chapter 5). This preparation should be done well before the presentation. Knowing you are prepared is a great confidence builder. Preparing the night before often gives you the jitters and is self-defeating.
5. Develop an alternate plan in case something does not work right. What do you do if the audiovisual equipment does not work or the participants do not ask questions when you want them to?
6. Practice making your presentation. If you have the time and resources, video- or audiotape it and play it back. Practice keeping your hands at your side. Do not hold your notes. It is okay to glance at them when needed, but do not be tied to them. If this is a topic you do not know well use overheads or some other visual aid. This will ensure you do not miss any key points and people will look at your visual aide a good part of the time taking some of the pressure off you.

The "Do Nots" of a Presentation	The "Dos" of a Presentation
Do not play with chalk like dice.	Do smile and move about.
Do not put your hands in your pocket or use some other distraction with your hands.	Do reinforce key points.
	Do let the audience know you are a credible speaker on the topic.
Do not say "I don't know this area very well" or "I don't know why I was asked to cover this."	Do use visual aids as appropriate.
	Do show an aura of confidence.
Do not get tied to a podium or your notes.	Do make eye contact.

The Presentation

1. Clarify what you will cover—what are your objectives? Students or clients will learn more if you make it clear what you want them to get out of your presentation. Speak at an appropriate level but do not be patronizing.
2. Present your information clearly, repeating important points.
3. Whenever possible check to be certain the audience is understanding your message. Always remember you are lecturing to reach your objectives. You are not there to only entertain. You are a health educator hoping to influence lives. Use humor if it helps achieve your objectives.
4. Review key points and prepare for the next step in your program. What do you want participants to do? What is the next step?

METHOD/INTERVENTION 16: MASS MEDIA

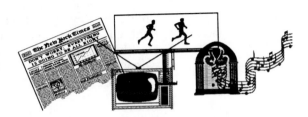

The term mass media refers to the use of media to reach large audiences or the use of available mass media materials to educate a target group. These materials include television, newspapers, magazines, pamphlets, billboards, and radio. Be certain to consider local media such as ethnic publications and community-based publications. Developing your own mass media program is generally expensive and requires special skills. However, many publications will provide free access for worthy causes and may even make their professional staff available. Generally, we recommend the use of specialists for such work. These specialists need not be Park Avenue firms, but can be local businesses or local community college or university staff personnel.

Another way to use media is to utilize available media examples through videotaping or copying. Often formal permission can be granted for educational programs. Many of the voluntary health agencies such as the American Cancer Society have high-quality materials.

An important issue is often preparing groups to analyze media messages and to examine fallacies.

Advantages

1. Can reach a large number of individuals.
2. Can reinforce important ideas.

3. Can create a positive environment for change.

Disadvantages

1. Difficult to change complex behaviors through short messages.
2. Can be very expensive.
3. Can require special personnel.

Who to See

1. Newspapers—the education or medical science editor if they have one, otherwise the appropriate news editor.
2. Television—the public service director or the program director.
3. Radio—the public service director or the program director.

Examples

1. American School Health Association, Marketing Kit—A Healthy Child: The Key to the Basics, available from ASHA, P.O. Box 708, Kent, OH 44240. 216-678-1601.
2. Health Education Advocacy Kit, available from Association for the Advancement of Health Education, 1900 Association Dr., Reston, VA 22061. 703-476-3437.

METHOD/INTERVENTION 17: MODELS

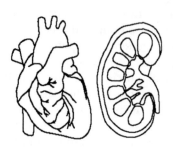

Models are useful visual aids for instruction. Examples of models include anatomical facsimiles, breast models for self-examination practice, model communities, car models, and any variety of materials to make a point or draw people visually into a discussion.

Advantages

1. Can provide variety.
2. Can be used to provide "hands-on" experiences.
3. Are very attractive and good attention-getters.
4. Seeing a facsimile can be much more meaningful than a picture in a text.

Disadvantages

1. Equipment required.
2. Can be expensive.
3. Require extra setup.

Examples

1. Mannequins to teach CPR.
2. Heart model for teaching heart attack prevention and care.

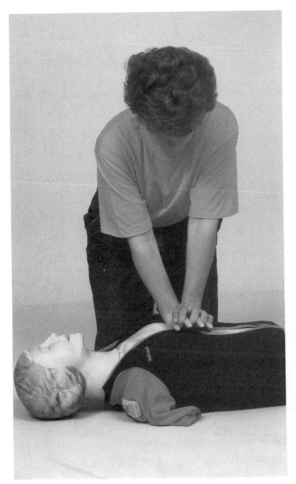

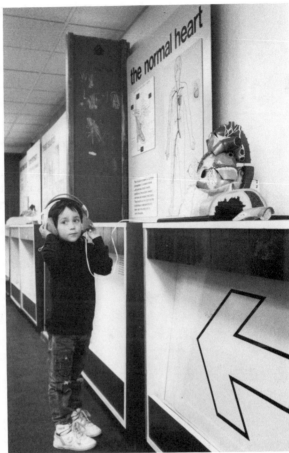

3. Model breasts for instruction in breast self-exam.
4. Model testicles for teaching testicular self-exam.

METHOD/INTERVENTION 18: MUSIC

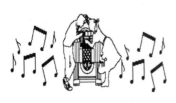

Music can be used in several ways. It can be used as a method or as part of a method. Music is a powerful mood setter. Music can be used in the background as a way of setting the mood for a skit or role play. It can be used for the message found in the lyrics. Students can make up their own lyrics. Music affects us all. We can select music to help us create a special mood or capture the interest of a group.

Advantages

1. Low cost. You can always sing without any equipment.
2. Often can help to discuss affective issues.

3. Excellent for setting a mood.
4. Can allow for individual expression.

Disadvantages

1. Equipment is often required. For example, a piano is sometimes difficult to obtain and move.
2. Sometimes difficult to find correct music.
3. Difficulty in appealing to variety of tastes.

Examples

1. Sing songs with health messages.
2. Develop songs to reinforce health messages.
3. Start a group chant:

> "No matter what you say about me, I'm still a worthwhile person."

> Walk around room making negative statement about each person. Group continues chanting and ignores the mean and harsh statements.

> Use chants to reinforce a message.

4. Play a funeral march to lead into a discussion about funeral customs and the purposes of a funeral.
5. Ask students to make up health lyrics to popular songs.
6. Ask students to bring in a sample of music which might express something personal or special to them.
7. How are relationships expressed or depicted in popular songs? Bring in examples to discuss.

METHOD/INTERVENTION 19: NEWSLETTERS

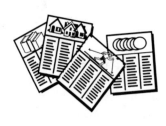

We are all familiar with newsletters, but often do not consider them as an intervention. Newsletters can be an important component of an educational intervention. They can provide important information to target groups, such as location, set a climate for an upcoming workshop or class, serve to reinforce concepts presented in a workshop, or act as a reminder for action. The newsletter is often a very cost-effective way to deliver information, reinforce information, encourage compliance, or increase the likelihood of attendance. The availability of personal computers makes this method accessible to many groups today.

Advantages

1. Have the potential for providing a considerable amount of information at relatively low cost.

2. Can target specific needs.
3. Can reinforce information presented in a program.

Disadvantages

1. Mailing costs and production costs sometimes prohibitive for some organizations.
2. Some equipment required. Generally need access to a personal computer.
3. Can be very time consuming to construct.
4. Require at least a minimal level of expertise.

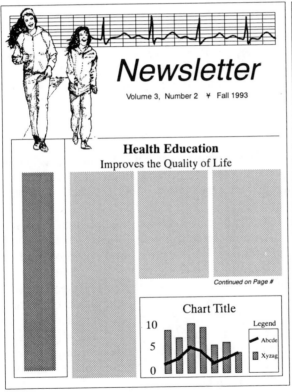

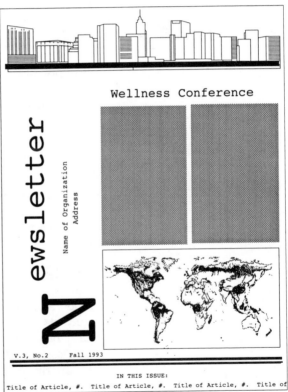

METHOD/INTERVENTION 20: PANELS

A panel is a useful way for an audience either to explore differing opinions about the same topic or to examine varying issues within the same subject area. A panel can be used in both the school and community settings where the panels can be made up of members of the local community (or class) or "experts" brought in from outside agencies. In the school setting a panel is an innovative way to motivate students to research an area and present their findings to the class in the context of a panel. The school health educator should always ensure that the school administration has full knowledge of any panels that include outside speakers. Using a panel in the community is a little more complicated, and great consideration must be given to certain factors when matching panel members with the community setting. For example, will the community members view the panel members as legitimate? Will the community give credence to "outside opinions"? Can the community members relate to the panelists in any way? These are all basic questions that must be considered with great care by the community health educator.

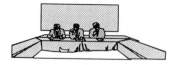

Advantages

1. Allow for a diversity of opinions about the same subject.
2. Have the potential for critical debate between the panelists, allowing the audience to observe the issues in greater depth.
3. Hearing more than one speaker decreases the likelihood of boredom which might occur when listening to one poor speaker.

Disadvantages

1. The right "mix" is often difficult to achieve. For example, one of the panelists might dominate the proceedings, or the members might be so antagonistic toward one another that nothing meaningful gets accomplished.
2. A moderator is a necessity as panelists have the potential of getting off track, either individually or collectively. Rules, such as allowed time to speak, opportunities for questions, and so on, should be considered before beginning.
3. Panels have the potential to lack some sort of closure and a good moderator can help alleviate this situation. In the classroom setting students might be asked to write a paragraph about what they have heard, or their feelings about a topic in light of the panel discussion. In the community setting the moderator might briefly summarize the discussion or allow a few minutes for each panelist to review his or her position.

Examples

You are a health educator who has been asked to organize a meeting for expectant teenage mothers and fathers to help them anticipate problems they might encounter. You decide that rather than give a lecture the group would be better served by being exposed to a variety of "experts." To that end, you might invite the following individuals:

- A teenage mother and father who have already been through the process and could describe their experiences.

- A representative of a local agency who could explain the available program resources, both financial and otherwise.
- A member of the local school system who could give information related to finishing school.

This list is not exhaustive and yet such a panel would be much more useful than a lecture from a single "expert" who has probably never experienced this particular problem. A link to local resources alone would make this panel a worthwhile and valuable health education strategy.

METHOD/INTERVENTION 21: PEER EDUCATION

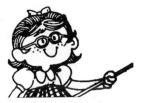 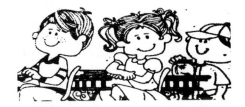

The peer education model of presenting health education information has become very popular over the past few years. This model, which consists of individuals or groups presenting workshops for their peers, can be a very effective and productive means by which to disseminate information. This method is commonly used on college campuses and in school and community settings. Peer education is a particularly useful method to use when funding for professional personnel is limited and/or when it is particularly important for the audience to be able to relate to the presenters. (See the example at the conclusion of this section.)

Advantages

1. Individuals often learn through modeling. Because peer educators are extremely similar to their audiences, the opportunity for modeling to occur is enhanced.
2. The effect of, for example, 10 peer educators on a population is likely to be greater than that of a solitary health educator. The peers have many more points of entry into a population than a professional and can potentially reach more people.
3. Peers have a greater opportunity to perform informal education. They will become known in the community as sources of information and referral and have the opportunity to educate even when they are not offering a structured presentation.
4. Peers can be "gatekeepers" to a population that many professionals cannot reach. The peers' values and interests are similar to

those of their potential clients, and this can provide an effective entrée which might otherwise have been missed.

5. Peer programming affords an incredible opportunity for the personal growth and development of the peers themselves. We should not ignore this potentially positive effect by simply concentrating on the recipients of the programming efforts (Goodhart, 1989).

Disadvantages

1. Because peer educators are not perceived as "professionals," they might sometimes lack credibility in the eyes of the audience.
2. Unless the peer educators are well trained and their programming is closely monitored, the peers could provide inaccurate information and/or perform poorly, resulting in the loss of program credibility.
3. Programs requiring a high degree of sophisticated and technical information should probably not be peer based. There is a danger of the peer educators' being asked to do more than they are capable of performing.

Example

You have just been appointed community health educator at a college with an enrollment of 15,000. You are the only health educator on staff, and your supervisors would like you to begin implementing programming around issues of alcohol abuse, sexuality, and stress management as soon as possible. Hopefully, after educating your supervisors as to what is humanly possible, you set about planning your strategy.

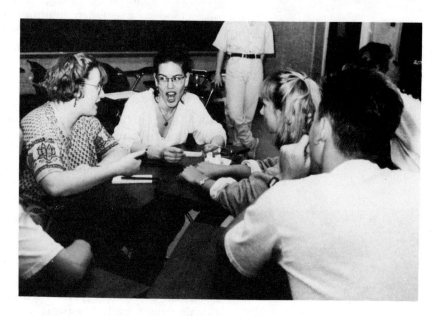

Peer education can be an incredibly valuable programming strategy, particularly when staffing levels are low. Although finding interested, enthusiastic students to help is not usually a problem, training them to high standards of performance can be demanding. High standards, however, are crucial in order to avoid fellow professionals' questioning the wisdom of using "mere students" in a paraprofessional role. Once the programs are up and running, an additional suggestion would be to formalize the program by investigating the possibility of obtaining course credit for the students. Independent studies and/or internships through sympathetic academic departments is one possibility, but the health educator must ensure that the programs are sufficiently well developed to survive academic scrutiny and sometimes cynicism!

METHOD/INTERVENTION 22: PERSONAL IMPROVEMENT PROJECTS

This type of project can be an incentive to make a positive personal change in a targeted health behavior. The objective is to provide clients with an opportunity to gain a good knowledge of proper techniques for changing health behaviors such as diet and nutrition practices and to enable them to incorporate these skills into their chosen lifestyle.

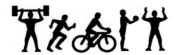

Components

1. Establish a contract with realistic objectives.
2. Chart these realistic objectives.
3. Chart actual progress.
4. Maintain some type of diary to explain progress.

Advantages

1. Low cost.
2. Have the potential for actually influencing directly health behavior.
3. Can target specific needs including behavioral objectives.
4. Can reinforce information presented in a program.
5. Require active application of principles.
6. Personalize health for every participant.

Disadvantages

1. Require considerable individual attention.
2. Can be difficult to achieve.
3. Require considerable paperwork.
4. Some participants may not be sufficiently motivated. If this is a course you may wish to provide an alternate assignment.

Example 1: Weight Reduction Project

It is not the intention of this project merely to provide incentive for another crash-diet program. The objective is to provide you with an opportunity to gain a good knowledge of proper diet and nutrition practices and to enable you to incorporate them into your chosen lifestyle.

In order to ensure this, it is part of this assignment that you read proper background material and determine a course of action that fits your needs (this should include consultation with your physician if possible and for certain if any major weight reduction is contemplated). In your paper you should explain your selection of a diet plan, your goal, any problems you encountered, and include a graph of your progress (see Figure 4-1). Weight data must be made on the same scales and measured at the same time of day to be "officially accurate." Before undertaking this project you must have a conference with your instructor.

Progress toward the objective should be charted. A personal computer can make charting progress easy.

FIGURE 4-1

Personal Improvement Project
Weight Loss John Doe
Target 25 Pounds

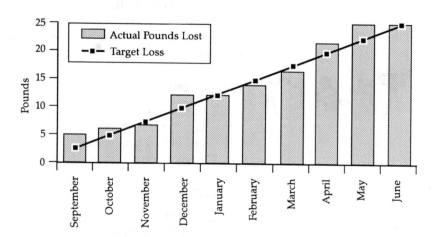

Other Sample Projects

1. Regular exercise program.
2. Increasing fruit and vegetable consumption.
3. Regular mental health breaks.
4. Smoking cessation.
5. Consistent seat belt use.

METHOD/INTERVENTION 23: PROBLEM SOLVING

The Problem Solution Technique

The problem solution technique requires scenarios that need a solution. These can be written or oral. Given the circumstances described, participants are asked to determine the best answer. Often there is no

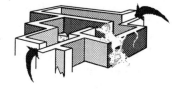

one acceptable answer, and the purpose is to stimulate discussion and to expose participants to multiple points of view.

Advantages

1. Can serve to create a questioning atmosphere.
2. Can demonstrate that often there is no one correct answer.
3. Sets the ground rules for participant interaction.
4. Develops questioning strategies.

Disadvantages

1. Can be time consuming.
2. Participants are sometimes uncomfortable with the notion that there is no one correct answer.

Example 1: "The Demise of Harvey Schwartz"

Cardiovascular Diseases

Harvey Schwartz, a fat middle-aged diabetic, was seated in front of the TV smoking and feasting on a meal of french fries, shrimp, strawberry shortcake, and beer when his wife Hilda came in screaming of his lazy habits. He jumped to his feet and began shouting in return when he collapsed on the floor holding his chest. His funeral was the following Monday. He was buried alongside his father and brother, who died of coronaries and strokes.

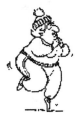 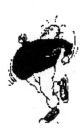 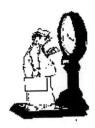

Which of the following do you feel contributed to Harvey's demise? Check the statements you agree with.

_____ 1. His understanding wife, Hilda Schwartz.
_____ 2. His fat body.
_____ 3. His culinary habits.
_____ 4. His choice of beverage.
_____ 5. His fine physical conditioning.
_____ 6. His use of tobacco products.
_____ 7. His genetic background.
_____ 8. His youthful appearance.
_____ 9. His foul-functioning pancreas.
_____ 10. His job as a taxi driver in Brooklyn, New York.

Example 2: **Violence**
"The Wrong Place
at the Wrong Time"

Lamon Thomas and Bruce Chen, wearing their gang colors, are attending a high school dance together when Lamon gets into a verbal argument with another student. The other student is offended when Lamon asks the other student's girlfriend to dance. All participants have been drinking. Bruce comes over to aid his friend when a gun appears. In the struggle Bruce is shot twice and later dies.

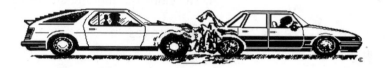

Which of the following do you feel contributed to Bruce's death? Check the statements you agree with.

_____ 1. Lamon's asking the young women to dance.
_____ 2. Bruce's getting involved with something that was not his business.
_____ 3. The way the young men were dressed.
_____ 4. Bruce's choice of beverage.
_____ 5. Lack of metal detectors at the entrance.
_____ 6. The availability of handguns.
_____ 7. Poor supervision.
_____ 8. Lack of parental control.
_____ 9. Lack of stated policies.
_____ 10. No police protection.

METHOD/INTERVENTION 24: PUPPETS

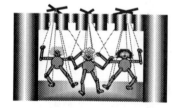

Puppets can be a very powerful tool in health education particularly with the young. Puppets can be purchased or made at low cost. Simply using a doll as a puppet can serve the purpose. Another easy-to-make puppet is the finger puppet. Each paper puppet is fashioned from a small paper drawing that is cut out of paper and held on a finger.

Advantages

1. Entertaining.
2. Can address difficult topics and the affective domain.
3. Can act out feelings without reprisals.

Disadvantages

1. May be difficult to get people to participate.
2. Can bring out unintended emotions or outcomes.

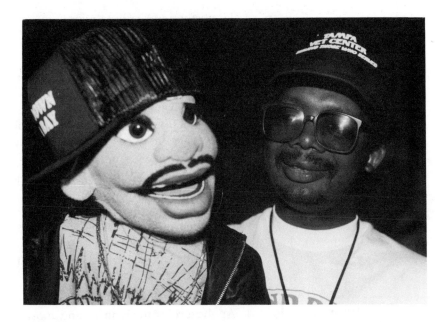

3. Facilitator must be well prepared due to uncertainty of outcome.
4. Can be threatening to some individuals.

Examples

1. Working with young people to express feelings. They will often talk to a friendly puppet but not an adult. This is used extensively with victims of child sexual abuse to elicit responses. This is an indication of how powerful a tool puppets can be. Be certain you choose your questions carefully.
2. Bring some entertainment to an adult group. Have a debate with your puppet. Tape a conversation and play the tape as you provide the answers.
3. Use paper dolls and put them on long sticks.

METHOD/INTERVENTION 25: ROLE PLAYS

Role plays are acting out assigned roles. There is no script as in a play, but participants are not free to act in any way. They are assigned parameters with limited flexibility.

Advantages

1. No equipment required.
2. Can address difficult topics and the affective domain.
3. Can act out feelings without reprisals.

4. Interesting and entertaining.

Disadvantages

1. May be difficult to get people to participate.
2. Can bring out unintended emotions or outcomes.
3. Facilitator must be well prepared due to uncertainty of outcome.
4. Can sometimes be difficult to control.
5. Participants may not take the activity seriously.

Rules

1. Actors are acting out *assigned* roles. It must be understood that they are not playing themselves.
2. No put downs of actors.
3. Do not stereotype casting.
4. Establish parameters for roles.
5. Should be understood that in real life it is rare that there is one clear-cut correct answer or role.

Debriefing Is Most Important

1. Analyze roles for realism and most common responses.
2. What are appropriate and realistic ways to handle the problems posed? Explore alternatives.
3. What are the likely consequences of each alternative?
4. How can we achieve positive outcomes?

Sample Debriefing Questions (should be outlined by facilitator before role play)

1. Was the situation realistic?
2. What would be the likely outcome of the actions of the big brother/sister?
3. What are other options?
4. What are the issues here? (drug use, dating older man, some unknown, sexuality, no supervision, etc.)
5. What are realistic objectives?
6. How can we reach these objectives?

Example Role Plays   **Drug Prevention/Drug Education**

1. Two parents discuss the marijuana joint one parent has found in their son's room. They must decide what action to take.
2. You (age 21 and a college student) walk into your home unexpectedly and find your younger sister (age 15) home alone with an older (age 19) boy. The couple is in the kitchen drinking beer and there are some red capsules on the table which are obviously illegal drugs. They both act nervously when you walk in and try to hide the drugs. Your mother (single-parent family) is working and will not be home for several hours.

3. Parents are teaching their child about drug abuse. You are sitting in the kitchen at home.
4. You find someone in the next dorm room smoking marijuana.
5. Intoxicated date wants to drive you home.
6. You are at a party and two friends urge you to try pot or LSD or some other illicit drug.
7. Your friend gives you his locker combination so you can retrieve the book you loaned him last night. While getting the book you notice several bags of drugs in his locker. This guy has been a pretty good friend and has never offered you or sold you drugs. What do you do?

Violence

1. A friend who lives in a very tough part of town has brought a handgun to school for protection. You spot it when you are having lunch together and he explains he needs it for protection. He says he does not need it at school but has no where else to hide it. You often bring your mom's car to school. He suggests leaving it in the trunk of your car during the day.
2. A good friend of your son is arrested for assault and carrying a concealed weapon (knife).

Sexuality

1. Parent finds diaphragm belonging to 16-year-old daughter.
2. Parent discovers condoms in purse of 14-year-old daughter.
3. Parent discovers condoms on dresser of 14-year-old son.

Ecology Social Responsibility

1. Your son or brother pours oil into the street drain after changing your oil.
2. Your friend dumps trash out of the car window.

METHOD/INTERVENTION 26: SELF-APPRAISALS

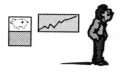

Self-appraisal is a technique to encourage personal assessment as an important step in personal behavior change. It involves some form of personal assessment which can range from a checklist of a few items to a diary and computer analysis kept for a long time. The key element is to encourage self-inspection as a first step in behavior change. Self-appraisal is sometimes coupled with personal improvement projects.

Advantages

1. Allow individual assessment.
2. An important first step in personal behavior change.

3. Provide excellent focus to start a workshop or class.
4. Interesting and entertaining.

Disadvantages

1. Many require computer.
2. Require development of instruments.
3. Can be misinterpreted.
4. May require medical testing.
5. Can be expensive if using a commercial vendor.

Examples

1. Self-tests.
2. Health risk appraisals.
3. Food intake—24-hour recall.
4. Post-workshop assessment.

METHOD/INTERVENTION 27: SIMULATIONS

Simulations are activities that take on the appearance of some real-life phenomenon. Simulations take on the appearance in a real-life way so that we can observe and perhaps participate in the event without the risk of injury in a very controlled manner. Common examples include injury simulation kits with realistic wounds and blood. Participants can treat injuries as they would in real-life situations.

Definition   According to Cruickshank (1972), a simulation is "the end product, the model resulting from the process of simulating. The simulation is contrived experience used to expose someone to a certain prescribed set of circumstances based on a model. It is usually to teach a role, function, or operation. By using simulation, it is possible to attain the essence of something without its reality."

Rationale   Simulated situations can be an asset to any emergency care program for the following reasons:

1. They provide examples of real-life emergency care situations.
2. They provide an opportunity for the practical application of skills covered in the classroom.
3. They provide practice in the analysis and evaluation of emergency situations without the risk of injury resulting from judgment errors.
4. They provide an alternative teaching strategy for the instructor.
5. They can provide an evaluation technique for instructors.

6. They provide students with practice in performing skills under stress and thus increase self-confidence.

Advantages

1. Provide an element of realism.
2. Can address some difficult-to-teach issues such as comfort levels of performance.
3. Provide variety.
4. Can provide opportunities for repetition of important skills.

Disadvantages

1. Generally are time consuming.
2. Can be expensive.
3. Often difficult to use with large groups.

Examples

1. First-aid instruction.
2. Fire alarm and building evacuation.
3. Application of CPR.
4. Simulation games where community member roles are simulated.

Example 1: First Aid[4]   Instructions for Participants

1. You must treat this *like a real-life situation*. Nothing will be assumed—you must *do* all that you would in a real-life situation. To receive credit for any procedure, it must actually be completed. The only exceptions to this are procedures that cannot be done in the classroom such as making a phone call, and they must be explained.
2. You may use only material *provided* in the testing area.
3. You may *not* use any notes or cards.
4. For assistance you may use only those people provided, and you *must give them explicit directions* for any aid they administer. No undirected assistance or information is to be given by other students or victims.
5. *Time will be an important factor in life-threatening situations*. A reasonable time will be allowed for less severe injuries, but do not waste time. (After using a situation several times, an instructor will have an idea of how long it should take to complete and may wish to set a time limit.)

---

[4]From G. G. Gilbert, *Teaching First Aid and Emergency Care* (Dubuque, IA: Kendall/Hunt, 1981).

SAMPLE SIMULATION SITUATION 1

Information supplied to first-aider.

Situation:

> You are home with your younger sister (age 11) when you hear her crying. You find her on the front porch.

Where:

> Your home.

Miscellaneous Information:

> No one else is home.

Position of Victim:

> Seated.

Special Instructions for Victim:

> Cry, but answer questions. You fell and scraped your knee. You have no other injuries.

Supplied Materials:

> Home materials box.

Tags:

> 1. Moderate bleeding (1)–knee.

6. In situations where you want to take a pulse, you must actually take a reading. (Victims will be taking their own pulse so that assessment can be properly made.)
7. Bleeding tags will be marked mild, moderate, or severe. Mild bleeding will require direct pressure and elevation for credit. Moderate bleeding will require the same plus proper use of pressure points where appropriate. Severe bleeding will require the use of all three aforementioned techniques plus proper use of a tourniquet. This is done only as a grading convention and is not meant to imply that proper first aid would be guided only by estimates of blood flow.

SAMPLE SIMULATION EVALUATION 1

Scraped Knee

Name of First-Aider   Grader

	Yes Well Done	Yes Adequate	No
1. Was the victim properly examined and questioned for all possible injuries?	4, 3	2, 1	0
2. Was the victim given verbal encouragement?	2	1	0
3. Was moderate bleeding controlled and bandaged properly?	7, 6, 5, 4	3, 2, 1	0

a. Direct pressure (2)
   b. Elevation (2)
   c. Proper bandage (3)			

4. Was proper shock treatment given?	2	1	0
Comments:			

Add _____

Deductions _____

Total _____

Possible _____ 15 _____

The evaluator circles the appropriate point value and adds the points up for grading. These can be used to determine pass or failure or a letter grade. Multiple situations must be developed prior to class (see Gilbert, 1981) so all participants have different situations.

SAMPLE SIMULATION SITUATION 2

Information supplied to first-aider.

Situation:

>   You are the first to arrive at the scene of a single-car automobile accident.

Where:

>   Freeway (interstate).

Miscellaneous Information:

>   Several other people stop, but no one has first-aid training. There appears to be no danger of fire.

Position of Victim:

>   Victim is face down on front seat (use two chairs).

Special Instructions for victim:

>   You are unconscious and will remain so.

Supplied Materials:

>   1. Coats.
>
>   2. Bandaging materials.
>
>   3. Water.
>
>   4. Splints.

Tags:

>   1. Moderate bleeding (1)–forehead.
>
>   2. Moderate bleeding (1)–nose (nose bleed).

SAMPLE SIMULATION EVALUATION 2

Bleeding

Name of First-Aider _____   Grader _____

	Yes Well Done	Yes Adequate	No
1. Was the victim examined carefully for all injuries?	4, 3	2, 1	0
2. Was moderate bleeding of the forehead controlled properly? a. Direct pressure (4) b. Bandaged properly (3)	7, 6, 5, 4	3, 2, 1	0
3. Was victim removed from car? (If removed–give credit if good explanation for removal given and proper technique applied.)	0	0	4
4. Was note made of possible head injury (medical personnel notified and movement minimized?)	5, 4, 3	2, 1	0
5. Was proper aid sent for?	2	1	0
6. Was the victim treated for shock?	3, 2	1	0
Comments:			

Add _____

Deductions _____

Total _____

Possible _____ 25 _____

METHOD/INTERVENTION 28: VALUE CLARIFICATION

Value clarification is a method designed to help people clarify and understand how they have reached decisions. It has the potential of teaching rational decision-making skills. This method had great popularity in the 1960s and 1970s. It fell into disfavor under charges it taught no values and allowed free choice even when the choice was clear to "any rational person." The method was often misused and this contributed to its being banned in some settings. It is a useful tool if used properly. Many of the principles can be applied well under the title developing decision-making skills.

Values Clarification

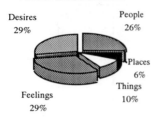

Desires 29%

People 26%

Places 6%

Things 10%

Feelings 29%

Advantages

1. Low cost.
2. Can deal with feelings and emotions.
3. Allows for individual and group expression.

Disadvantages

1. Can be controversial.
2. Instructor must be prepared to deal with emotional responses.
3. Responses can be unpredictable.

Rules for Conduct of Activities

1. No put downs.
2. Respect rights of others to different opinions.

According to Raths, Harmin, and Simon (1966), page 30, true values are those which do the following:

Choosing	1.	Freely
	2.	From alternatives
	3.	After consideration of the consequences of each alternative
Prizing	4.	Cherishing, being happy with choice
	5.	willing to affirm the choice publicly
Acting	6.	Doing something with the choice
	7.	repeatedly, in some pattern of life

Example: Health Education Decision

1. List five major factors that influenced you to go into health education. These can be people, places, things, feelings, or desires.
2. Draw a large circle.
3. Divide the circle into pie slices for each of your "influencers" and make the proportion of each slice appropriate to the amount of influence.

Discussion

1. Are these rational and positive ways to make a decision?
2. How would the pie chart look if you went about this decision the best most rational way?
3. Are you proud of your decision?

METHOD/INTERVENTION 29: WORD GAMES AND PUZZLES

Word games are entertaining and are very useful in increasing vocabulary. They are commonly used with elementary school children, with people studying English as a second language, or with any area that introduces a considerable number of new vocabulary words. These activities include crossword puzzles, anagrams, and other word games.

Advantages

1. Low cost.
2. Fun.
3. Good productive filler for individuals who finish work fast or need additional stimulation.
4. Excellent for improving vocabulary.

Disadvantages

1. Generally only address cognitive domain.
2. Require time to develop.
3. Require equipment to reproduce.

Example 1: Crossword Puzzle

Methods Sample Puzzle

Methods Vocabulary

ACROSS

3 a classification of national background can be from any ethnic group.

5 a precise statement of intended outcome and must be stated in measurable terms.

8 An orderly self-contained collection of activities educationally designed to meet a set of objectives.

9 Belief or expectation by an individual that they can carry out the desired behavior.

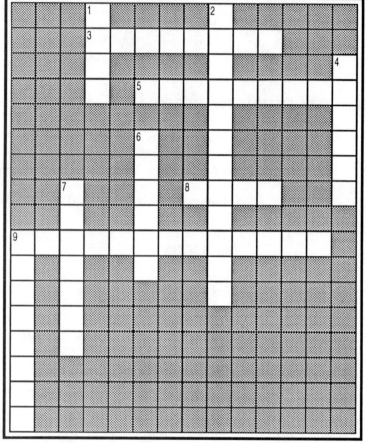

Created using Crossword Creator, Centron Software Technolgies, Inc., Version 1.12, 1992.

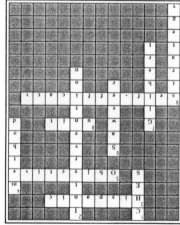

DOWN

1 Certified Health Education Specialist

2 The overall strategy to achieve stated objectives.

4 One component of intervention - can be used interchangeably with strategy.

6 Author of text.

7 Author of text.

9 One component of the intervention. Can be used interchangeably with method.

Example 2: Anagram   Change the following names into drug classifications.

Name	Drug Classification
Minee Haptma	Amphetamine
Bet Arbitura	Barbiturate
Lum Stanti	Stimulant
Ant Pedress	Depressant

See the methods selection matrix in Chapter 3.

PROMISING METHODS BY TOPIC

As we have stated many times, we encourage you to consider all methods that might meet your objectives. The following is a list of methods by topic which have either had some success or the authors recommend the exploration of this method for the listed content area.

Drug Education

Debates

Experiments and demonstrations

Mass media

Panels

Peer education

Role plays

Value clarification

Human Sexuality

Debates

Guest speakers

Panels

Peer education

Puppets

Role plays

Value clarification

Environmental Health

Debates

Experiments and demonstrations

Field trips

Guest speakers

Panels

Consumer Health/Nutrition

Computer-assisted instruction

Guest speakers

Mass media

Personal improvement projects

Self-appraisals

First Aid

Computer-assisted instruction

Guest speakers

Simulation

EXERCISES

Take a look at the following situations. Construct *one* behavioral objective for each situation and then select *one* appropriate method to fulfill the objective. Give a brief justification as to why you selected a particular method and how the method would facilitate achieving the objective.

1. You are teaching the first class in a five-part unit on nutrition for approximately 25 seventh-grade students.
2. You are conducting a one-hour, once-only workshop for a community group of women (approximately 20 women aged 35 to 45) on the subject of menopause.
3. You are facilitating the first in a series of eight workshops on smoking cessation for a community group of 10 adults.
4. You are teaching the final class in a five-part unit on HIV/AIDS for a group of 25 tenth-grade students.
5. You are facilitating the second of six one-hour workshops for approximately 10 college students on the subject of body image/weight management.
6. You are teaching the first in a three-part unit on environmental health for an eighth-grade class of approximately 20 students.

SUMMARY

This chapter has reviewed 29 categories of methods that can be employed by a health educator. Each has advantages and disadvantages which should be taken into account when making a selection for inclusion in any health education program.

REFERENCES

Ames, E. E., L. A. Trucano, J. C. Wan, M. H. Harris. 1992. *Designing School Health Curricula: Planning for Good Health.* Dubuque, IA: W. C. Brown.

Arends, R. I. 1991. *Learning To Teach.* New York: McGraw-Hill.

Bates, I. J. and A. E. Wider. 1984. *Introduction to Health Education.* Palo Alto, CA: Mayfield.

Bedworth, A. E. and D. A. Bedworth. 1992. *The Profession and Practice of Health Education.* Dubuque, IA: W. C. Brown.

Carroll, L. 1946. *Alice in Wonderland and Through the Looking Glass.* New York: Grosset and Dunlap.

Cruickshank, D. 1972. Simulation and gaming. Unpublished mimeographed handout.

Davis, W., K. Feller, and M. Thaut. 1992. *Introduction to Music Therapy.* Dubuque, IA: W. C. Brown.

Feldman, R. H. L., and J. H. Humphrey. 1989. *Advances in Health Education: Current Research,* vol. 2. New York: AMS Press.

Galli, N. 1978. *Foundations and Principles of Health Education.* New York: Wiley.

Gilbert, G. G. 1981. *Teaching First Aid and Emergency Care.* Dubuque, IA: Kendall/Hunt.

Gilbert, G. G. and M. Ziady. 1986. *Experiments and Demonstrations in Smoking Education.* Washington, DC: U.S. Department of Health and Human Services, Office on Smoking and Health.

Gold, R. S. 1991. *Microcomputer Applications in Health Education.* Dubuque, IA: W. C. Brown.

Goodlad, J. I. 1984. *A Place Called School: Prospects for the Future.* New York: McGraw-Hill.

Greenberg, J. S. 1988. *Health Education: Learner-Centered Instructional Strategies.* Dubuque, IA: W. C. Brown.

Greene, W. H., and B. G. Simons-Morton. 1984. *Introduction to Health Education.* New York: Macmillan.

Gronlund, N. 1991. *How to Write Instructional Objectives.* 4th ed. New York: Macmillan.

Hellison, D. 1978. *Beyond Balls and Bats: Alienated (and Other) Youth in the Gym.* Washington, DC: AAHPER Publications.

Hoff, R. 1988. *I Can See You Naked.* New York: Andrews and McMeel.

Joyce, B., and M. Weil. 1986. *Models of Teaching.* Englewood Cliffs, NJ: Prentice-Hall.

Krathwohl, D. R., B. S. Bloom, B. B. Masia. 1964. *Taxonomy of Educational Objectives: The Classification of Educational Goals. Handbook II: Affective Domain.* New York: David McKay.

Lazes, P. M., L. H. Kaplan, K. A. Gordon. 1987. *The Handbook of Health Education.* Rockville, MD: Aspen.

Loya, R. 1984. *Health Education Teaching Ideas: Secondary.* Reston, VA: American Alliance for HPERD.

Mayshark, C., and R. Foster. 1966. *Methods in Health Education.* St. Louis: C. V. Mosby.

Goodhart, F. 1993. Generating enthusiasm among peer educators. *Journal of American College Health* 41(6):295.

Pfeiffer, J. W., and J. E. Jones. 1970. *A Handbook of Structured Experiences for Human Relations Training,* vol. 2. Iowa City, IA: University Associates Press.

Pfeiffer, J. W., and J. E. Jones. 1971. *A Handbook of Structured Experiences for Human Relations Training,* Vol 3. Iowa City: University Associates Press.

Popham, W. J., and E. L. Baker. 1970. *Establishing Instructional Goals.* Englewood Cliffs, NJ: Prentice-Hall.

Raths, L., H. Harmin, and S. B. Simon. 1966. *Values and Teaching.* Columbus, OH: Charles E. Merrill.

Read, D. A., S. B. Simon, and J. B. Goodman. 1977. *Health Education: The Search For Values.* Englewood Cliffs, NJ: Prentice-Hall.

Rubinson, L., and W. F. Alles. 1984. *Health Education: Foundations for the Future.* Prospect Heights, IL: Waveland.

Scheer, J. K. 1992. *HIV Prevention Education for Teachers of Elementary and Middle School Grades.* Reston, VA: AAHE/AAHPERD.

Scott, G. D., and M. W. Carlo. 1979. *On Becoming a Health Educator.* Dubuque, IA: W. C. Brown.

Sculley, J., and J. Byrne. 1987. *Odyssey.* New York: Harper and Row.

Suess, Dr. [Theodor S. Geisel and Audrey S. Geisel]. 1973. *The Lorax.* New York: Random House.

Taffee, S. J. 1986. *Computers in Education,* 2nd ed. Guilford, CT: Dushkin Publishing Group.

U.S. Department of Health and Human Services. 1980. *Promoting Health Preventing Disease Objectives for the Nation.* Washington, DC: U.S. Public Health Service.

U.S. Department of Health, Education, and Welfare. 1979. *Healthy People: The Surgeon General's Report on Health Promotion and Disease.* Publication 79-55071. Washington, DC: U.S. Public Health Service.

Willgoose, C. E. 1972. *Health Teaching in Secondary Schools.* Philadelphia: W. B. Saunders.

Zannis, M. A. 1992. Health educators' use of microcomputer technology in graduate programs. Unpublished Doctoral Dissertation. University of Maryland.

Chapter 5

Using Media and Common Audiovisual Equipment

Entry-Level Health Educator Competencies Addressed in This Chapter

Responsibility III: Implementing Health Education Programs

Competency A: Exhibit competence in carrying out planned educational programs.

Competency C: Select methods and media best suited to implement program plans for specific learners.

Responsibility VI: Acting as a Resource Person in Health Education

Competency A: Utilize computerized health information retrieval systems effectively.

Competency D: Select effective resource materials for dissemination.

Responsibility VII: Communicating Health and Health Education Needs, Concerns, and Resources

Competency C: Select a variety of communication methods and techniques in providing health information.

Taken from *A Framework for the Development of Competency-Based Curricula for Entry Level Health Educators,* National Task Force on the Preparation and Practice of Health Educators, Inc., 1985. Reprinted by permission.

Method Selection in Health Education

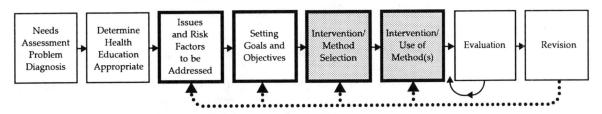

Heavy-bordered boxes indicate subjects addressed in this text; shaded boxes indicate subjects(s) of current chapter.

Case Study   *The room was hot and dark. Jason was trying to count the number of dust motes as they slowly passed in front of the projector's rays of light. At a subconscious level, he could hear the narrator's voice droning on interminably about the effects of alcohol on the liver, but even a pictorial switch from a talking head to a grossly abused and swollen liver was insufficient to disturb Jason's reverie. Sure, he saw the offending organ, glistening on the marble slab . . . sure, he could hear the narrator listing the dangers of an intemperate lifestyle . . . but Jason wasn't actually in the room. The warmth and darkness had transported him to a far more interesting place . . . his imagination. The football game this weekend . . . the party at Scott's place . . . catching that new movie . . . much more interesting than the talking head who had just returned to the screen. The visual switch was enough to make Jason briefly wonder why all talking heads wore white coats and sported haircuts from the 1960s . . . not that it really mattered, it was back to the party for him! Boy, the party was crowded—was everyone in the room counting dust motes and partying? . . . an alarming prospect!*

This is an alarming prospect indeed, but unfortunately an all too common one. As modern technology has become more sophisticated and available, the use of educational media has increased in both the school and community setting. Unfortunately, this increased usage has not always proven to be beneficial to program participants. Too often the materials being used are outdated, of poor technical quality, too heavily laden with facts, inappropriate for the audience, and perhaps the greatest sin of all . . . they are often excruciatingly boring! Modern-day individuals like Jason, who have been nurtured on extremely high quality productions from national television, movie studios, and MTV, have developed the uncanny ability of being able to identify such examples of suspect health education media within a matter of seconds. The classic clues, for example, on a film or videotape might include an extremely dated soundtrack, characters wearing flared pants and giving the "peace" sign, no sign of any automobiles built since 1978, and the talking head in the form of a physician wearing the ubiquitous white coat listing information at the camera. Any or all of these attributes are guaranteed to encourage Jason and his peers to leave their bodies in search of greater stimulation!

After studying the chapter the reader will be able to:

- describe the major advantages and disadvantages of using each media method
- justify a rationale for using a particular form of media, including how it complements the overall learning objectives
- develop a personal checklist for media evaluation
- describe the major steps involved in media development

MAJOR TYPES OF MEDIA

Film (usually 16 mm)   Before the rapid development of the videotape, film usage with the standard film projector was perhaps the most common form of audiovisual aid used in both school and community health. However, since the advent of the videotape, the use of the film projector has become much less common. It is important to realize that although fewer films and projectors are being used today, many instructional materials are still being filmed in 16 mm, before being transferred to the videotape format for distribution.

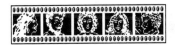

Advantages

1. Film is easy to show to relatively large audiences.
2. Film tends to be a more emotive medium than videotape.
3. Film projectors tend to be somewhat more portable than a VCR and television monitor.

Disadvantages

1. Films tend to be very expensive, often nearly double the price of videotapes.
2. Fewer and fewer films are available in a 16-mm-film format; consequently, many existing materials are out of date.
3. Many individuals find loading a projector somewhat intimidating, and a projector is usually more difficult to use than a VCR.
4. Projector maintenance can be very expensive, particularly on older machines which are more prone to mechanical failure.
5. Film can be a fragile material and after a great deal of use it can become easily damaged. The care and repair of film are important factors to consider before spending large amounts of money on this format.
6. The use of film necessitates finding an available screen or very white wall.
7. This is a technology that will see little use in the future, and most groups understand that fewer and fewer films will be made and equipment will become less available.

CLOSE TO HOME   JOHN McPHERSON

© 1993 John McPherson/Distributed by Universal Press Syndicate

JANE FONDA

3-22   McPHERSON

"Here's the problem! The workout tape has been on fast-forward the whole time!"

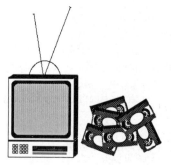

Videotapes The most common form of videotape used today is the one-half-inch VHS. Three-quarter-inch VHS tapes are more frequently used in high-quality professional settings where production values are essential, and Beta-type tapes are rarely used anywhere today. Always be sure, however, that if you are using a videotape in a presentation or class, you check ahead of time that you will be using the correct type of machine!

Videotape usage has enjoyed an incredible expansion over the past 10 years. Videotapes are widely used in school and community health settings, and many private households now also have VCRs. The medium of videotape has clearly supplanted the 16-mm film as the most commonly used form of audiovisual aid in education today.

Advantages

1. Videotapes are very easy to use, and because many individuals use videotapes at home, professional use has become simplified.

2. Videotape prices are cheaper than 16-mm film, usually costing from $125 to $350 for a 20- to 30-minute tape.

3. If a videotape has actually been shot in a 16-mm-film format and then transferred to videotape, the videotape will then have most of the quality of film without the expense.

4. Health education videotapes are becoming more plentiful, and so the information depicted is more likely to be current.

5. Video cameras are now becoming more affordable, and when such technology is available in health education settings the potential for incorporating self-generated videotapes is immeasurable (e.g., videotaping presentation styles, modeling the behavior of saying "no" to drugs, or negotiating safer sex).

Disadvantages

1. Unless a video projector is available, showing videotapes to large groups is very difficult. Multiple monitors can be used, but setting

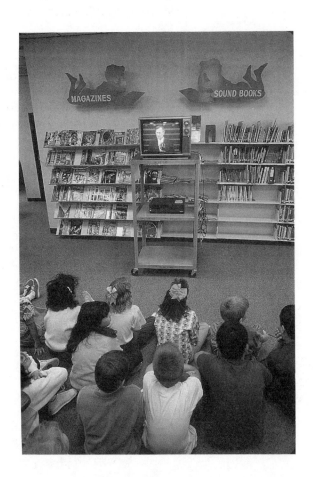

up the machines becomes complicated and time consuming and often results in a less than satisfactory performance.

2. Videotape players and television monitors are not very portable, and so the health educator is dependent on such equipment's being available at the site of the presentation. Such equipment is not always available!

Videodiscs

The most recent technological advancement that has tremendous potential in enhancing health education delivery is the interactive videodisc. Although current use is limited, this form of media may well eventually supersede the videotape as the most commonly used audiovisual instructional aid. Currently, many users are only using the videodisc player which has some advantages over the VCR but does not take advantage of the full potential of the technology. Schools are major users, but shifts in technology are generally slow because budgets do not allow for major changes in paradigms. Teachers are often excited to simply have access to an Apple II computer. The number of schools with full interactive video are limited but growing.

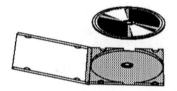

Advantages

1. The instructor has more options of how to use the videodisc than he/she would have with a regular videotape. For example, the disc can be stopped and then restarted at any point the instructor selects often in less than a second. Fast-forwarding or reversing a videotape to find a certain spot can be a lengthy and often frustrating experience, but the speed of the videodisc is amazing and getting faster. Many are equipped with bar-code-type readers to simplify organizing programs in the manner you wish.

2. Quite often the videodiscs are designed to encourage frequent pauses to allow for discussion. This is particularly useful for reinforcing cognitive information, permitting process of affective ideas, and a major advantage for instructors dealing with groups who have short attention spans! The picture quality is much better than most videotapes.

3. Perhaps the greatest advantage of the videodisc is its interactive nature. This allows learning to be less of a spectator sport and more of a mutual endeavor. Groups can interact with the program in a community or classroom setting, or programs can be utilized which focus on the individual. The individual focus is particularly useful when dealing with sensitive, personal issues such as human sexuality and drug abuse.

4. Because this technology is relatively new, the programs that exist tend to be more current than some of the other forms of instructional materials.

Disadvantages

1. Like most new technology, the cost of the equipment can be quite expensive. However, as this medium becomes more commonly used, the cost of purchase is likely to decrease. Costs have been dropping.
2. Some individuals may be a little intimidated at first about operating the videodisc player. However, after becoming familiar with the equipment and materials, most instructors report few problems with using videodiscs.
3. As with the videotape player and television monitor, this equipment is not very portable.
4. Lesson/presentation plans will have to be changed and updated. This is time consuming.

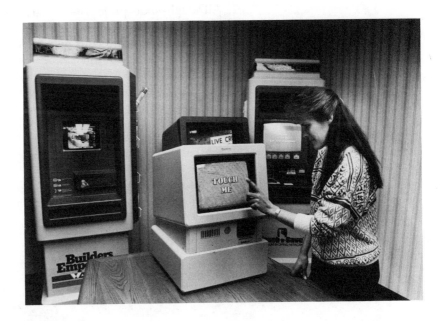

Slide Projectors

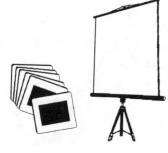

Slide projectors have been around for quite some time and continue to be an extremely useful way to disseminate information. To a major extent, this particular medium has taken the place of the filmstrip. (See the next section.)

Advantages

1. Perhaps the greatest advantage is that you can develop your own slides to suit your particular purposes. This allows you to tailor presentations specifically to your goals, rather than adapting less suitable material.

2. Written material and tables can be displayed on a large screen, making visibility for the audience very easy.
3. The order of presentation can be easily changed, and previous slides can be revisited with little difficulty.
4. Slides of just about anything can be made, and so information from books, magazine advertisements, newspaper headlines, and so on can all be used in a very creative manner.
5. Slide projector use is very common, and there are many pre-packaged slide programs available.
6. Slide projectors are usually light and therefore extremely portable. This is an obvious advantage when moving from classroom to classroom or traveling to a community presentation.

Disadvantages

1. Although slide projectors are usually reliable, maintenance and repair costs can be quite high.
2. Although preparing your own slides has great potential value, the cost of slide preparation can be very high, particularly if slides are being made from magazine advertisements or graphics, and so on.
3. Some people find using a slide projector fairly difficult, particularly in getting the image to be the right way up! Ideally, you should load your slides and test that you have them correctly positioned in the slide carousel before beginning the lesson/presentation. This will also allow you to appropriately focus the projector.
4. Slides do have the potential of being very boring, and with the lights necessarily being lowered, the potential exists for behavior

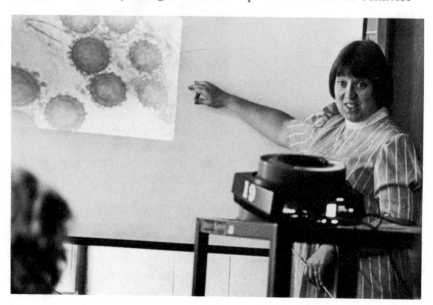

problems in a classroom setting or disinterest in a community setting.
5. The need for a screen is an added complication.

Filmstrips

Filmstrips were commonly used in the school setting until more sophisticated media like the slide projector became more readily available. They are now used sparingly and are most likely to be found in the elementary school setting.

Advantages

1. Usually come complete with teaching guides and often include accompanying audiotapes that provide a narration.
2. Filmstrip projectors are small, light, and very portable.
3. Filmstrip projectors are usually very simple to use.

Disadvantages

1. Many of the filmstrips available today are not very current.
2. Many of the filmstrip projectors in use are very old and do not provide projection of a very high quality.
3. As with the slide projector, the static nature of the filmstrip and surrounding darkness of the room can have a high potential for boredom, particularly if the filmstrip is old and not very inspiring.
4. Again, the need for a screen is an added complication.

CD-ROM and Photo-CD

CD-ROM stands for compact disc read-only memory, which are small compact discs with an amazing storage capacity. They can store over 600 megabytes of information. The size of storage allows access to a large amount of information at high speeds since the information is read by a laser. For example, two sets of standard encyclopedias could fit on one disc. The entire United States Library of Medicine might fit into a couple of suitcases! Because of the large memory, sight and sound can be used, allowing impressive presentations. Encyclopedias are now available that include numerous quick-search capabilities, and by a simple command selected people might talk with you or you might observe an animal in its natural habitat. It is possible that in the near future you may be able to carry on a conversation with a person from history (or a health educator), for example, whose image is projected using a hologram that is observable from 360 degrees. The technology will continue to advance; the challenge is how to make good use of it to meet your health education objectives.

Photo-CDs use the same technology as CD-ROMs to store photo images that generally are made from standard photographs taken with a 35-mm camera. These images are transferred to a photo-CD which can be shown on a photo-CD player attached to a monitor or on a CD player with the correct software and shown on a computer monitor. They can then be shown on a very large screen or projection system.

Advantages

1. Vast amount of memory.
2. Small and very portable.
3. Potentially entertaining because materials can include sight, sound, and motion.
4. Low cost for the amount of material.

Disadvantages

1. Special equipment required including a computer.
2. Few discs available with useful health information.
3. Not yet commonly available at health education sites.
4. Equipment is expensive.

Personal Computers

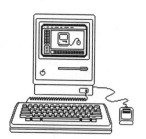

Personal computer technology has advanced at an incredible rate over the past 20 years, and so the computer has become a legitimate health education instructional tool in both the school and community settings. Computer applications are diverse and can include small-group or individualized usage. They span a full range of interest areas from health assessments to health education games and puzzles to statistical analysis. Many applications now include sight, sound, and motion and can be highly entertaining.

Gold and Duncan (1980) stress the usefulness of the personal computer as a motivational device:

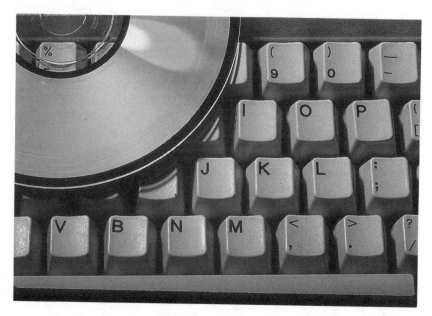

One of the most basic ways in which the computer may serve as a motivational device is through the use of self-assessment programs. Widely used among such approaches are the computerized dietary analysis models. These programs allow the student to input information concerning what they eat (on a single day or combination of days) and receive in return some output which identifies how well they have met some set of dietary standards. Such programs can provide an excellent introduction to the study on nutrition by developing and focusing student interest. We have made similar use of a life stress measurement program to introduce a unit on stress and life expectancy prediction.

Advantages

1. Computers offer an incredibly diverse set of possibilities for use in health education, ranging from complicated statistical analysis to elementary-school-level health education games.
2. Many modern personal computers are now much easier to use than previous models, allowing access to children and fearful adults.
3. Computers can be fun to use and are of particular value in the classroom as a motivational tool.
4. Computers can allow individual usage which permits working on personal programs where privacy might be a concern.
5. With the use of a modem or some connector to international computer systems such as Bitnet, the user can access an array of databases and expertise that is truly worldwide in scope.
6. Use of the computer opens up desktop publishing which allows low-cost target-specific high-quality publications.
7. Multiple technologies can be integrated using the computer. This is sometimes referred to as hypermedia. The computer can allow the integration of videotapes, text, music, and other images. This can be done for a specific target population at relatively low cost if the equipment and software are available.

Disadvantages

1. Although greatly reduced in price compared to a few years ago, computers are still relatively expensive, and therefore accessibility will be limited.
2. The format of one computer per person is often not possible, and having three or four individuals crowded around one monitor can become frustrating and disruptive.
3. Computer equipment can vary greatly from one machine or piece of software to the next. Some individuals may be comfortable on one type of machine and yet total novices on another type. Learn-

ing can be difficult with such differing levels of skill and experience.

4. Some health educators rely on the technology to accomplish health education instead of viewing it as an additional tool in their arsenal.

Quick Health Promotion Software Review[1]

1. Have you conducted an appropriate needs assessment and determined that this program meets your needs?

How Much Are Health Educators Using Computers?

A doctoral study by Zannis in 1992 looked at the use by graduate faculty of health education programs around the country. Five hundred fifty-six faculty members participated. More than half of respondents used word processing, mainframe statistical packages, on-line databases, and spreadsheets. Almost all used computers for word processing while a much smaller number used them for electronic mail, bulletin boards, health risk appraisals, or simulations. Uses include word processing (92%), spreadsheets (51%), databases (46%), on-line databases (58%), electronic mail (44%), bulletin boards (23%), simulations (16%), health risk appraisals (39%), dietary analyses (30%), drill and practice (23%), mainframe statistics (64%), and personal computer statistical packages (47%) (Zannis, 1992).

Availability of Software

A masters study by Lisa Gilbert in 1991 looked at the use of microcomputers in instruction in the 50 largest undergraduate health education programs in the country. Gilbert found a significant number of titles available mostly for Apple II series computers (188) and IBM compatibles (184) (Gilbert, 1991, p. 38). However, most were old and difficult to purchase. The most commonly used were health risk appraisals and nutrition analysis programs. Most instructors were interested in obtaining quality software. Barriers to use included lack of access to hardware and software, lack of knowledge regarding sources of programs, lack of computer access, absence of motivation; and inadequate training.

---

[1]G. G. Gilbert, in *Microcomputer Applications in Health Education,* by R. S. Gold (Dubuque, IA: Wm. C. Brown Publishers, 1991).

2. Is there evidence of a good health education basis for the software? (Author's credentials in health, appropriate advisory help, etc.)
3. Is the manual easy to follow, and have you been able to find answers for two or three questions without difficulty?
4. Have you personally tried the software, or do you have recommendations from more than two people whom you trust and who have similar needs?
5. Is the cost reasonable for what you will receive?
6. If the program costs $100 or more, is there a help line, and have you called it to see what kind of help is available?
7. Does the program use the capabilities of the computer, or would it be just as effective as a book or other medium?
8. Has the program been pilot-tested with an audience comparable to your intended audience, with good results?
9. Will the program run on your system, or does it warrant purchase of special hardware?
10. Are you reasonably certain that this is the best program you can find to accomplish this task? (It is very upsetting to find another, better, program at lower cost a few weeks after making an important purchase.)

If you cannot answer yes to all questions, it is time to reevaluate your selection. Do not make a purchase until you can answer yes to all questions.

Overhead Projectors

The overhead projector has been used for many years in both the school and community settings. As a means to display both text and graphic information, this instructional medium has proven to be both effective and enduring.

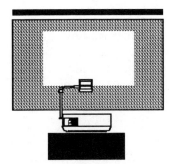

Advantages

1. Allows the instructor to display detailed information to relatively large groups.
2. Information being displayed can be changed or modified while audience is watching.
3. Overhead projectors are very easy to use.
4. Overhead transparencies are easy and inexpensive to prepare and can even be made on most photocopying machines.
5. The newer overhead projectors are quite compact and easy to transport and maintain.

Disadvantages

1. Along with an overhead projector, the instructor will need to use some type of screen or find a very white wall.

2. Use of the projector necessitates semidarkness. This has the potential for cutting off the speaker from the audience, and in the classroom setting this can cause disruption.
3. Although overhead transparencies are easy to prepare, the preparation is somewhat of an art. Often individuals will try to place too much information on a single overhead or use print that is too small and difficult to read.
4. Poor transparencies and too much factual data can lead to boredom. To many students or workshop participants, overhead projectors and boredom are synonymous!

SELECTING AND EVALUATING MEDIA

The selection of films, videotapes, and other media forms is crucially important, particularly in health education. All too often audiovisual materials are used for the wrong reasons. For example,

- the film that has always been used for a certain topic
- to fill a blank space on the schedule
- because a particular videotape is the only one available
- because a film is the only one that can be afforded
- because the topic is applicable, even though the level of the material is inappropriate

As obviously inappropriate as these reasons for using audiovisual materials may seem, they occur all too frequently. Historically, very little systematic thought has occurred in the selection and evaluation of media. Campeau (1974), in a review of research on the uses of audiovisual materials, bemoans the rather dubious criteria for selecting such programs:

> All indications are that decisions as to which audiovisual devices to purchase, install, and use have been based on administrative and organizational requirements and on considerations of costs, availability, and user preference, not on evidence of instructional effectiveness. (Campeau, 1974, p. 31)

There have been some early attempts to somehow objectively evaluate media, particularly in the area of drug education. The Audiovisual Group of the Addiction Research Foundation (ARF) provided a rating of films based on the following nine criteria:

1. the scientific accuracy of information presented
2. its merits as a teaching aid
3. whether or not it is contemporary
4. the clarity of message

5. whether or not it could influence attitudes
6. if it appeared believable
7. its technical merits
8. whether or not it maintained interest
9. whether or not it was applicable to individuals from different social strata (Fejer et al., 1972)

Although this early effort at least provided some basic guidelines for audiovisual material selection, the ambiguity of its components is obvious. It is not within the scope of this text to document further specific audiovisual research in health education, but a review of the literature clearly denotes a paucity of meaningful evaluation . . . a sad commentary, particularly in the light of how frequently such materials are used today.

To aid the health educator in choosing the most appropriate media materials, a helpful evaluation checklist has been designed (see Figure 5-1). This checklist is by no means exhaustive, and additional categories can be added where appropriate. However, the checklist does include some important basic principles to consider when selecting media materials.

It is important to note that this checklist concentrates on some basic principles and intentionally employs no specific rating techniques. For a more comprehensive and complicated media rating system, health educators should examine a scale called "An Analysis Checklist for Audiovisuals" developed by Martin and Stainbrook (1986).

Media Objectives

Will the materials used fulfill or facilitate achieving the objective(s) of the presentation? All too often materials are chosen because they are topic appropriate and yet they may do little to achieve objectives. For example, in AIDS education, films depicting factual information about the disease or those showing interviews of people with AIDS have traditionally been shown in school and community settings in an attempt to elicit attitude and sexual behavior change. Using cognitive information may well improve knowledge levels, but such an approach will do little to influence attitude or behavior. If attitude change is an objective, perhaps in this case in dealing with AIDS education, the objective might be to increase perceived susceptibility to HIV, then the film selected should be affective in nature and be far less didactic. If a simple increase in knowledge is the objective, then the factual film is appropriate. Clearly, an awareness of specific objectives is crucial to media selection. (One condition that has exacerbated this problem is that until relatively recently the vast majority of available media materials have been of the factual variety, thus perpetuating the axiom of, "if that's all there is, then we'll have to use it!" On many occasions

MEDIA EVALUATION CHECKLIST

Media objectives	_____
Level	_____
Language	_____
Content	_____
Culture/Ethnicity	_____
Time/Duration	_____
Cost	_____
Interest Level	_____
Production Quality	_____
Evaluation	_____
Availability	_____
Format	_____
Approval	_____
Others _____	
_____	

FIGURE 5-1

using nothing is more appropriate than using ineffective, inappropriate materials!)

Level

Is the level of the material suitable for the audience? It is important to consider the learning styles and levels of the audience when considering media materials. If the material is either too complex and difficult or too simplistic, the audience may become frustrated and disinterested. Again, the availability of level-appropriate materials might be limited, and the health educator must make a decision as to the material's potential utility. As stated earlier, inappropriate materials may well do more harm than good.

Language

Is the language used in the materials appropriate for the audience. This can be viewed on two levels. Is the language used offensive in any way and possibly inappropriate, particularly in school settings? Perhaps more important, is the language intelligible to the audience? For example, can you use a film in English in a predominantly Hispanic setting? There are no easy answers to these questions and solutions may be different in each case. For example, if the only film available on a certain topic is in English, showing such a film to an Asian or Hispanic group is not necessarily out of the question. The group's level of English may be quite sufficient to understand the meaning of the film. Health educators should consider both the language capabilities of the group and the language complexity of the media materials.

Content

Is the content of the materials accurate and up to date? Here is where the "we've always used this film!" doctrine can be dangerous. Many health issues change so quickly that as new information transposes the old, media materials can become outdated, and even worse, inaccurate in relatively short periods of time. The high cost of some materials makes updating media libraries a difficult task, and, again, the health educator may be faced with the decision of not using media materials rather than risking the dissemination of inaccurate information. It is perhaps useful to note that affective materials less concerned with cognitive information probably have a longer "shelf life" than their more factual counterparts.

Culture/Ethnicity

Are the media materials culturally sensitive? Are they appropriate for a specific audience? These questions are probably two of the most difficult to address in a satisfactory manner. In an ideal situation the health educator would be able to choose media materials that are topic specific and completely culturally appropriate. For example, when considering a drug education film, the health educator could choose from affective to factual films, with alternative versions for each different ethnic group—predominantly black, Hispanic, Asian, white, and so on. But would we then also have to include even more versions which would be appropriate for not only race, but socioeconomic status? It would certainly seem insensitive to assume that individuals within races are all the same! To that end, achieving this utopia would necessitate the development of literally hundreds of new media materials, each culturally specific and appropriate. Given the cost of media development, this situation will never exist, and the health educator is again left with deciding upon some type of compromise. The search for media materials that will satisfy the needs of every group is both futile and unreasonable. The health educator must make every effort to obtain materials that are as inclusive as possible and that will not patently offend groups or individuals. A decision that no useful or appropriate materials were available to be used in certain contexts would not be unusual.

Time/Duration

Just how long does it take to show specific materials? Is it reasonable to take up the entire 50-minute classroom period to show a film? In the community setting while facilitating a 90-minute workshop, what length of videotape would be reasonable to show? Is it reasonable to show a film in two parts because the film is too long to complete in one session? Again, each situation must be evaluated individually, with both the context of the presentation and the objectives of using specific media materials being of paramount importance in making a decision. What should be avoided is the selection of media materials because they happen to fit the presentation time frame. If some materials are deemed to be valuable but too lengthy, perhaps with careful preparation crucial pieces can be substituted for the whole. Many health education materials are of a sensitive nature and can often elicit powerful reactions. An important rule of thumb is to always allow enough time in the presentation for adequate process and discussion of media materials. This basic principle is becoming increasingly important as more emotive, affective materials are being produced with the specific intent of group process.

Cost

No matter how useful some educational materials may be, there will always be the question of cost. As with anything related to consumerism, you tend to get what you pay for. High-quality, well-produced, interesting, educationally sound media materials are usually expensive. As production costs continue to rise, the price of the finished media products also increases. As mentioned earlier, the average cost of a high-quality 20-minute videotape will range from $125 to $350. With ever-diminishing budgets in both the school and community settings, media selection must be made very carefully, with an eye to longevity and maximized usefulness of the materials. It is perhaps sad to note that with all the important factors incorporated in media selection in an effort to maximize the educational experience, the single greatest factor determining the final decision may well be the issue of cost.

Interest Level

How interesting are the materials? Will students in the classroom find the materials so dull that they mentally absent themselves from the experience, making the time and expense of using such materials futile? Will the community health smoking cessation group find the videotape "talking head" to be so technical and boring that participants begin to question continuing their involvement in the program? Perhaps the single most common criticism of health education materials has been their dull, lifeless, and uninspiring format. No matter how important and useful the health information may be, if individuals have "tuned out," then the whole experience has achieved nothing. When seeking out media materials, attempt to find something to which the audience can closely relate. For example, some of the best health education films for middle and high school levels have been the ABC network's "After School Specials." However, would this material be applicable to college students, or would they dismiss the information as being irrelevant? Is the most effective approach for changing the sexual behavior of college students to show a predominantly young, heterosexual, non-drug-using population a film depicting middle-aged drug abusers or homosexual men describing how they contracted AIDS? Palmer (1990) believes that such strategies ensure low interest levels and decreased potential for learning.

> When students do not see the connection between subject and self, the inducement to learn is very low. (Palmer, 1990, p. 14)

Health education materials have certainly improved over the past few years, but in selecting such products, health educators should never underestimate the importance of interest levels in making their final decision.

Production Quality

How good are the production levels of health education materials? Historically, health education materials, particularly films, have been of very poor quality. Over a decade ago, health education leaders were complaining about the appalling quality of educational materials. These materials were being produced to combat the much more sophisticated and glossy materials originating on Madison Avenue which promoted "unhealthy" products. The criticism of the health education productions was that they tended to be boring, preachy, and unimaginative and that by making such films, health educators were wasting the most powerful medium of all. Today's youth, in particular, has become accustomed to a high-tech, high-quality level of media, typically found in contemporary television. To present health education materials in a form any less sophisticated is to risk a total loss of credibility and usefulness. High-quality, interesting health education materials are now becoming more common, but, as mentioned earlier, they come at a significant cost. Health educators may well be faced with deciding between using materials of poor quality or using nothing at all . . . and it would not be unreasonable to choose the latter.

Evaluation

Have the materials under review ever been evaluated in any way? It would probably be safe to say that the vast majority of media materials have never been evaluated. Films and videotapes may have been reviewed by other health educators, but often these reviews are very subjective and are prey to the vagaries of personal opinion. Little or no quantitative evaluation exists which examines the effects of specific forms of media (Sawyer and Beck, 1991). Most evaluation that has occurred tends to center around the effects of specific programs or courses of study, giving scant attention to the individual components of media. With such little objective data available, the health educator should take great care to always preview new materials prior to use and, if necessary, seek out additional opinions from colleagues.

Availability

In selecting educational materials, the health educator needs to be concerned with the issue of availability. Do companies provide preview copies of materials? How long can you keep the materials? Is renting expensive products an option? If so, how much notice is needed for reservations? If you want to purchase materials, how long will it take to receive them? Although these questions appear to be fairly obvious concerns, the importance of planning ahead and gaining all possible relevant information cannot be overemphasized. If, for example, a film is a crucial part of a presentation, then the presenter should begin planning to obtain the film well in advance of the presentation. All types of complications are possible, and the simple process of determining the availability of materials can alleviate many of these potential problems.

Format

This is a particular concern in the area of film, videotape, and computer usage. As discussed earlier, film is used much less frequently than videotape. To that end, many productions are no longer available on film or have become prohibitively expensive. When considering videotape, the vast majority of tapes are one-half-inch VHS format, but three-quarter-inch VHS and Beta tapes are also available. Health educators need to be clear before ordering as to what type of format they can use. Ordering software for computer usage also presents some choices. Most software is still not yet compatible with other types, so if educators see software programs that they want to order, they must be careful that the program is available in the correct format.

Approval

Being able to use specific media materials in an educational setting may well be determined not by the individual health educator but by outside agencies. For example, in most public school settings any materials used in the classroom must be preapproved by a board or committee in the school system. This is particularly common when teaching "sensitive" topics such as human sexuality. A school health educator would obviously be well advised to ensure that materials he/she intends to use are "approved" or, if not, that approval is sought. Individual teachers may not always agree with a committee's opinions on which materials are acceptable, and yet ignoring this approval process invites professional sanctions. The community health educator is less likely to confront such formal approval procedures. Nevertheless, the educator should take every precaution to ensure that he/she selects materials that will be deemed appropriate by the community. Consultation with professional peers and community leaders would certainly reduce the possibility of embarrassment.

MEDIA DEVELOPMENT

One of the major problems of applying rigorous evaluation standards when previewing media materials is that, given the limitations of many of the products currently available, the health educator may be unable to find anything that suits his/her needs. Some individuals may be able to compromise and use the materials despite their obvious limitations. Others may decide that the price of compromise is too high and will choose not to use media materials. Finally, a very few individuals may decide, in the absence of useful materials, to develop their own! Historically, health education materials, particularly film and videotape, have not been developed by health educators. These materials have been invariably designed by media production companies, and health educators have used them because the subject matter has been health related . . . a sort of marriage of convenience. This has often resulted in high-quality production levels, but levels achieved at a cost to the effectiveness of the health education message. Conversely, many of the productions that have been designed by health educators have adhered more closely to principles of health education, but have incorporated such low production qualities that they are viewed as boring, amateurish, and ineffectual. To that end, the development of high-quality, credible health education materials, which can compete with glossy and sophisticated commercial productions, is of paramount importance. Health educators know better than anyone else the types of materials they need and feel would be effective to enhance programming efforts. Unfortunately, their lack of technical expertise has often caused health educators to feel too intimidated to embark on media development. Although the development of new, exciting, high-quality materials is not easy, the process is well within the grasp of many educators. Figure 5-2 provides an outline of some important points to consider when contemplating media development. Once

MEDIA DEVELOPMENT

Objectives   _____

Present Resources   _____

Format   _____

Expertise   _____

Cost   _____

Financing   _____

Marketing   _____

Production Quality   _____

Evaluation   _____

Others _____

_____

FIGURE 5-2

again, this list is not exhaustive but provides some useful fundamental questions that you the health educator should consider.

Objectives

What do you specifically want to accomplish? The development of specific objectives or learning outcomes is the first crucial step in material development. From which domains are the objectives derived: cognitive, affective, or psychomotor? Do the objectives include components from more than one domain? Before even deciding what type of media to produce, think through and commit to paper no more than three behavioral objectives. A common mistake is expecting to be able to accomplish multiple objectives from one production . . . an incredibly difficult task irrespective of the elaborate nature of the materials. You may well limit yourself to one major objective.

Present Resources

Does a vehicle already exist that will meet your desired objective(s)? Although this might sound like an obvious concern, before embarking on what is usually a very time-consuming and often expensive venture, you need to be absolutely certain that such materials have not already been developed. This is of particular concern if you intend to market your materials in an effort to recoup production costs.

Format

What will be the most effective format for the new materials? Slides, overhead transparencies, videotape? Unfortunately, the most effective format is not necessarily the most practical. For example, a film might be considered the most effective way to lessen the fears of adolescents before they experience their first pelvic examination. However, the production of a high-quality film can be quite involved and very expensive. The health educator might then decide that the development of a high-quality set of slides, accompanied by a well-written script, would be a more practical strategy. The sequence of brainstorming here is important. Begin by thinking through the most effective format, regardless of cost and impracticality, and do not compromise until you have explored every possibility to develop your first choice. Talk to others in your field or individuals who have expertise in media development. You may be surprised by what is possible!

Expertise

Do you have the knowledge and level of expertise necessary to develop your own materials? For most of us in health education the answer to this question will be a resounding "No!" You may be an expert in health education, but probably your skills and knowledge concerning the intricacies of media production are limited. The recognition of individuals who are skilled in production is an absolutely vital component in the successful development of quality materials. Such individuals can be found in many settings, from the very expensive professional film production company to university students who are studying film and television, graphics, art, journalism, or other related fields. Develop your ideas for media materials, shape them into a preliminary proposal, and then seek out some individuals who can react to your ideas. There are many individuals in the university setting who would be delighted to be involved in media development. Some will be looking for payment, students in particular might be interested in course credit, and other individuals might simply be interested in the experience. The key point here is to pursue your ideas with enthusiasm. You will not know what is possible unless you try!

Cost

How much will the development and production of your materials cost? The answer is nearly always "too much!" In most cases the cost of production will be the critical determining factor in deciding on the media format. Once again, as a health educator you might have little idea as to production costs, and the necessity of consulting the media professional becomes obvious. For example, if your initial objective is to produce a videotape, in order to obtain a fairly accurate estimate of cost, you would need to develop a rough script and outline. If money is no problem a production company could even do this for you, but a more likely scenario is to collaborate with someone who has an interest in this area. The film/video producer can then give you a fairly accurate estimate of cost given your project requirements.

The sequence of events is fairly similar for all media formats—think through your ideas, focus on specific objectives, develop an outline and proposal, and then research cost. Obviously, selecting a less involved format means that you can do more of the production yourself and be less concerned with cost. Once you feel that you have a fairly accurate estimate, the next step is to seek financing.

Financing

Can you access sufficient sources of funding to develop your materials? Now that you know what you would like to produce and how much this is going to cost, you need to work out if you can fund the materials. If you feel that your intended materials might fill a need shared by others, then with some persistent searching you may be able to find some financial help. Collaboration with several groups, organizations, or departments will certainly reduce individual burdens. Investigate the possibility of funding through grant writing. There are many federal, state, and private organizations that offer grants for health-related issues, and the development of educational materials is certainly a legitimate avenue. Again, consulting with individuals who are knowledgeable in obtaining grants would be very useful. Approach private companies that may manufacture products relevant to your topic. Although you would need to tread carefully in the area of sponsorship, the development of useful new educational materials can sometimes be facilitated by collaboration with the private sector. Media distributors that also produce their own materials may be receptive to a proposal, leading to their producing the educational materials. Often the key to confronting the cost of media development is a combination of creativity and sheer persistence. Before you decide that the cost of developing your materials is too prohibitive, make sure that you have solicited every source!

Marketing

Do you intend to develop your materials for personal use, or would you consider marketing your product at the local or national level? One important point to consider is that if you are developing materials because a void exists in what is currently available, there is a good chance that other health educators are experiencing the same problem and may be interested in your product. This whole issue is integrally linked to obtaining initial funding. If you can provide a very strong proposal which includes evidence of a widespread universal need for your materials, the chance of obtaining some type of funding is greatly enhanced. If individuals or groups are likely to recoup their initial investment and even perhaps make a profit, they are far more likely to help finance a project than if they perceived their support as a donation. Health educators could certainly distribute their own materials, but without any real expertise in this area, their success would be limited. Professional organizations could be helpful in this process, either in distributing the actual materials or providing mailing lists of fellow professionals (at a cost!). Examples of such organizations include the American College Health Association (ACHA); the American Alliance for Health, Physical Education, Recreation, and Dance (AAHPERD); the American School Health Association (ASHA); and the American Public Health Association (APHA). In addition to professional organizations, commercial media distribution companies are only too glad to distribute high-quality products, but at a large cost to the developer. For example, commercial distributors of videotapes will customarily take 70 to 75 percent of the selling price of each tape sold, leaving the producer with a much lower 25 to 30 percent of the share. However, although the rates might seem unreasonable, a good, aggressive distribution company can potentially sell many more videotapes than could the producer, thus compensating for offering a smaller share of the profits. As with sponsorship discussed in the previous section, association with commercial distribution companies should be thoroughly investigated, often with legal advice, before any commitment is made. Finally, publishing companies which previously had concentrated only on printed materials have begun to broaden their horizons. In the light of diminishing book sales, these companies are becoming more progressive and are demonstrating a firm interest in alternative or supplementary educational materials, in particular, videotapes, interactive videodiscs, and computer software programs.

Production Quality

What level of production quality do you anticipate developing? A good part of this question will have already been answered by considering the factors of cost and marketing previously mentioned. These factors are inextricably linked and probably should almost be considered simultaneously. Obviously, if national marketing is anticipated, then production qualities must be of the highest order. This, in turn, will ensure that production costs are fairly high. On the other hand, there is absolutely nothing wrong with setting your sights lower, keeping production costs to a minimum, and confining the use of the materials to yourself and local colleagues.

Evaluation

Although the vast majority of media materials have not been exposed to rigorous outcome evaluation, many of the products currently available have at least been developed through some type of professional and/or student validation. When developing media materials it is often useful to involve the intended target audience in the production. Small focus groups to test various components of the materials can provide invaluable feedback, as can input by fellow professionals. Changes and alterations can easily be made along the way, whereas attempting to change completed materials can be expensive, time consuming, and sometimes impossible.

EXERCISES

1. You are a high school health teacher and have just been told by a friend about a new videotape on HIV/AIDS. You are scheduled to teach a unit on AIDS in a few weeks and would potentially like to use the videotape. Carefully describe all the steps you would take to achieve this goal.

2. You have the opportunity to obtain what you consider to be an outstanding film on alcohol abuse and youth. You must choose between a 16-mm-film format or a videotape format. Cost is no problem! Make the decision about format and briefly explain the reasons for your choice.

3. You are a school or community health educator who has received a $500 grant to purchase media materials related to heart health. Make a detailed budget list of the materials you will purchase. (Do not just make up a fictitious list! Do some research and consult some audiovisual catalogs, film, videotape, and audiotape libraries, bookstores, health professionals etc.) You must reference all items, for example, the name of a videotape, its distributor, address, cost and so on. You may be surprised how little you get for $500!

4. You are a school or community health educator who is interested in media materials. Thinking of your particular area of expertise or interest within health education, what sort of media materials could be developed that would really enhance education in this area? Where do you consider the gaps in available media to be when related to your area of particular interest? Do some initial research to ensure that materials do not already exist and then write a descriptive outline of *your* proposed new media materials. Be creative! Do not worry about budget or lack of previous experience. What do you think would really enhance your teaching or presentations? What type of media would you develop? What would your goals and objectives be? What type of approach would you use? Give it a try!

5. Select two films or videotapes from the same subject area and, utilizing Figure 5-1 (or, if you prefer, a similar instrument), evaluate the films/videotapes. Include in your evaluation what you would consider the goals and objectives of each film/videotape and whether or not you would use either of them in your work.

SUMMARY

1. The use of media materials in health education has become extremely common. Unfortunately, much of the early materials were of poor production quality, reflected low levels of interest, and generally did little to enhance health education programming.
2. A recent trend in media materials is a move away from the fact-filled production to a more affective, process-oriented approach.
3. There is an obvious need for health educators to use high-quality, polished productions in order to counteract the same levels of

quality used by commercial agencies that often promote "unhealthy" lifestyles.

4. Health educators need to be aware of the advantages and disadvantages of the various forms of media discussed in this chapter.

5. Health educators would be well advised to develop a basic operating knowledge of the media equipment described in this chapter.

6. Selecting media materials should be based on more than cost, availability, and personal preference. Selection should be based on the goal of achieving behavioral objectives formulated before the review process begins.

7. Media selection is a multifaceted process and should be based on a combination of sound principles described in this chapter.

8. The decision to use no media material rather than something of dubious quality will usually be the right decision. Poor-quality, outdated, or boring materials will usually have a detrimental effect on the presentation.

9. Media materials should be viewed as vehicles to enhance learning, not products that will stand in isolation. Process of materials is an essential part of the educational process.

10. New media development should always be considered an option when existing materials are deemed to be insufficient. The production of media should be based on sound principles of development as discussed in this chapter.

REFERENCES

Campeau, P. L. 1974. Selective review of the results of research on the use of audiovisual media to teach adults. *Audio-Visual Communications Review* 22:5–40.

Fejer, D., P. Hawley, E. Kuchar, D. Lucitis, and C. Webster. 1972. *Assessing Audiovisual Aids for Drug Education: Preliminary Study*. Ontario: Addiction Research Foundation.

Gilbert, G. G. 1983. Concerns about the use of microcomputers in health education: An editorial. *Health Education*, vol. 6, no. 6.

Gilbert, L. K. 1991. A survey of computer assisted instruction in selected undergraduate health education programs. Unpublished Masters Thesis. University of Maryland.

Gold, R. S. 1992. *Microcomputer Applications in Health Education*. Dubuque, IA: W. C. Brown.

Gold, R. S., and D. Duncan. 1980. Computers and health education. *Journal of School Health* 50:503–505.

Martin, C., and G. L. Stainbrook. 1986. An analysis checklist for audiovisuals when used as educational resources. *Health Education* 17(4):31–33.

Palmer, P. 1990. Critical thinking. *Change* (January/February):14

Sawyer, R. G., and K. H. Beck. 1991. The effects of videotapes on the perceived susceptibility to HIV/AIDS among university freshmen. *Health Values* 15(2):31–40.

Zannis, M. 1992. Health educators' use of microcomputer technology in graduate programs. Unpublised Doctoral Dissertation. University of Maryland.

Chapter 6

Curriculum
Development

Taken from *A Framework for the Development of Competency-Based Curricula for Entry Level Health Educators,* National Task Force on the Preparation and Practice of Health Educators, Inc., 1985. Reprinted by permission.

Method Selection in Health Education

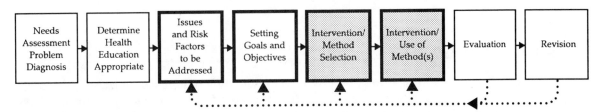

Heavy-bordered boxes indicate subjects addressed in this text; shaded boxes indicate subjects(s) of current chapter.

Case Study   *Shane is ill and asks a colleague at his agency to take over for the day. On his agenda is a presentation to students at Hillsboro Public High School regarding HIV infections. Mary, the colleague asked to fill in, is well versed in HIV and AIDS issues, having formerly worked for the State Public Health Epidemiology Division. Mary can find only brief notes so she grabs some slides on Kaposi's sarcoma and other diseases associated with AIDS and heads to the high school. She provides a very graphic presentation on homosexual avenues of transmission and, of course, a very visual show on the effects of the diseases. Shane is surprised some days later when he is reprimanded for the presentation and told he is no longer welcomed at the high school.*

Shane and Mary have made numerous errors in planning. Shane has failed to construct an appropriate lesson plan with clear objectives, methods, and content. Mary made several inappropriate decisions regarding content and format. Shane failed to make the school standards clear to his substitute for the day. The regular teacher at the high school should also assume some of the blame since she failed to share the school standards with the substitute. Generally, the regular teacher is held accountable for the presentation of any guest speaker and that means she must communicate the standards of the school and school district to any speaker.

This chapter will discuss the components of lesson/presentation plans and unit plans in curriculum development.

After studying the chapter the reader will be able to:

- develop an appropriate lesson/presentation plan for a given setting
- construct a unit of instruction for a given setting and population
- describe the strengths and weaknesses of using lesson/presentation plans and unit plans for instructional organization

Key Issues   Preparing a Lesson Plan   Strengths and Weaknesses of
            Preparing a Unit Plan   Lesson Plans and Unit Plans

LESSON/PRESENTATION PLANS

Preparing properly for a presentation requires organization. You must take into account all the issues used to select or write your objectives and carefully review what objectives are appropriate for your workshop, presentation, or class. Lesson/presentation plans should be written in a format that any health educator could use and present the

LESSON/PRESENTATION PLAN FORMAT

Name: _____

Grade Level/Comm. Setting: _____

Date: _____ Topic/Unit: _____

Lesson Title: _____

Age of Target Population: _____

Introduction (a statement of what you will be doing and why):

_____

_____

_____

Objectives (Consider cognitive, affective, and action or psychomotor):

_____

_____

_____

Initiation (Method/description of transition into the content):

_____

_____

_____

_____

(continued on page 182)

materials well. If properly constructed the presentation should capture the essence of what the author intended.

There are many suggested formats for lesson/presentation plans. Check with your agency or school to see if there is a required or recommended format. All suggested formats include the basic components of background information, introduction, objectives, initiation, developmental section (body or core), culmination, and evaluation. It is also recommended that you try to anticipate problems by preparing an alternative plan (often referred to as plan B).

Background   This initial section includes basic information that will assist in determining strategy selection: the setting for the presentation (community or school), the presentation topic, the approximate number of participants, and as much demographic information about the participants as can be obtained (age, ethnicity, socioeconomic status, etc.)

Developmental Section (this section may be several pages):

Content Outline	Method/Strategy	Estimated Time Needed	Materials Needed

I. XXXX
  A. XXX
  B. XXX
  C. XXXXX
	Name Game	20 minutes	None

II. XXXXXXXXXX
  A. XXXX
  B. XXXXX
  C. XX
    1. XXXXXXXXXXXXXXXXX
      XXXXXXXXXXXXXXXX
    2. XXXXXXXXXX
    3. XXXXXXXXXXXXXXXX
	Lecture/
	Discussion
		15 minutes	Overhead projector

III. XXXXXXXXXX
  A. XXXXX
  B. XXXX
    1. XXXXXXXXXXXXXX
    2. XXXXX
    3. XXXXXXXXXXXX
    4. XXXXXX
    5. XXX
	Guided Imagery—see attachment	30 minutes	Tape recorder
			Tape of sounds
			Script—see attachment

XX. XXXXX
  A. XXXXXXXXXX
  B. XXXXX
    1. XXXXXXXXX
    2. XXXXX
	Game Bingo—see attached for rules	20 minutes	Bingo cards
			Pencils
			Questions
			Prizes

Culmination (Summary of this lesson and what will happen next):

_____

_____

Anticipated problems and possible solutions:

_____

_____

Evaluation (How will you determine if you have been successful):

_____

_____

_____

Introduction This is where you capture the interest of the target audience. Give a welcome and provide reasons for covering the information. Include some local statistics, if appropriate, and logical statements regarding the issues addressed that will get the group enthusiastic about the topic.

Objectives These are the specific objectives you hope to achieve with this lesson/presentation. They must be stated in specific terms (see Chapter 2). You may have only one objective or you may have several. However, contact time must be taken into account since you cannot achieve some objectives in a short time frame. You must be realistic in what you set out to achieve. You might be able to achieve several cognitive objectives in a short time or one or two psychomotor objectives but generally not both. It is important to review educational principles and remember some important issues such as the need to repeat key points and the need to use multiple approaches to accommodate differences in learning styles.

Initiation This is the transition between the introduction and getting into the lesson. It is the link between the introduction and the first major activity or learning strategy. It should provide a bridge between the introduction and the developmental section.

Developmental Section This is the core of the lesson plan and includes all strategies and the appropriate information to carry them out. Sufficient information must be supplied in outline or text format so *any health educator given some preparation time could conduct the lesson or presentation.* Time estimates and needed materials should be included. This section is often multiple pages. All the information needed for any health educator to conduct the lesson should be included. Content materials or directions might be attached especially if photocopying materials is easier than rewriting the information.

Culmination This is the ending of the lesson/presentation and should include a summary of the key issues covered (reinforcement) and directions for the next meeting. If this is a one-time workshop or the final workshop of a series, it should include a thorough review and an opportunity for feedback and questions. This would also be the time to administer an evaluation questionnaire.

Anticipated Problems

We can never anticipate every problem that might occur when making a presentation, but we can often anticipate certain problems through good planning. It is important that we learn to do this as well as possible. Good planning will increase our self-confidence, allowing us to focus on the lesson. We should consider audiovisual failures and a group's unwillingness to participate, for example, as very common problems. We should develop the best alternate plan possible.

Some common problems often encountered in lesson/presentation preparation include the following:

1. Not enough material (people often speak faster when nervous or anticipated group discussion does not materialize).
2. Methods inappropriate for group.
3. Little variety in methods employed.
4. No evaluation or feedback system built in.

Evaluation

The evaluation is an integral part of any lesson plan. If our objectives are well stated and achievable, evaluation should be straightforward. Short time frames influence evaluation in that we must often use the majority of time for the intervention. However, it is always important that we conduct as much evaluation as possible. Contact time will have a major impact on evaluation time. If this is a one-time, one-hour presentation, a simple anonymous evaluation form or even a few oral questions may be all that is necessary. If this is the final presentation in a series, then a much more elaborate assessment tied to your objectives is in order. The type of evaluation techniques employed will be a function of the objectives, available time, type of group, and resources. Consider outcome and process evaluation techniques.

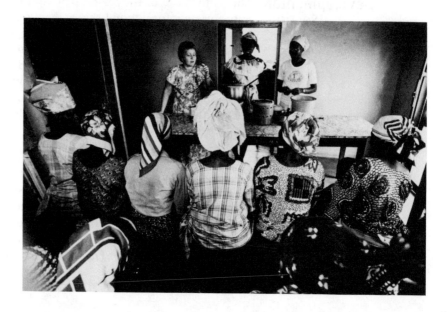

Case Study   *Michael, a young, enthusiastic health educator, had recently been hired by the local health department. His first assignment was to plan and implement a series of five one-hour workshops on general health issues for a senior citizens' community group. In college Michael had taken a methods and materials course, but he had put little effort into studying the construction of lesson/ presentation planning or unit development. He had argued that only school health majors needed that knowledge, and the last thing that Michael wanted was to be a teacher! Michael asked all the right initial questions related to group size, demographic background, location, time, available equipment and so on. He then jotted down a few notes for the first meeting, grabbed an available videotape, arranged for the use of a VCR, and was on his way to the first workshop. Michael's first presentation left a lot to be desired. He lectured far too long, boring many of the participants, and was unable to show the videotape on the VCR that the group had gone to great pains to borrow. When asked what the ensuing workshops would cover, Michael was unable to answer, mumbling something about covering whatever the group wanted. The following week only one of the group's members showed up and eventually the series of workshops was canceled. Not surprisingly, Michael was asked to meet with his supervisor!*

Michael's attitude that school and community health educators need to develop different sets of skills is all too common among many health education students. When planning for a presentation/ intervention/lesson, regardless of what we call the "entity," the planning and delivery is virtually the same for both school and community health educators. When Michael stands up in front of a community group for an hour-long presentation and then declares that he does not teach, one has to wonder what he has been doing!

Presenting/teaching successfully require the same skills; it is simply the setting that is different. Why do we assume that the community health educator who has to plan five one-hour workshops on drug prevention will not have to follow the same sound principles of planning and methods delivery as the teacher who has to prepare a five-lesson unit also on drug prevention? Yes, the rules and constraints in the school classroom might influence the teacher's planning, but the fundamental principles remain the same in the school and community settings. To be an effective health educator, particularly at the entry level, good presentation skills are essential. In order to optimize these presentation skills and deliver good presentations, sound and thoughtful planning must occur at both the individual lesson/presentation level and at the series or unit level. Anyone who has sat through a stunningly boring presentation in the classroom or in the community should consider how much time the presenter spent on thoughtful planning and method selection . . . probably very little! This important phase of health educator preparation involves us all, regardless of where we work.

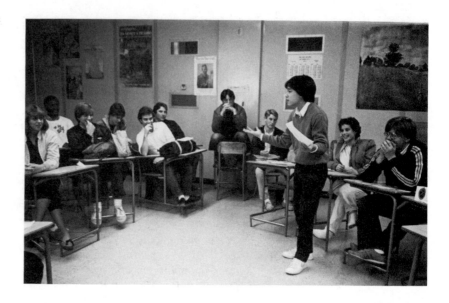

UNIT PLANS

There are many ways to organize for instruction. Whenever you have more than a few hours of contact time with a target population group, you should consider organizing for instruction in a unified manner. These systems are called curriculum plans, modules, strands, units, or any number of other titles. We will use the term unit plan to describe an orderly self-contained collection of activities educationally designed to meet a set of objectives. All such systems seek to organize materials so that they are more than the sum of their parts and have a high likelihood of achieving the stated objectives. All such systems are meant to be more than a collection of lesson plans. They are coordinated activities that build on one another and together may be able to influence even challenging issues such as attitudes or behaviors. Depending on the time and other resources available, the unit plan can be a powerful tool if implemented as constructed. The unit plan is appropriate where there is a significant amount of contact time—usually over five hours and a fairly consistent participating group. Otherwise a lesson/presentation plan might be more appropriate since you may only be working with a group of people for an hour at a time.

You may be planning a major three-day community workshop or 20 hours of classroom contact time in a school setting. The common thread is that you have a significant amount of contact time for your intervention and therefore can build one component onto another.

Summary Components of a Unit Plan

1. Overview
2. Statement of Purpose

3. Long-range goals or general objectives or key concepts
4. Behavioral objectives of the unit
5. Outline of the content to be presented
6. Methods/strategies/learning opportunities
7. List of materials
8. Evaluation activities
9. List of available resources and materials
10. Block plan

*The greatest medications are
those swallowed by the
mind.
—Mohan Singh*

UNIT CONSTRUCTION GUIDELINES FOR HEALTH EDUCATION COMPONENTS

1. Overview
Begin with a paragraph or two that describes the setting. Include the ages of participants or grade level, number of meetings and duration, economic situation, and cultural setting. Name the actual location(s) where the health education program will be conducted. Pertinent demographics should be included.

2. Statement of Purpose
This is a description of why this content is part of the curriculum for this target population. Footnote any statistics or generalizations used to support the need for this unit. Write this section as if you were trying to convince an outsider of the need for this unit. Use statistics whenever possible to support the need for this specific target population. Supporting statistics should always be included if available.

3. Long-Range Goals or General Objectives or Key Concepts
These are the very broad outcome intentions for the unit. These are optimal behaviors you hope to achieve and need not be easily measurable. See Chapter 2.

4. Behavioral Objectives of the Unit
The objectives are stated in behavioral terms (cognitive, affective, and psychomotor) according to recognized authority or as covered by the instructor. Often your agency, hospital, or school will have a specific format. These are the specific objectives to be achieved and should include an indication of how they will be measured. See Chapter 2.

5. Outline of the Content to Be Presented
This section should include all items to be covered in outline format. This detailed outline can be supplemented by an appendix with more detail or copies of the overheads to be used. This is all the content to be covered and should be presented in a logical order but not necessarily in the order of presentation to be followed in the unit plan.

6. Methods/Strategies/Learning Opportunities

These involve a series of suggestions (teaching strategies) capable of implementing the objectives. Each method should be selected with your objectives in mind. *List after each activity which objective(s) it will implement/achieve.* Include enough information so that the reader could carry out the strategy. All directions and rules should be included. You may refer to a handout included in an appendix.

7. List of Materials

Include a list of materials needed by the *facilitator* (i.e., overhead projector) and those needed by each *participant* (i.e., paper).

8. Evaluation Activities

These are based on your stated objectives (your *complete* evaluation activities for the unit). For example, you might include five quizzes, 10 multiple-choice questions each, and one final, an essay variety worth 40 percent and so on. Include activities to measure *knowledge, attitudes,* and *behavior.* There should be a variety of assessment techniques appropriate for the target population. Be certain to include *teacher/ facilitator evaluation* activities.

9. List of Available Resources and Materials

The list should include only those materials known to be of good quality and availability, that is, books, articles, and/or films. Include complete titles, costs, and where available.

Let the health educator be as a coconut floating upon tropic seas and letting down roots on a foreign strand, that others may harvest their own nuts.
—Mohan Singh

10. Block Plan

This is a breakdown of your suggested sequence including the amount of time to be spent on each activity. Since learning opportunities are explained in detail in component 6, they need only be listed here. Give consideration to the proper sequence for the material including the appropriate amount of time.

UNIT PLAN SAMPLES

Unit plans can be and often are, hundreds of pages. The following samples are only representative of the type of information to be included and are incomplete for even a short unit plan. It is suggested that the reader review complete unit plans developed by professionals as well.

1. Sample Overview (Well-Baby Program)

This unit plan is targeting pregnant women who have applied for the "HELP NOW" program of King Sam County of Anystate. The program will work with the first 50 women who sign up. Based on county statistics, it is estimated that the group will range in age from 13 to 40, with the majority of participants being under 20 years of age. Most will be English speaking, and approximately two-thirds can read at above a fifth grade level. Approximately half will be African American and half are estimated to be white. Group size will be approximately 25, and participants will self-select their group according to their schedule. Only a very small number of participants are working, and the site will be in the community where transportation is not expected to be a problem. Day care will be an issue since 50 percent of the participants have one or more children and less than 25 percent have a spouse or partner living with them.

This section will generally be less than one page and lays out the estimated demographics of the group.

2. Sample Statement of Purpose (Drug Prevention Program)

This unit was developed because of an identified need in the community and because we have identified a program that has proven to be successful in other communities similar to ours. Anytown has shown rather dramatic increases in drug use by school age children. According to the Anytown Department of Health annual survey,[1] the number of students using marijuana was as follows:

	1985	1990	1991
4th Grade	2%	6%	9%
6th Grade	3%	8%	9%
8th Grade	11%	13%	16%
11th Grade	14%	14%	18%
12th Grade	13%	16%	27%

Cocaine use has shown a similar trend as follows:

	1985	1990	1991
4th Grade	1%	2%	3%
6th Grade	1%	3%	3%
8th Grade	2%	5%	8%
11th Grade	1%	7%	10%
12th Grade	2%	8%	14%

Alcohol use has remained a serious problem:

	1985	1990	1991
4th Grade	11%	12%	13%
6th Grade	11%	13%	13%
8th Grade	22%	25%	38%
11th Grade	21%	27%	40%
12th Grade	32%	48%	64%

[1]These are phony studies for the purpose of illustration.

State studies[2] have indicated a strong relationship between the use of these drugs and the increase in violence, unwanted pregnancies, AIDS, and low school performance. Studies indicate that 90 percent of cases of unprotected intercourse occurred during the use of drugs, including alcohol, by both males and females. Last year three seniors scheduled to graduate died in an alcohol-related auto accident three weeks before commencement. This unit is needed in our schools and should be implemented as part of our comprehensive school health education program.

Local statistics should be used when appropriate. The U.S. Health Goals for the Year 2000 are often helpful as are local newspaper reports.

3. Sample Goals (Child Abuse Prevention)

1. Participants will acquire a set of workable and practical stress management techniques.
2. Participants will develop good parenting skills.
3. Participants will develop efficacy in the presented parenting skills.

Three or four general goals are usually adequate to express the general nature of a program unless it is a very long unit. Many units are 10 hours or less in total contact time. Schools often have longer units which might average 20 contact hours each.

4. Sample Objectives (Stress Management)

Cognitive

1. Participants will be able to identify personal sources of stress according to the guidelines presented in the program.
2. Participants will be able to define stress, eustress, and stress management according to the handouts provided.

Affective

1. Participants will show a willingness to learn more about stress management by voluntarily signing up for future programs.
2. Participants will show increases in self-efficacy in self-ratings of utilization of presented stress management techniques.

Psychomotor

1. Participants will be able to demonstrate Jacobson progressive relaxation as shown in class.
2. Participants will be able to demonstrate the Jones breathing techniques as presented in class meeting 4.

The number of objectives will depend largely on the contact time and resources available. The number is really not important. The important consideration is that they be appropriate, achievable, and clearly stated. Most units of 20 hours or more have 15 or 20 objectives.

---

[2]All statistics should be referenced, be as local as possible, and be as recent as available.

5. Sample Outline (Nutrition)

I. Dietary Guidelines for Americans

  A. Recommendations to help people maintain good health and/or improve it.

  B. A good diet is based on variety and moderation.

  C. Moderation means not eating large amounts of foods high in fat (saturated fatty acids and cholesterol).

  D. A risk factor is a condition that may increase the chance that something (usually negative) might be experienced by someone.

  E. For some people, certain types of diets are risk factors for chronic health conditions, such as heart disease, cancer, and high blood pressure.

  F. The Seven Dietary Guidelines

    (1) Eat a variety of foods.

      (a) No one food can supply all the essential nutrients needed for maintaining good health.

      (b) Should include foods from a variety of food groups.

      (c) Creates a balanced diet.

    (2) Maintain desirable weight.

      (a) Desirable weight will vary according to many factors such as age, health, gender, and so on.

      (b) Avoid sudden, potentially dangerous, aggressive dieting.

      (c) Calorie intake and expenditure must be balanced to maintain weight.

    (3) Avoid too much fat, saturated fat and cholesterol.

      (a) A small amount of fat is needed in your diet.

      (b) Risk of heart attack is increased by diets high in fat.

      (c) How foods are prepared will influence the fat content of food.

    (4) Eat foods with adequate starch and fiber.

      (a) starch is a complex carbohydrate.

      (b) Carbohydrate-rich foods provide many essential nutrients and fiber.

      (c) Dietary fiber is plant material which humans cannot digest.

      (d) Grain products and starchy vegetables are good sources of starch.

      (e) Whole grain products, fruits, vegetables, nuts, and dry beans contain fiber.

      (f) How the food is prepared will affect the fiber content.

    (5) Avoid too much sugar.

      (a) Sugars are carbohydrates; some present in food naturally, some added.

(b) Added sugars provide calories/energy, but almost no nutrients.

(c) High-sugar diets can increase the risk of developing tooth decay.

(d) High-sugar foods often take the place of more nutritious foods in your diet.

(e) Through careful food selection and preparation, you can control sugar levels.

(6) Avoid too much sodium.

(a) Sodium is an essential nutrient.

(b) Helps the body maintain normal blood volume and pressure, helps muscle function.

(c) High sodium increases risk of hypertension, heart attacks, strokes, and so on.

(d) Sodium is added to many foods as a flavor enhancer.

(e) Food labels can help to identify high-sodium foods.

(f) Through careful food selection and preparation, you can control sodium levels.

(7) For teens: avoid alcoholic beverages.
For adults: if you drink alcohol, do so in moderation.

(a) People who drink alcohol and drive increase their risk for unintended injuries.

(b) Heavy alcohol use can contribute to liver disease and some forms of cancer.

(c) Alcohol can add calories to your diet, but almost no nutrients.

(d) There are many nonalcoholic beverage alternatives.

II. Reading a Nutrition Label

A. Found on food package/container. . . .

This section should include all items to be covered in outline format. This detailed outline can be supplemented by an appendix with more detail or copies of the overheads to be used. This is all the content to be covered and should be presented in a logical order but not necessarily in the order of presentation to be followed in the unit plan. If the contact time is 20 hours, this section may be 30 or 40 pages.

6. Sample Methods (Nutrition Unit)

1. Lecture 1
Will cover outline parts I and II.
Overheads will be used for reinforcement.

Objectives addressed
Cognitive objectives 1, 2, 7, and 8

2. Lecture 2
Guest speaker who is a registered dietitian will cover outline parts III and V, including food labeling.

Objectives addressed
Cognitive objectives 2, 3, and 4
Affective objectives 1

3. Nutrition relay
See appendix D for rules and questions.

Objectives addressed
Cognitive 1, 2, 3, 4, 6, 8, 9, 10, 11, and 12

4. Demonstration and cooking
See appendix E for recipes and list of ingredients.

Facilitator will demonstrate proper cooking of vegetables followed by an opportunity for all to enjoy a meal that they have prepared. Prior notification required and special material needed.

It is most important that activities be selected with achieving objectives in mind. This is the most crucial component of a unit, assuming the objectives are appropriate and well stated. The number of methods is dictated by the contact time and the objectives to be achieved. A variety of learning styles should be addressed as well as the characteristics of the target population.

7. Sample Materials (Any Unit)

Facilitator

1. Extra pencils and paper
2. Blackboard
3. VCR and monitor (VHS format)
4. Chalk

Participant

1. Paper and pencil

8. Sample Evaluation (HIV/AIDS Workshop)

Outcome Evaluation

1. Pretest and posttest on content of workshop.
2. Post-workshop survey of behaviors.
3. Postconference short survey of health behaviors in six months.

Process Evaluation

1. Post-workshop evaluation of facilitator performance and rating of workshop components.

The quantity and to some extent the quality of evaluation strategies will depend on the contact time for the workshop and for evaluation. Evaluation strategies should be tied to the objectives.

CLOSE TO HOME   JOHN McPHERSON

**Every high school student's worst enemy:
the essay question.**

CLOSE TO HOME copyright 1993 John McPherson/Dist. of UNIVERSAL PRESS SYNDICATE. Reprinted with permission. All rights reserved.

9. Sample Resources (First Aid)

1. Doe, John. 1995. *First Aid.* J&J Publishers, Anytown. $29.95
2. American First Aid Society Film Series (five short videotapes)
   National Headquarters, Anytown U.S.A.
   Cost $1,250 set or $15 rental each
3. First Aid Chart
   American First Aid Society Film Series
   National Headquarters, Anytown U.S.A.
   800-222-2222
   $49.95

List only those materials you know to be very useful and important to the success of the unit.

10. Sample Block Plan (Any Topic)

Day 1	Day 2	Day 3	Day 4	Day 5
Introduction Statement of Purpose Lecture 20 minutes	Introduction Review of last meeting What we will do today 10 minutes	Introduction Review of last meeting What we will do today 10 minutes	Introduction Review of last meeting What we will do today 10 minutes	Introduction Review of last meeting What we will do today 10 minutes
Get-acquainted activity Get it off my back 20 minutes	Skit Communications 10 minutes	Lecture Discussion on communication strategies 25 minutes	Role play Communications Stop and discuss as needed 45 minutes	Videotape on communication strategies 20 minutes
Lecture Discussion on the need for communications 25 minutes	Debriefing Overview of communication strategies 45 minutes	Problem-solving activity 15 minutes	Debrief review methodology 10 minutes	Debriefing of videotape 10 minutes
		Debriefing 10 minutes		Role play Communications 20 minutes
Summary review next meeting 10 minutes	Summary review next meeting 10 minutes	Summary review next meeting Self-assessment 15 minutes	Summary review next meeting 10 minutes	Summary review next meeting Evaluation 15 minutes

The health educator who plays roulette must first invent the wheel.
—Mohan Singh

The block plan is how the total intervention fits together. Use of educational principles should be evident including pacing, variety, and reinforcement.

EXERCISES

**Exercise One–
You Be the Judge!** Take a look at the following lesson/presentation plans and critique them. Consider the appropriateness and feasibility of the objectives, the variety of the teaching methods, and the general "completeness" of the lesson/presentation plan. (Please note that in the interests of time and space the "content" section of the plans are highly abbreviated. A greater depth of information would ordinarily be required.)

Lesson/Presentation Plan 1

Group: 25 seventh-grade students, mixed ability

Unit: Addictive behaviors (four sessions)

Topic: Cigarette smoking (first session)

Time: 50 minutes

Objectives

1. Students will understand that smoking is an unhealthy habit.
2. Students will understand the harmful effects of smoking.
3. Students will decide to stop or not begin cigarette smoking.

Initiation of Lesson/Presentation

Students will write down all the reasons why people their age begin smoking cigarettes.

Development of Lesson/Presentation

Content	Method	Time	Materials
1. Reasons why people begin smoking	Q & A	10 minutes	None
2. Physical effects of smoking	Lecture	20 minutes	Overhead
3. Smoking and addiction	Lecture	15 minutes	Slides

Conclusion

Verify that students have understood the basic concepts of the lesson by asking them questions about the material covered in class. Students will respond orally.

Lesson/Presentation Plan 2

Group: 35 older adults (aged 60 to 65) in community group setting

Topic: Healthy nutrition (one session only)

Time: 1 hour

Objectives

1. Participants will be able list the four major food groups.
2. Participants will be able to describe the contents of a well-balanced meal.
3. Participants will appreciate the relationship between nutrition and health and make a commitment to improve their diets.

Initiation of Lesson/Presentation

Facilitator will uncover four dishes at the front of the room to reveal four meals. Each dish will be held up and described, and participants will be asked to rank-order each dish according to its nutritional value.

Development of lesson/presentation

Content	Method	Time	Materials
1. Describe the four major food groups	Lecture	15 minutes	None
2. Discuss suggested daily caloric intake	Q & A	15 minutes	Pamphlets
3. Suggested healthy food preparation	Videotape	25 minutes	TV and VCR
4. Question time	Respond to questions	5 minutes	None

Conclusion

Distribute pamphlets related to nutrition and healthy food preparation.

Critique–Lesson Plan 1

Objectives

The first problem with this lesson plan is that the objectives are very poorly stated. The first two objectives are more like goals in that they are written in a very general and nonmeasurable sense. The verb *understand* is not very appropriate for use in objective writing unless it is followed by another verb that reflects the degree or specificity of "understanding," such as *list* or *describe*. The problem with the third objective, "Students will decide to stop or not begin cigarette smoking." is that it is completely unreasonable. Again, as a goal for a lesson, this type of statement would not be out of place. However, to suggest that a 50-minute lesson could have such a dramatic impact on health behavior is both unrealistic and potentially harmful. By including possibly profound behavior change in the objectives, the health educator and the program are immediately set up for failure. When individuals begin smoking or fail to stop smoking, the behavioral objectives have not been met, and critics of the program might justifiably question the validity of continued support for such an ineffectual program.

Development

The lesson has a promising beginning by quickly involving the students in the learning process. They write down reasons why people their age begin smoking cigarettes, and then through question and answer the responses are verbalized. Unfortunately for the teacher and the students, that is the end of student involvement! For the majority of the lesson (35 minutes) the teacher intends to lecture to this class of seventh graders . . . good luck! In addition, the use of audiovisual equipment such as the overhead and slide projectors, which require semidarkness and are not traditionally known for scintillating lessons, could exacerbate the problems. When developing a lesson/presentation plan, the instructor needs to pay particular attention to the target population. In this case, seventh-grade students require teaching methods far more diverse than simply lecture. Break up a 35-minute block by using methods that are more interactive and interesting and yet still permit the dissemination of important information (see Chapter 4).

Conclusion

The teacher has allowed for some type of summary or wrap-up. In this case, verbal responses to questions might allow the teacher to get a sense of how effective the lesson has been. This type of method is often used and yet could be criticized as being somewhat haphazard. The teacher could allow a little more time for this section and finish with a very brief pencil and paper test. Alternatively, teams could be organized and some type of game format utilized to review the information (see Chapter 4).

Critique of Lesson Plan 2

Objectives

The first two objectives are quite good in that they are measurable, fairly precise, and seemingly achievable. They could be improved if a "qualifier" of standard was added . . . "list four major food groups *according* to . . ." or "describe the contents of a well-balanced meal *according to* . . ." Now the parameters and criteria of the objectives are specifically stated. There are a few problems with objective 3. First, the verb *appreciate* is too vague and would need to be followed by an additional verb that could quantify the objective. For example,

> Participants will appreciate the relationship between nutrition and health by listing five positive effects that a sound diet can have on health, according to the workshop.

Also, the third objective is actually two objectives within one. This is not an uncommon problem with individuals who are inexperienced in objectives design, but must be corrected to prevent confusion. We have already discussed the difficulty with using ambivalent terms like *appreciate,* but now the facilitator has added another objective related to committing to an improvement in diet. Such a commitment is not a bad objective if a "qualifier" is added:

> Participants will make a commitment to improve their diets *by voluntarily joining a relevant support group.*

However, this objective cannot simply be tacked on to the end of another; it must be given its own space. It is quite possible that participants will be able to list five positive effects of a good diet and yet will refuse to join a support group. In this case, has the instructor succeeded or failed to achieve the objective? Keep objectives simple and beware of linking two objectives together by use of the word *and.*

Initiation of Lesson/Presentation Plan

The intended initiation is an excellent attention getter and is a practical and effective way for the facilitator to both gain the audience's attention and lead into the subject matter of the workshop. Unfortunately, the presentation plan shows no evidence of any follow-up of this introduction in the development section. Warm-up exercises in the classroom and introductions in the community presentation are going to be most effective when they are innovative and capture the attention of the participants. However, the introductory exercises should be more than merely attention grabbers. There needs to be some form of follow-up in the development section of the lesson/presentation, so that the relevance and connection of the introduction become obvious. In this specific instance, the facilitator planned an extremely innovative introduction by bringing actual meals to the workshop to enable a practical comparison. After being rank-ordered, the meals could have been incorporated into the discussion of the major food groups and the preparation of nutritious meals. This inclusion would add a real-life feel to the workshop, and the presentation would tie together more effectively.

Development

The greatest concern when looking at this presentation plan is the "passivity" of the learning process. The participants are simply not actively involved in the workshop and concerns about boredom and distraction must be considered. If the facilitator is an outstanding speaker who can hold the attention of audiences, then these concerns might be minimized. The question-and-answer period is the only part of the plan that calls for group participation, and even this method affords only a mediocre level of participation.

The facilitator intends to show a 25-minute videotape. Unlike the school setting where the discipline issue could be problematic, with this population fatigue might be a concern. Will the videotape be riveting enough to even keep the audience awake, especially after several minutes of lecturing preceding the videotape? Health education films are often dull and boring and should only be used if they impart important information, are relevant to the audience, and are at least minimally interesting. A more fundamental question might be, is a 25-minute videotape too long to use in a one-hour workshop? Many experienced presenters might feel that unless the videotape is of incredible importance, it is in fact too long to be used in such a brief workshop. A more effective approach might be to view only parts of the videotape, so that at least some of the value of the tape could be utilized.

Allowing five minutes to answer questions is almost certainly not enough, particularly in the light of so much information being disseminated without any substantial discussion. The videotape would undoubtedly raise issues and concerns and allowing only five minutes for responding to questions is simply poor planning.

Conclusion

There is none! The facilitator has allowed no time to bring the workshop to an effective conclusion or perform any type of evaluation. In an attempt to perhaps reinforce the material covered in the workshop, the facilitator plans to distribute pamphlets. Distributing pamphlets is common practice and can be an effective means to achieve several goals. This process, however, should not replace the summary or conclusion of a presentation and obviously plays no part in evaluation. In addition to some type of evaluation (however informal) dealing with what the audience has learned and how the facilitator has performed, the facilitator should also be concerned about the effectiveness of the videotape and whether or not using nearly half the workshop time showing the videotape is worthwhile. Obtaining participant feedback on the videotape is one way to achieve this end.

This particular presentation plan has some obvious problems, and the intended workshop has the potential to be extremely boring and ineffective. Hopefully, these two brief examples of less than perfect lesson/presentation plans provide a clear sense of how crucial thoughtful planning is to the success of any presentation. Think about the type of class or workshop you would like to be involved in as a participant and, conversely, remember some of the characteristics of the most boring and ineffective classes or presentations you have sat through. Do not perpetuate poor presentation methods! Thorough planning and method consideration can minimize your chances of boring someone else to death!

Exercise 2: Now You Try!   Using your new-found knowledge of lesson/presentation planning, consider the following scenarios and develop an appropriate lesson/presentation plan for each. Remember to include sound, achievable objectives and a variety of methods.

1. You are teaching the first of a four-session unit on cigarette smoking to a class of 25 seventh graders of mixed ability. The class period is 50 minutes long.
2. You are conducting a single, once-only workshop on hypertension for a group of 20 older adults (age 50 to 65). The group is racially

diverse, includes both men and women, and the workshop lasts for one hour and fifteen minutes.

3. You are teaching the final session of a three-session unit on sexuality and communication/date rape to a group of 20 tenth-grade high school students. The class period is 50 minutes long.

4. You are completing a two-session workshop on bicycle and traffic safety for a group of 18 ten-year-old children from a local youth group. Each session is one hour long, and all the children have brought their own bicycles with them.

REFERENCES

Ames, E. E., L. A. Trucano, J. C. Wan, M. H. Harris. 1992. *Designing School Health Curricula; Planning for Good Health.* Dubuque, IA: W. C. Brown.

Arends, R. I. 1991. *Learning to Teach.* New York: McGraw-Hill.

Bates, I. J., and A. E. Wider. 1984. *Introduction to Health Education.* Palo Alto, CA: Mayfield.

Bedworth, A. E., and D. A. Bedworth. 1992. *The Profession and Practice of Health Education.* Dubuque, IA: W. C. Brown.

Carroll, L. 1946. *Alice in Wonderland and Through the Looking Glass.* New York: Grosset and Dunlap.

Galli, N. 1978. *Foundations and Principles of Health Education.* New York: Wiley.

Goodlad, J. I. 1984. *A Place Called School: Prospects for the Future.* New York: McGraw-Hill.

Greenberg, J. S. 1988. *Health Education: Learner-Centered Instructional Strategies.* Dubuque, IA: W. C. Brown.

Greene, W. H., and B. G. Simons-Morton. 1984. *Introduction to Health Education.* New York: Macmillan.

Hellison, D. 1978. *Beyond Balls and Bats: Alienated (and Other) Youth in the Gym.* Washington, DC: AAHPER Publications.

Hoff, R. 1988. *I Can See You Naked.* New York: Andrews and McMeel.

Joyce, B., and M. Weil. 1986. *Models of Teaching.* Englewood Cliffs, NJ: Prentice-Hall.

Lazes, P. M., L. H. Kaplan, and K. A. Gordon. 1987. *The Handbook of Health Education.* Rockville, MD: Aspen.

Mayshark, C., and R. Foster. 1966. *Methods in Health Education.* St. Louis: C. V. Mosby.

Rubinson, L., and W. F. Alles. 1984. *Health Education: Foundations for the Future.* Prospect Heights, IL: Waveland.

Scott, G. D., and M. W. Carlo. 1979. *On Becoming a Health Educator.* Dubuque, IA: W. C. Brown.

U.S. Department of Health and Human Services. 1980. *Promoting Health Preventing Disease Objectives for the Nation.* Washington, DC: U. S. Public Health Service.

U.S. Department of Health, Education, and Welfare. 1979. *Healthy People: The Surgeon General's Report on Health Promotion and Disease.* Publication 79-55071, Washington, DC: U. S. Public Health Service.

Willgoose, C. E. 1972. *Health Teaching in Secondary Schools.* Philadelphia: W. B. Saunders.

Chapter 7

Special Challenges

Taken from *A Framework for the Development of Competency-Based Curricula for Entry Level Health Educators,* National Task Force on the Preparation and Practice of Health Educators, Inc., 1985. Reprinted by permission.

Method Selection in Health Education

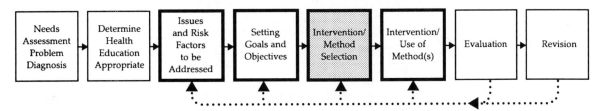

Heavy-bordered boxes indicate subjects addressed in this text; shaded boxes indicate subject(s) of current chapter.

Case Study   *Susan is a community health educator who has recently been planning and implementing presentations related to increasing the number of women receiving pelvic examinations. She has been asked to present a program to a women's group on the east side of the city. Having performed several of these presentations before, Susan gives little thought to preparation and arrives with her materials at the appointed time and place. Susan quickly realizes that this will not be a "standard" presentation as the audience is predominantly Asian, with almost no grasp of English. The group leader graciously offers to translate, and the presentation moves laboriously along despite the translator's obvious discomfort at having to translate graphic information related to sexuality. The presentation finally concludes with both audience and presenter feeling uncomfortable and dissatisfied.*

Susan had been presenting her important information to very homogeneous groups and had not stopped to consider the culture of this latest group. Had she discovered the ethnic background of the participants beforehand, Susan could have identified levels of language, knowledge, and specific perceived needs of this population. Statistically, most health educators today are both white and middle class. As opportunities for ethnic minorities and special populations increase, the discipline will become more multicultural and sensitivity to the specific needs of others will increase. However, health educators currently practicing in the United States need to make great efforts to gain information about individuals and/or groups with whom they will be working. Sometimes this information will make little difference to how a presentation is made, and yet in other situations radical change is necessary. The key to successful teaching and presentations in any discipline is preparation, and this chapter is intended to give the reader a glimpse into the lives of different populations. Wherever possible, suggestions are made for facilitating this process, but as the reader will discover, for many of these minority populations little research has been performed to even identify specific health needs, and documented methodologies for health education interventions are scarce.

After studying the chapter the reader will be able to:

- list some populations that might require the health educator to prepare material differently for presentation
- describe health concerns unique to specific populations
- define terms related to disability and exceptionality
- compare the impact of various health problems among ethnic groups

The authors would like to thank Judy Ratner, a special education teacher/health educator for Anne Arundel County Schools, and Susan Karchmer and Jennifer Morrone-Joseph from Gallaudet University for their advice and expertise in writing this chapter. Their collective suggestions proved invaluable.

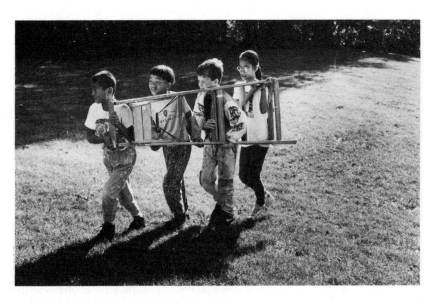

- list the most common mistakes in attempting to work with special populations
- describe the extent of research related to health and some of the special populations
- describe strategies to enhance presentations for special populations

Key Issues

Race	Disability
Ethnicity	Health Knowledge Levels
Culture	Sources of Health Information
Literacy Levels	Political Awareness
Language	Community Gatekeepers

MINORITY HEALTH

The United States of America has often been described as a "melting pot" in reference to the diverse ethnic backgrounds of its population. This country is indeed heterogeneous, and along with the richness and vitality that such diversity brings comes an intriguing complexity.

Here are some important questions to consider:

- Are all ethnic groups affected in the same way by specific health problems?
- Do we even have data that will enable us to generalize about the health problems of certain ethnic groups?
- Will an educational intervention that seems to be successful with one group work with another?

- Can only health educators who are themselves from an ethnic group work successfully with that particular group?
- Do ethnic groups trust "outside" sources of information?
- Is ethnicity the real key to planning health behavior interventions, or is socioeconomic status a more powerful factor?

In 1985 the U.S. Department of Health and Human Services published an important series of documents called the *Report of the Secretary's Task Force on Black and Minority Health* (TFBMH). This report clearly demonstrated that a major discrepancy exists between the health status of ethnic minorities and their white American counterparts. The report, in defining social characteristics of minority populations, categorically points to four important variables or characteristics which are believed to be especially significant: demographic profiles, nutritional status and dietary practices, environmental and occupational exposures, and stress and coping patterns. The following discussion is intended to afford the reader a brief overview of the social characteristics of minority groups within the context of these four variables. This summary is based on the *Report of the Secretary's Task Force on Black and Minority Health (1985)* and data collected in the 1990 Census. For up-to-date information related to the composition of the U.S. population and trends in growth, see Figures 7-1 and 7-2.

African Americans

African Americans are the single largest minority group in the United States, accounting for over 12 percent of the population. In 1990 about 59 percent of all African Americans lived in central cities and one-third lived in the southern region of the country (TFBMH, 1985).

The median age of African Americans is 24.9 years, and the life expectancy in 1983 was 65 years for men and 74 years for women, compared to 72 and 79 years for white men and women, respectively (TFBMH, 1985).

Childbearing among African American women is higher than among their nonminority peers, 2.3 births per woman versus 1.7 in

FIGURE 7-1
U.S. Population by Ethnicity, 1990
Source: U.S. Census Bureau, 1993.

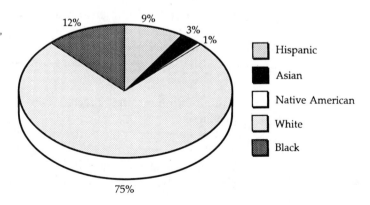

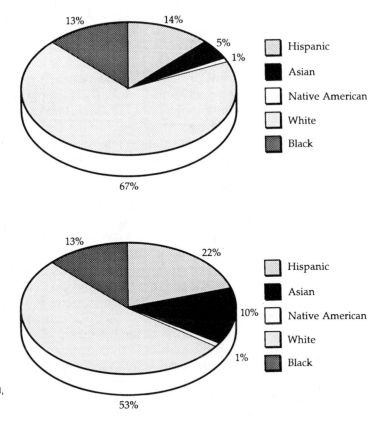

FIGURE 7-2
Projected Percentage of
Population 2010 (*top*)
and 2050 (*bottom*)
Source: U.S. Census Bureau,
1993.

nonminority women. Data related to households headed by women reveal a major difference between ethnic groups. African American women head 37.7 percent of all households, more than three times higher than that of nonminority households headed by women (10.9 percent) (TFBMH, 1985).

In 1981 one out of every three African Americans (34 percent) lived below the poverty level, which was comparable to other minorities such as Hispanics and Native Americans, but substantially higher than nonminorities (11 percent). Seventy-nine percent of African Americans have completed high school, and 13 percent are college graduates (U.S. Census, 1990).

Within the African American community, there are a variety of dietary patterns which tend to be mostly influenced by demographic variables: southern areas of the United States versus northern areas, urban versus rural, and native-born versus foreign-born. There do not appear to be any data that would reflect significant differences between African Americans and nonminorities with regard to calories consumed from proteins, carbohydrates, and fats. However, one significant nutritional risk is the prevalence of obesity among African

American women compared with nonminority women (U.S. Census, 1990).

Health Trends

African Americans experience higher rates of morbidity and mortality from unintentional injuries, drownings, and housefires than do nonminority individuals (TFBMH, 1985).

African American men die from strokes at twice the rate of men in the general population, and they also experience a higher risk of cancer than white males (TFBMH, 1985).

Diabetes is 33 percent more common among African Americans than whites (TFBMH, 1985).

The rate of AIDS among African Americans is more than triple that of whites. Over 50 percent of AIDS cases among women and 54 percent of pediatric AIDS cases are found in the African American community (CDC, 1992).

Infant mortality is twice as high in the African American population as it is in the white population (TFBMH, 1985).

Violence is a major risk factor in the African American community where men are seven times and women four times more likely to be victims of homicide than their white counterparts (TFBMH, 1985).

Hypertension is more common in both genders in the African American community compared to the total population (TFBMH, 1985).

Births to teenagers are more common in the African American community than the white teenage population—three times higher in girls aged 15 to 17 years and nearly five times more common in girls younger than 15 years old (TFBMH, 1985).

AIDS is the leading cause of death in African American women of childbearing age (Ellerbrock et al., 1991).

Although African American women exhibit higher rates of compliance for pap and pelvic examinations than Hispanic or white females, they experience a higher rate of cervical cancer than other races (Harlan, Bernstein, and Kessler, 1991).

Family and kinship ties play a major role in emotional and social support in the African American community, and for many individuals the church is also an important source of strength. Families can be broad and extend from the immediate family to very distant relatives. Children tend to be the focus of the family, and mothers and grandmothers are traditionally the core influences for young children (TFBMH, 1985).

Hispanic Americans

The Hispanic American population in the United States is a rapidly growing community, increasing in numbers by 53 percent from 1980 to 1990. In 1990 Hispanic Americans constituted 9 percent of the U.S.

population. It is expected that by the year 2015 Latin Americans will be the largest minority in the United States. (Census, 1990) Data collections related to Hispanics can be confusing, particularly when categories such as White, Black, and Hispanic are used. Hispanics can be of *any* ethnic group, and the term Hispanic is actually a classification of national background.

Nearly two-thirds of Hispanics are Mexican Americans. Central/South Americans (14%) are the second largest subgroup, followed by Puerto Ricans and Cubans (see Fig. 7-3).

Demographically, 70 percent of all Hispanics live in Texas, Florida, New York, and California. New Mexico has the largest share of Hispanics, California second, and Arizona third; one in three residents of New Mexico is Hispanic, one in four Californians and one in four Texans are also Hispanic (U.S. Census, 1990).

The median age of Hispanic Americans is 23 years. Data on life expectancy are unreliable due to a basic problem in data collection. Few states require a Hispanic identifier on the death certificate and so data collection for this ethnic minority is typically incomplete (TFBMH, 1985).

Hispanic Americans have a relatively high fertility rate, 2.3 children per family. Twenty-three percent of Hispanic households are headed by women, and among Puerto Rican families the rate is 40 percent. The rate of high school graduation for Hispanic Americans is about 58 percent, nearly 20 percent lower than that of the African American population. Approximately 10 percent of Hispanic Americans have a college degree (TFBMH, 1985).

Diet and nutritional patterns strongly reflect the diversity of backgrounds within this subculture. Although fiber and fat contents tend to be high, most food consumption and preparation are thought to be nutritionally adequate (TFBMH, 1985).

Hispanic Americans are overrepresented in jobs associated with manufacturing and construction, two industries that report high proportions of work-related injuries. This association is certainly a factor

FIGURE 7-3
Hispanic Americans in the United States Subgroups in 1990
Source: U.S. Census Bureau, 1993.

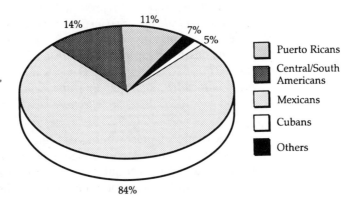

to consider when realizing that Hispanic Americans report rates of severe disability almost twice that of nonminority Americans (TFBMH, 1985).

Health Trends

Death rates from heart disease and cancer are lower than for non-Hispanics. Diabetes is especially prevalent in Mexican Americans.

Forty-three percent of Hispanic men smoke cigarettes, and both male and female Hispanic teenagers smoke at higher rates than their non-Hispanic counterparts (TFBMH, 1985).

The rate of AIDS for Hispanics is three times higher than for non-Hispanic whites, with rates among Puerto Rican–born Hispanics nearly seven times higher. Incidence among Hispanic women is about eight times higher than among non-Hispanic women, with the rate of pediatric HIV infection over six times higher than for non-Hispanic children (CDC, 1992).

Hispanic Americans tend to have very strong family ties, which extend to the local community. The male is usually the head of the household and can be a dominant, authoritarian figure. Responsibility in caring for the sick usually rests with another family member, and approaches to illness may be of a fatalistic nature. Modesty, particularly in females, is highly valued. The church and community are often the social center for many individuals (TFBMH, 1985).

Case Study   *Denise, a community health educator, had been asked to speak with representatives from several local Hispanic women's groups to explore their perceived needs concerning preventive health services. Eager to be prepared for the encounter, Denise thoroughly researches health issues relevant to Mexican Americans and on learning that fluency in English among the women is very limited, she persuades a good friend visiting from Madrid to accompany her in the role of translator. Denise's confidence that she is well prepared is short lived as the workshop begins! Denise had made the seriously wrong assumption that all Hispanic people are alike and come from the same culture. The women at the workshop represented group members from Mexico, South America, Central America, Cuba, and Puerto Rico. Although the women had some similar concerns, they were offended that Denise was making broad assumptions based on information that was foreign to their particular cultures. To make matters worse, Denise's interpreter friend was experiencing major difficulties understanding and being understood! This exploratory session was rather less than effective.*

Although Denise's motives were laudable, she made some obvious mistakes based on erroneous assumptions. If a health educator has any doubts at all about a group or population with which he/she is unfamiliar, questions should be directed whenever possible to individuals within the group in question. Denise could have contacted some of the women leaders beforehand to familiarize herself with the groups and assess what would be required to make the workshop successful. If this is not possible, perhaps there are fellow educators who have worked with these individuals or groups before who could provide information and advice. Working with diverse populations is not a simple matter, and we should all definitely avoid making assumptions based on what is often less than reality.

Asian/Pacific Islanders

This subgroup of the population grew by 107.8 percent between 1980 and 1990 and represent approximately 2.9 percent of the U.S. population. Asian/Pacific Islanders include a large percentage of foreign-born individuals (58 percent), which is a larger percentage than any other minority group (U.S. Census, 1990).

This minority group is represented by over 20 countries, the three most common countries of origin being: China, the Philippines, and Japan (U.S. Census, 1990).

The majority of Asian/Pacific Islanders live in the western region of the United States, although this trend has started to change as settlement in other areas of the country has increased (U.S. Census, 1990).

The median age of the Asian/Pacific Islander population is 28.7, which is higher than the other three largest minority groups. Fifty-eight percent of Asian/Pacific Islander women are in the workforce, and only 11 percent of women in this population are heads of households, a rate lower than nonminority women (TFBMH, 1985).

Educational levels are similar to the nonminority population—seventy-five percent have completed high school, and approximately 33 percent have earned a college degree (TFBMH, 1985).

Rice, prepared in many different ways, represents the primary source of calories for most Asian/Pacific Islanders. Consumption of fruits, vegetables, and fish tends to be higher than nonminority groups, while intake of animal protein and dairy products is lower. Many individuals gradually change to a more traditional American diet, increasing the amounts of animal protein, fats, and refined sugar consumed. Obesity and heart disease are more common in Asians in the United States compared with individuals in their countries of origin (TFBMH, 1985).

Health Trends

Two infectious diseases that have accompanied immigrant Asian and Pacific Islanders to the United States are tuberculosis and hepatitis B.

Smoking is a risk factor for many Asians. For example, among Californian immigrant groups, smoking rates among men are 92 percent for Laotians, 71 percent for Cambodians, and 65 percent for

Vietnamese versus approximately 30 percent in the general U.S. population (TFBMH, 1985).

Trends in Asian/Pacific Islander occupations show a higher-than-usual proportion involved in white-collar work—19 percent of Chinese, 15 percent of Japanese, and 14 percent of Filippinos versus 13 percent of nonminorities. However, a disproportionate number of Asian/Pacific Islanders work well below their educational levels (TFBMH, 1985).

The family is extremely important to Asian/Pacific Islanders, and very often seeking help outside the family confines is not encouraged. In addition, some individuals within these cultures take great pride in their independence and may be reluctant to seek help from health agencies. Family units are often an extended family with three or four generations living together. The oldest male is the head of the household and great importance is placed on father-son relationships. Asian American parents traditionally take an active role in their children's learning activities and generally are strict in controlling their children's behavior (TFBMH, 1985).

Native Americans

This category includes American Indians, Aleuts, Alaskan Eskimos, and Native Hawaiians. However, available data used here refer primarily to American Indians. American Indians are the smallest minority group in the United States, comprising less than 1 percent of the population. American Indians have a birth rate that is nearly double that of other groups, with an average family size larger than any other minority or nonminority group. The median age of American Indians is 22.4 years, with a life expectancy six years less than other minority groups (U.S. Census, 1990).

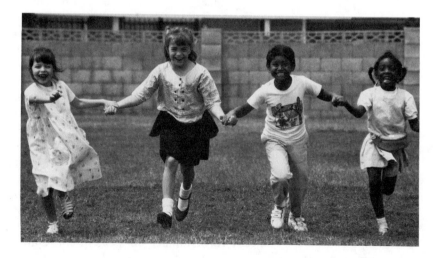

Nearly 50 percent of American Indian women work outside the home, and approximately one out of four households is headed by a woman.

The educational levels of American Indians are the lowest of all the minority groups. Less than one-third of this population have completed high school, and only 7 percent have graduated from college (TFBMH, 1985).

Fifty percent of American Indians live in the West or Southwest of the United States. Nearly one-quarter live on reservations, most of which have populations less than 1,000 (U.S. Census, 1990).

The diet of American Indians is extremely varied according to tribal custom. In general, diets tend to be high in refined carbohydrates, fat, and sodium, and low in meat and dairy products, indicating a potential problem with protein deficiency (U.S. Census, 1990).

Health Trends

There is a disproportionate incidence of high weight for height in American Indians, in addition to a problem of obesity in adult American Indians. This may explain, at least in part, the high incidence of diabetes in this population (TFBMH, 1985).

A large proportion of this population die before age 45. Most of the excess deaths are caused by unintentional injuries, cirrhosis, homicide, suicide, pneumonia, and complications of diabetes (TFBMH, 1985).

The homicide rate is 60 percent higher than that of the general population. Alcohol is again believed to play an important role in this health risk (TFBMH, 1985).

Suicide among Native Americans occurs at a rate 28 percent higher than that of the general population. Once again, alcohol is believed to play a major role.

Native Americans share with African Americans the highest rates of injury and death from nondisease causes. Alcohol-related motor vehicle accidents are particularly high in this population, as are injuries related to industrial accidents. Alcoholism rates are high and contribute to family violence, motor vehicle accidents, assaults, accidental injury, suicide, depression, and obesity. The leading cause of death among Native American men aged 43 years and younger is unintentional injuries, 75 percent of which are alcohol related and 54 percent of which involve motor vehicle accidents (TFBMH, 1985).

American Indians traditionally revere the family, their tribe, and the land. Respect for elders is a primary element of Native American culture. An individual's rights and the importance of noninterference in another's personal life unless requested are also basic tenets of Native American life.

For some American Indians the traditional medicine men play an important role in healing the body and the mind. Any health interventions should certainly take into account this influence (TFBMH, 1985).

One factor that many novice health educators tend to overlook is that ethnic minorities do not all have the same health problems and needs. Even a cursory glance at Figures 7-4 and 7-5 clearly indicates that the death rates by both race and gender are very different.

When the leading causes of death in the United States are considered by race the discrepancy between the majority and minority populations becomes even more apparent. See figure 7-6 and 7-7.

In addition to higher rates of death from heart disease and cancer in the African American community, other health problems are clearly

FIGURE 7-4

Average Annual Age-Adjusted Death Rates for All Causes, 1979–1981
Source: National Center for Health Statistics, Bureau of the Census, and Task Force on Black and Minority Health.

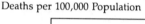

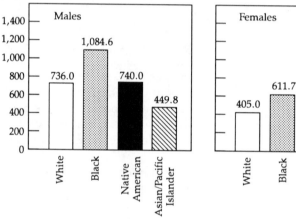

Note: Death rates for Hispanics are not available. Death rates for Native Americans and Asian/Pacific Islanders are probably underestimated due to less frequent reporting of these races on death certificates as compared with the U.S. Census.

FIGURE 7-5

Life Expectancy at Birth, According to Race and Sex: United States, 1950–1983
Source: National Center for Health Statistics.

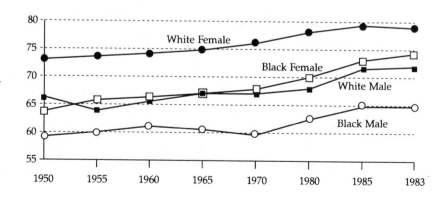

Deaths per 100,000 Population

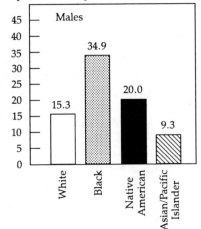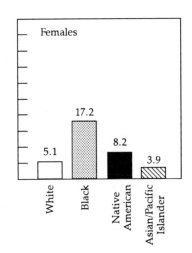

FIGURE 7-6
Average Annual Age-
Adjusted Death Rates for
Heart Disease for Persons
Under 45 Years of Age,
1979–1981
Source: National Center for
Health Statistics, Bureau of
the Census, and Task Force
on Black and Minority
Health.

Note: Death rates for Hispanics are not available. Death rates for Native Americans and Asian/Pacific Islanders are probably underestimated due to less frequent reporting of these races on death certificates as compared with the U.S. Census.

FIGURE 7-7
Average Annual Age-
Adjusted Death Rates for
Cancer, 1979–1981
Source: National Center for
Health Statistics, Bureau of
the Census, and Task Force
on Black and Minority
Health.

Deaths per 100,000 Population

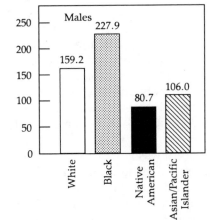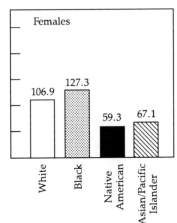

Note: Death rates for Hispanics are not available. Death rates for Native Americans and Asian/Pacific Islanders are probably underestimated due to less frequent reporting of these races on death certificates as compared with the U.S. Census.

Tuskegee: A Legacy of Doubt

One of the major issues discussed in this chapter is the difficulty experienced by health educators attempting to plan and effectively implement programs when viewed as "outsiders." Although most young health education students will probably be unaware of research begun in the 1930s, the Tuskegee syphilis study provides an excellent example of why a community, in this case the African American community, might exhibit a pervasive sense of distrust of public health agencies.

In the late 1920s, the Public Health Service (PHS) was completing a study of the prevalence of syphilis in the black population in Mississippi. In order to expand syphilis research in the rural South, the PHS was awarded a grant from the Julius Rosenwald Foundation, a philanthropic organization located in Chicago. The research was to study the testing and treatment of syphilis in five rural counties in the South: Albemarle County, Virginia; Glynn County, Georgia; Pitt County, North Carolina; Macon County, Alabama; and Tipton County, Tennessee (Parran, 1937).

The depression, beginning in 1929, played havoc with the research funding, and the treatment phase of the study was never completed. In Macon County, Alabama, the prevalence of syphilis had been reported as high as 35 to 40 percent of all age groups tested. It was this community in Alabama that was to serve as the proving ground for the effects of untreated syphilis. A PHS physician, Dr. T. Clark, stated simply, "the Alabama community offered an unparalleled opportunity for the study of the effect of untreated syphilis" (Jones, 1981).

One of the great ironies of this study was the astonishingly thorough and textbook approach taken by the PHS in implementing the program. Prestigious black institutions were persuaded to cooperate, several black churches added their credibility, and individual black community leaders ensured participation (Thomas and Quinn, 1991). The research continued and little concern was voiced that anything questionable was taking place. However, in addition to not treating the infected individuals, the PHS team also chose not to provide any education about syphilis (Jones, 1981). No mention was made of the disease by name. It was simply referred to as "bad blood," a rural, southern term descriptive of many health problems at that time. Individuals were not told that the disease could be sexually transmitted or that infants could be born infected (Thomas and Quinn, 1991).

United States involvement in World War II began in 1941, and so desperate was the PHS not lose its subjects to the war that it pressured the draft board into not drafting these men. In 1943 the recently developed "miracle drug" penicillin was being widely used, including in the treatment of people infected with syphilis. This effective form of treatment was withheld from the men in the study. Clearly, treatment of the infected individuals would end the study and future research, something the PHS did not want to occur. The study and the withholding of treatment continued until 1972 when the *Washington Star's* front-page exposé created enormous public outcry, finally stirring health officials into ending the study (Parran, 1937).

What are the implications of the Tuskegee study for health educators? What can we learn from this obviously inhumane and unethical research? Thomas and Quinn (1991) draw a powerful connection between the Tuskegee study and the current AIDS epidemic. The authors point out that the legacy of Tuskegee is a legitimate and understandable fear and distrust of the "health establishment." They cite the fears of some African Americans who believe that AIDS is an agent of white forces developed as a form of genocide. Dr. Mark Smith from Johns Hopkins University described the African American community as "already alienated from the health care system . . . and somewhat cynical about the motives of those who arrive in their communities to help them" (National Commission on AIDS, 1990, p. 19). A health educator from Dallas, testifying before the National Commission on AIDS commented, "So many African American people that I work with do not trust hospitals or any of the other community health care service providers because of that Tuskegee experiment. It is like . . . if they did it then they will do it again" (National Commission on AIDS, 1990, p. 43).

As health educators we must not underestimate the importance and power of past events. Twenty years after the study ended, and over 60 years since it began, the Tuskegee study is still with us. It would be easy to dismiss as preposterous the notion that AIDS is a deliberate attempt at genocide. Yet, in the light of Tuskegee, is that type of fear so farfetched? Thomas and Quinn (1991) make a forceful point when they describe the necessary ingredients for a successful community-based HIV education program that are ethnically acceptable and culturally sensitive: (1) the use of program staff indigenous to the community, (2) the use of incentives, and (3) the delivery of health services within the target community. The authors comment however, that these were the exact methods used in the Tuskegee study and that health educators will have to work hard to ensure that these sound strategies are not diminished by their association with this fateful study (Thomas & Quinn, 1991).

a major concern for some ethnic groups. For example, AIDS disproportionately affects minority groups. As of July 1992, over one-quarter of all men with AIDS were African American, and over 16 percent were Hispanic. The imbalance is even more evident when data describing AIDS in women are examined. African American women account for 53 percent of all female cases, with Hispanic women accounting for 21.1 percent. Obviously, these figures far exceed the proportion of minorities found in the general population (CDC, 1992).

Suggested Health Promotion Strategies when Planning Programs for Diverse Cultures (TFBMH, 1985)

Channel efforts for minority communities through local leaders who could represent a powerful force for promoting acceptance and reinforcement of the central themes of health promotion messages.

Data suggest that health messages are more readily accepted if they do not conflict with existing cultural beliefs. Where appropriate, messages should acknowledge existing cultural beliefs.

Involve family, churches, employers, and community organizations as a support system to facilitate and sustain behavior change to a more healthful lifestyle. For example, although hypertension controls in African Americans depend on appropriate medical therapy, blood pressure control can be improved and maintained by family and community support of activities such as proper diet and exercise.

Language barriers, cultural differences, and lack of adequate information on access to care can complicate health maintenance and treatment. Health educators must ensure that culturally sensitive information is available in many forms within a specific community. This should not only be subject specific, but also include basic information on *how* to access services.

Assess the suitability of existing information and materials and/or develop new culturally sensitive materials. Enlist the participation of professional and lay members of each minority group to assess the suitability of the materials.

Encourage private organizations, such as religious and community organizations, clubs, and schools, to participate in developing minority support networks and other incentive techniques to facilitate the acceptance of health information and education.

Important Points to Consider Before Teaching and/or Presenting to Diverse Populations

What is the precise ethnic mix of the class or audience? A description of *Hispanic* or *Asian* is probably not precise enough. Obtain as much specific information as possible.

Find out more about the demographics of the group. Where do they live—in an urban, suburban, or rural setting? Do you have any information about educational levels or socioeconomic status?

Consider the language proficiency of the class or group. Is there a high proportion of recent immigrants who speak little English? Is a translator necessary and, if so, can you find one?

Are there any health problems unique to this group of which you should be aware? Research the health status of the group.

Identify and consult individuals, perhaps school and community leaders, who are from, or at least familiar with, a specific race or culture.

Adopt teaching or presentation strategies that will be culturally sensitive to specific groups. Your presentations will be much more effective and better accepted if the students/audience can closely relate to your style and content.

Be aware of strong cultural influences within specific cultures, such as the family and the church. Gaining support and even cooperation from both these areas will add much credibility to the learning experience.

Case Study

Monica is a young and inexperienced community health educator presenting a workshop to a group of middle-aged Hispanic (Mexican American) women. The topic of the workshop is the importance of having a regular pelvic examination. Monica has been told that Hispanic women tend to report low rates of pap smear screening, and Monica's main objective is to increase compliance to this important test. Monica believes that many women feel uncomfortable with their own bodies and has decided to begin the workshop with an exercise designed to reduce this discomfort. To the amazement of the group of Hispanic women, Monica lays down on the table at the front of the room, lifts up her dress, pulls off her underwear, and proceeds to identify her cervix with the aid of a mirror. Meanwhile, an assistant moves around the audience slowly, handing out similar mirrors to the stunned and silent group. Once the audience realizes the intention of the instructor, there is a mass exodus toward the nearest exit . . . the workshop is over.

Monica's rather radical introduction to the workshop is a great example of poor method selection! This type of activity might have been problematic in many settings, and, had Monica carried out the necessary research on this particular target population, she would have realized that such a strategy was entirely inappropriate. Although Monica's intention was understandable, this type of overt and direct activity could not be successful with a population that is generally modest and self-conscious about sexuality. This rather disasterous workshop illustrates the necessity for thoroughly researching the characteristics of specific populations before designing intervention strategies.

One question that is often raised with regard to health education and race is, Should the race of the health educator always be the same as the race of the intended audience? This often becomes a moot point in that there are simply insufficient numbers of minority health educators to serve all populations. However, all things being equal, does the race or culture of the presenter make a major difference when considering the effectiveness of a class or program? The consensus about this question would seem to suggest that wherever possible a presenter/ teacher of similar culture would be preferable. Obviously, familiarity with a culture would avoid some major pitfalls in sensitivity, as, for example, were committed by the overzealous Monica in the case study. The issue of trust must also be considered. The Tuskegee study is an excellent illustration of why some cultures are suspicious of "external" interference. A more recent study seems to confirm the continuing suspicion of certain populations toward "outside influences." In a study of African American women attending a public health clinic, the researcher found that 21 percent of the women did not trust the federal government's reports on AIDS and 54 percent were uncertain about them. In addition, when questioned as to whether they considered AIDS to be an act of genocide against the black race, only 52 percent disagreed with the notion (Sharon, 1992). Given this issue of mistrust, a same-race health educator would seem to be optimal. Ironically, when asked if the race of the information "messenger" was of any consequence, 70 percent of the women in the previously mentioned study responded that race was not an issue.

EXCEPTIONAL POPULATIONS

A much underserved and underconsidered population with regard to health education is one often labeled as *exceptional.* Mainstream health education students may be justifiably confused by descriptive labels related to this area, so some definition is necessary. Mandell and Fiscus (1981) offer three fairly straightforward clarifications of often-used labels:

Exceptional—atypical; a performance which deviates from what is expected, either a higher or lower performance.

Disability—total or partial behavioral, mental, physical, or sensorial loss of functioning. All disabled people are exceptional, but the reverse is not necessarily true.

Handicap—environmental restrictions placed on a person's life as a result of a disability or exceptionality. (Mandell and Fiscus, 1981, p. 3)

To illustrate the endless possibility of variations of exceptionality, the same authors describe a case study of a six-year-old boy named James. James was born with spina bifida, a condition where the spinal column fails to close and where the extent of disability can be extremely varied. He has limited use of his legs and has no bowel or bladder control. With regard to academic potential, James has been identified as gifted, and he attends a regular first-grade class. How would James fit into the preceding definitions?

Label	Corresponding Behaviors
Exceptional	James deviates from the norm (below average) with regard to physical performance and exceeds the norm in intellectual performance.
Disabled	James is unable to walk or control bowel and bladder functions.
Handicapped	James cannot move physically through his environment without assistance. In addition, he requires educational programs for the academically talented. (Although giftedness is not considered by most to be a handicap, it is the authors' opinion that the gifted are handicapped in that their superior abilities, for the most part, are not developed in most traditional educational programs.)

Beware, for the most sacred cow may become the tiger's breakfast.
—Mohan Singh

This profile clearly illustrates how labeling can be applied to specific conditions. However, although labeling serves a useful purpose in identifying the type of educational interventions that might prove optimal for individual development, the procedure is not without criticism. Meyen (1978), for example, believes that labeling or classifying an individual can be problematic for the following reasons:

1. All too often the label emphasizes the negative instead of stressing the positive. This stresses the individual's limitations not his/her strengths . . . what the person *cannot* do rather than what he or she *can* do. This may become a self-fulfilling prophecy.
2. The accuracy of the label may be questionable. Often labels are simplistically given on the basis of single factors which may conceal a more complex causation.
3. Labeling does not accurately account for differences within individual classifications. A broad range of disability can be found within any classification, a good example of this being hearing loss.
4. The conditions of individuals rarely remain static, and classifications do a poor job of including this temporal concept. Individuals tend to change over time, as will their educational needs. Specific labeling therefore may no longer be accurate for some individuals over a long period of time.

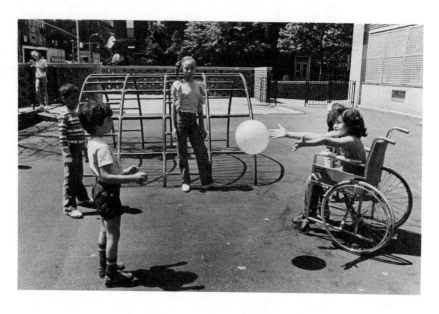

As a result of this type of concern and criticism, there are some educators who would abandon completely the practice of labeling. In its place, they would substitute a more precise description of each individual, with a focus on the implications for learning strategies (Goldstein et al., 1975).

Categories of Exceptional Children

The passage of Public Law 94-142 (PL 94-142) in 1975 codified the rights of all exceptional children and youth to a free, appropriate education. Exceptional children who are eligible by law for services through special educational placements are categorized as follows: mentally retarded, deaf and hard of hearing, speech impaired, visually impaired, emotionally disturbed, orthopedically and other health impaired, and learning disabled. These descriptors or labels are very broad, and to fully understand the population served by this law, a more precise definition is needed. The *Federal Register* of August 1977 contains the rules and regulations of PL 94-142 and defines the labels listed previously as follows:

Deaf means a hearing impairment which is so severe that the child is impaired in processing linguistic information through hearing, with or without amplification, which adversely affects educational performance.

Deaf-blind means concomitant hearing and visual impairments, the combination of which causes such severe communication and other developmental and educational problems that they cannot be accommodated in special education programs solely for deaf or blind children.

Hard of hearing means a hearing impairment, whether permanent or fluctuating, which adversely affects a child's educational performance but which is not included under the definition of "deaf" in this section.

Mentally retarded means significantly subaverage general intellectual functioning existing concurrently with deficits in adaptive behavior and manifested during the developmental period, which adversely affects a child's educational performance.

Multihandicapped means concomitant impairments (such as mentally retarded–blind, mentally retarded–orthopedically impaired etc.), the combination of which causes severe educational problems that cannot be accommodated in special education programs solely for one of the impairments. The term does not include deaf-blind children.

Orthopedically impaired means a severe orthopedic impairment which adversely affects a child's educational performance. The term includes impairments caused by congenital anomaly (e.g. clubfoot, absence of some member, etc.), impairments caused by disease (e.g. poliomyelitis, bone tuberculosis etc.), and impairments from other causes (e.g. cerebral palsy, amputations, and fractures or burns which cause contractures).

Other health impaired means limited strength, vitality or alertness, due to chronic or acute health problems such as heart condition, tuberculosis, rheumatic fever, nephritis, asthma, sickle cell anemia, hemophilia, epilepsy, lead poisoning, leukemia, or diabetes which adversely affects a child's educational performance.

Seriously emotionally disturbed is defined as follows:

(i) The term means a condition exhibiting one or more of the following characteristics over a long period of time and to a marked degree, which adversely affects educational performance:

   A. An inability to learn which cannot be explained by intellectual, sensory, or health factors.
   B. An inability to build or maintain satisfactory interpersonal relationships with peers and teachers.
   C. Inappropriate types of behavior or feelings under normal circumstances.
   D. A general pervasive mood of unhappiness or depression or;
   E. A tendency to develop physical symptoms or fears associated with personal or school problems.

(ii) The term includes children who are schizophrenic or autistic. The term does not include children who are socially maladjusted, unless it is determined that they are seriously emotionally disturbed.

Speech impaired means a communication disorder, such as stuttering, impaired articulation, a language impairment, or a voice impairment, which adversely affects a child's educational performance.

Visually impaired means a visual performance which, even with correction, adversely affects a child's educational performance. The term includes both partially seeing and blind children.

It is not practical or within the scope of this text to describe in great detail all the previously defined categories of "exceptionality." The majority of mainstream health educators will have extremely limited contact with individuals included in some of these categories. To that end, the remainder of this chapter will focus on the categories of exceptionality with which school and community health educators are likely to have the most frequent contact.

VISUALLY IMPAIRED

This term is used to describe individuals who have defective or impaired vision. Definitions of impairment or blindness can be either legally or educationally based. Legal definitions are based on a technical evaluation, whereas educational definitions tend to be more pragmatic and simplified, stating that the visually impaired are those people whose visual condition is such that special provisions are necessary for successful education (Meyen, 1978). This is an important population for the health educator to be familiar with, as many individuals with visual impairments are being mainstreamed in both the school and community settings.

Similar to the deaf population, the effects on the education of visually impaired people are dependent to a great extent on the age of onset, any degree of accompanying disability, and the availability of developmental opportunities. Identifying the extent of visual impairment is reasonably straightforward, and yet measuring the secondary effects of impairment such as language development and cognition skills is more difficult simply because most available instruments and standardized tests are written. Lowenfeld (1962) describes the primary effects of visual impairment as restrictions imposed on the individual in:

1. range and variety of possible experiences
2. ability to move about the environment

3. control of the environment and of the self in relation to it.

The ability to move about the environment is particularly important as it is this freedom which provides the sighted individual the opportunity for observation and experience. The absence of this opportunity will obviously impact the development of any individual. A concrete example of restricted experience is in the development of language. As most children develop, they take notice of what is happening around them. Children can then question a parent or other person about what they see . . . sometimes in an endless string of questions that only children can ask! A child who does not see a small animal or large gray rain cloud has a compromised ability to ask questions and learn about the world. Vocabulary may then become limited, as will comprehension of the environment.

Case Study   *Robert is preparing to present a workshop on nutrition and fitness for college students. He has ascertained that approximately 35 students will attend and in anticipation of a workshop filled with a great deal of information, he has prepared a large number of overhead transparencies to facilitate teaching. As Robert is adjusting the focus on the overhead projector, he notices two students with canes carefully entering the classroom. They are obviously significantly visually impaired. Robert has a sinking feeling as he stares at has pile of overhead transparencies and wonders what to do next.*

Robert could take the easy way out and just continue with his prepared lecture. Hopefully, Robert will demonstrate initiative and take steps to alleviate a possible problem. The most obvious initial step would simply be to welcome the visually impaired participants and before beginning the lecture ask them if there is anything that Robert could do to make the workshop more effective. Would seating arrangements make a difference? Perhaps he could seat them closer to the front of the room. Should Robert make a greater effort to verbalize the written material to facilitate understanding? Would written materials like pamphlets be useful to distribute after the workshop so that someone could read them to the visually impaired participants or perhaps even translate them into Braille? Obviously, there is a limit to what Robert can do at such short notice. However, by not panicking, Robert could take these simple steps in an attempt to accommodate *all* his workshop participants.

In its initial stages, motor development is dependent on vision. Seeing objects in the immediate environment stimulates an infant to raise his/her head or reach out a hand. If an infant is blind, the motivation to move may well be inhibited, and subsequently the visually impaired child cannot develop the experience of being able to move through his/her environment. The obvious lack of visual stimulation can lead some blind individuals to resort to *blindisms* or primitive movements—perhaps a rocking back and forth motion or excessive rubbing of the eyes. If an environment is provided that stimulates a child and encourages physical response, the child's motor development will probably progress within the typical chronologic range (Cratty, 1971).

Meyen (1978) suggests four important principles which the teacher of any subject should consider when instructing visually impaired people:

1. Because all visually impaired people are not the same, instruction should be *individualized* as much as possible.
2. Teachers should stress as much as possible relationships between things in the environment which are not discernible to the blind.
3. Stimulation of all types must be provided to attract and maintain attention.
4. Some visually impaired children must be taught to actively engage in the learning process. Children devoid of stimulae might tend to be somewhat passive and need to be taught how to become more involved.

Mandell and Fiscus (1981) also offer some invaluable suggestions to individuals who might be teaching visually impaired people:

- Explain about and allow individuals to explore their physical environment—classroom, meeting room, and so on.
- Maximize the remaining vision of the visually impaired—consider adequate levels of light, classroom seating, using larger writing, and so on.
- In the school setting, give non-visually impaired children the opportunity to discuss blindness with the students who have vision problems.
- Provide learning opportunities that will actively include people who are blind.
- Ask other involved professionals, or in the case of children ask parents, "What works?" Do not be afraid to ask for advice.
- In the classroom setting, be sure to orally repeat anything that is written on the blackboard.
- Verbally clarify any predominantly visual materials that you may be using—maps, charts, and graphs.
- If an individual is utilizing Braille, allow additional time.
- Encourage individuals to utilize any alternative techniques and or technology that might facilitate learning.

Learning Aids and Material for the Visually Impaired

Learning aids can basically be divided into two categories: optical and non-optical. Examples of optical aids might be glasses, magnifiers, and so on, while an example of a nonoptical aid would be the use of Braille. Simply stated, Braille consists of a series of raised dot patterns which represent elements of language. The dot patterns are placed within a six-dot cell to denote letters of the alphabet, numbers, and punctuation. See Figure 7-8.

The Braille characters are "read" by a person's fingertips. An important point for educators to remember is that Braille is more ambiguous than the printed word. Children who are blind and utilizing Braille might take longer to read material than a seeing child who is reading print. This discrepancy in reading speed is often continued into adulthood. For example, in a study comparing the reading speeds of blind and seeing high school seniors, the blind students using Braille averaged 90 words per minute versus 250 words per minute by students reading print (Myers, Ethington, and Ashcroft, 1958). This type of discrepancy needs to be acknowledged and included when planning presentations or lessons. Individuals who are blind can also write in Braille. The two major options to do this are: a braillewriter, a machine somewhat similar to a typewriter in appearance, which embosses paper with the Braille code; and a slate and stylus. The latter device consists of a hinged frame between which paper is clamped. The writer presses down with the stylus, pushing the paper on to the back of the frame which contains six depressions arranged like dots in the Braille cell. The writer thus creates the Braille cells by hand as opposed to using a machine, the braillewriter, which performs this function more easily.

An additional and frequently utilized nonoptical aid is the audiotape. Cassette audiotapes are relatively inexpensive and easy to record with and can provide the opportunity for the visually impaired to listen to a lecture, take a test from a tape, or simply listen to a best-selling novel which has been transposed onto tape.

Assisting the Partially Sighted

There are many individuals who are not blind, and although they have a vision impairment, they are still able to partially see. These individuals might be helped by taking the following simple steps to facilitate learning:

- Use specially adapted books with larger print. See Figure 7-9.

FIGURE 7-8

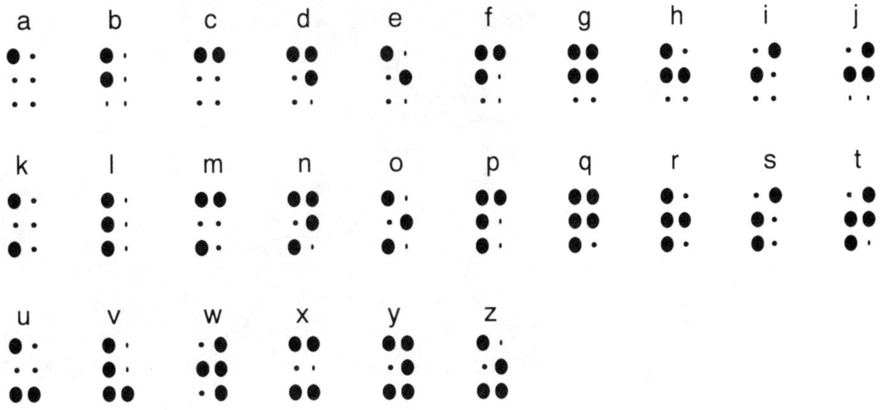

This is an example of the type of font size which is typically used in books and other written materials specifically designed for people with visual impairment.

Compare that font size to this smaller size, typically used for readers without any form of visual impairment.

- Carefully consider background colors when preparing presentation materials. Ensure that print and graphics are clearly defined against the background.
- Seating an individual at the front of the room might be helpful.
- Ensure that good levels of lighting are available.
- Allow extra time for completion of work.
- For some individuals listening might be a more effective learning device than reading. To that end, ensure that a quiet atmosphere exists which might be more conducive to learning.

FIGURE 7-9
Adapted from C. J. Mandell and E. Fiscus, *Understanding Exceptional People*, p. 213 (St. Paul, MN: West Publishing, 1981). Reprinted with permission

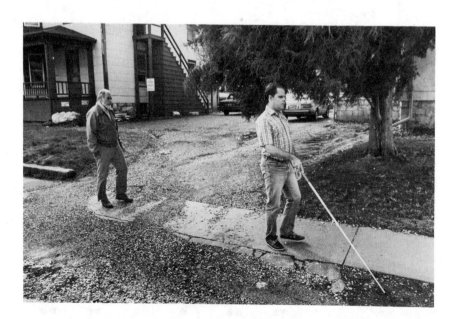

There are many agencies that provide resources for the visually impaired, the primary source of supplies being the American Printing House for the Blind in Louisville, Kentucky. For additional information, see the Appendix.

LEARNING DISABLED

The label of *learning disabled* has become a somewhat amorphous term, often utilized to describe students who do not succeed in school. Some definitions include "slow learners" or mentally retarded, and others incorporate emotionally unstable and blindness. Other experts in this field believe that the label learning disabled is much more specific and that failure to succeed in school is much too vague a definition. There are obviously many reasons why children might fail in school, which can hardly be designated as a learning disability— poor motivation and/or inappropriate or mediocre teaching methods, for example. Mandell and Fiscus (1981) suggest the yardstick should be that if learning difficulties can be overcome by a different type of instruction, then the child should not be considered learning disabled.

A national definition was established in 1977 as a result of PL 94-142 (*Federal Register,* December 29, 1977, Part 3):

> Specific learning disability means a disorder in one or more of the basic psychological processes involved in understanding or in using language spoken or written which may manifest itself in an imperfect ability to listen, think, speak, read, write, spell or to do mathematical calculations. The term includes such conditions as perceptual handicaps, brain injury, minimum brain dysfunction, dyslexial and developmental aphasia. The term does not include children who have learning problems which are primarily the result of visual, hearing or motor handicaps, of mental retardation, of emotional disturbance, or of environmental, cultural or economic disadvantage.

The *Federal Register* (1977) goes on to identify seven areas where a major discrepancy may exist between ability and achievement:

1. Oral expression
2. Listening comprehension
3. Written expression
4. Basic reading skill
5. Reading comprehension
6. Mathematics calculation
7. Mathematics reasoning

In order for a child to be eligible for special educational services, an evaluation team must agree to the following:

- The child must exhibit learning difficulties in at least one of the seven areas listed previously.
- The child has a severe learning achievement problem.
- The major reason for the discrepancy between achievement and ability is not other handicapping conditions or sociological factors.

In 1966 the Easter Seal Research Foundation, a federally sponsored task force, published a report which listed the 10 most frequently cited characteristics of learning-disabled children (Clements, 1966). Being aware of these more prevalent characteristics might be useful to the health educator as he/she considers health education methodology:

Hyperactivity is characterized by an inability to remain seated and constant movement from one point of the room to another.

Perceptual-motor impairments involve difficulty in reproducing information received through the senses: difficulty with copying, problems with written information, identifying letters of the alphabet, reading from left to right, and reproducing basic shapes. One of the better known learning disabilities in this category is *dyslexia*.

Attention is characterized by a problem with focus and holding attention for any length of time. Individuals might experience difficulty in completing tasks, are easily distracted, and often cannot remain seated for long periods of time.

Memory might involve difficulty in memorizing information over long and short periods of time. Indicators might include an inability to remember basic information like the family's address and telephone number or being unable to remember things learned the day before.

Speech and hearing are demonstrated in some children who have a form of communication disorder and might have a problem with using correct grammar and articulating words and thoughts. Another indicator might be a repetition of the same phrases, over and over, resulting from restricted language development.

Emotional liability is manifested in some children who have not developed emotionally and socially to an age-appropriate level. This may result in a low threshold for frustration, difficulty with social interaction, and, on occasion, a temper tantrum.

Coordination deficits might be identified as awkward or clumsy physical movements or problems with fine motor skills such as using scissors or pencil and paper.

Impulsivity is characterized by children rushing into reactions or responses without any thought for the consequences. This could include writing down the first answer that comes to mind in a test or running out into the street after a ball without regard for traffic.

Learning deficits in basic academic subjects are manifested in students who demonstrate a wide discrepancy in achievement between subjects. For example, a student might be a full grade level ahead in reading ability, but two years below in math. Relevant terms in this section include:

Dyslexia—problems in reading

Dysgraphia—problems in writing

Dyscalcula—problems with arithmetic

Reading disability

Word blindness

Equivocal Neurological Signs are characterized by the questionable or uncertain. For children in this category, there is no direct evidence of neurological damage, and yet the individuals might demonstrate characteristics such as hyperactivity, poor attention, problems with concentration, becoming easily distracted, impulsivity, and poor motor functioning.

With such a wide variety of potential problems, designing methods of instruction for this population can be extremely complicated and there are no simple solutions for planning presentations. Hammill and Bartel (1978) believe that when constructing materials for teaching learning-disabled students, instructors must consider three areas: design, methods, and practicality. The design component speaks to the basic organization of the material which the authors believe should be presented in logical, sequential building blocks. The method component considers whether the material should be used individually or in groups. In addition, because of the variety of existing learning levels, a diversity of presentation methods is necessary along with a willingness to be flexible toward varying student responses. Practical considerations dictate that materials be "durable" (able to stand the test of time) and that they can be utilized both independently and with supervision (Hammill and Bartel, 1978).

Aukerman (1972) suggests that when presenting written information to people with learning disabilities, the instructor should:

- Avoid figurative or symbolic language—use concrete, pictorial terms.
- Use pictures and diagrams to illustrate text.
- Turn written numbers into numerals.
- Use words that follow phonic rules.
- Avoid words with double meanings.

Some health educators believe that it is particularly important for learning-disabled students to receive sound information related to sexuality education. Gordon (1973) argues that people with learning disabilities need sex education for three major reasons: for the most part, they have the same desires as other people for companionship, love, and sexual activity; the passage from adolescence to adulthood is often intensified for this population; and learning-disabled individuals may have difficulty processing information and therefore remain dangerously uninformed. In the context of human sexuality, Haight and Fachting (1986) suggest the following principles for teaching learning-disabled students:

- Use printed materials that have a fairly low reading level.
- Use materials that have a mature theme. Many learning disabled students are of average intelligence and would be bored and feel patronized by immature content and approach.
- Use interactive teaching methods to actively involve students in the learning process (role play, games, skits, etc.).
- Make material as relevant as possible to real-life situations.
- With written materials, use simplified syntax, short sentences, and also short paragraphs with the main subject first.

DEAFNESS

Case Study *Jill was a community health educator who had been asked to present a one-hour workshop on safer sex to a group of 30 new students at a local community college. The organizer had mentioned the possibility that one or two students who were either deaf or hard of hearing might attend the workshop. Jill gave the matter little further consideration, feeling that if the students did attend they could be seated at the front of the room and that she would attempt to speak louder and enunciate more clearly. Two deaf students did indeed attend, and after seating them in the front row Jill proceeded with the workshop, taking great care to speak loudly and clearly, facing the deaf students as much as possible. Part of the workshop included a short videotape on safer sex practices, and when the two deaf students left the room five minutes into the film, Jill supposed that the students had been offended by the explicit nature of what they had seen. Jill completed the workshop oblivious to her mistaken assumptions and beliefs.*

Jill was fortunate enough to have gained the information that deaf students might be attending her workshop *before* the event took place. Had she done some basic research into the deaf population, Jill could have avoided some very basic mistakes. Her first thought should have been to find out if an interpreter was needed and, if so, seek help in making such an arrangement. The presence of an interpreter could have alleviated the whole problem. Jill also subscribed to the myth that if you speak loudly and clearly enough, a deaf person will understand you. As this section of the chapter will describe, lip reading is not an easy or efficient means of comprehension for the vast majority of deaf or hearing-impaired people. Jill made the assumption that the deaf students left during the videotape because of its sexually explicit nature. Although this could have been the case, a more obvious explanation would be that the students could simply not hear the narration and therefore had little understanding of what was occurring. This case study illustrates the need for a greater knowledge of special populations when planning health education interventions.

The deaf and hard of hearing are included in this chapter because they are truly minority populations in regard to language and culture. Many individuals might believe that people who are deaf or hard of hearing are exactly like hearing individuals, with the one obvious exception that they cannot hear. Is this a simplistic notion?

Here are some important questions that health educators must consider:

- Are the health needs of the deaf identical to the health needs of the hearing?
- Are the health knowledge levels of the deaf similar to the knowledge levels of the hearing?
- Is there any difference in health behavior between the deaf and hearing populations?
- How do knowledge levels, attitudes, and behaviors differ within the deaf and hard-of-hearing communities?
- Can health educators use the same methods of health education with deaf people as they do with hearing people?
- Can materials originally developed for hearing audiences be used effectively by deaf or hard-of-hearing audiences?

Before attempting to address some of these questions, it is essential for the health educator to understand at least a minimum of basic information related to deafness.

Deaf Culture

Like any true subculture or minority group, people who are deaf adhere to certain cultural norms which are passed on from one generation to the next. Most cultures pass on their culture within the family unit. However, the deaf community is unique in the way that its culture is perpetuated. Because 90 percent of deaf children have two hearing parents, only a minority of deaf individuals acquire their cultural identity and social skills in the home. The majority of deaf people learn about their culture in schools for the deaf, from other children, teachers, and houseparents (Gallaudet University, 1990).

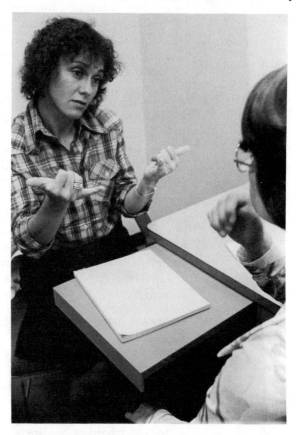

Study about the deaf culture has isolated and defined some characteristics and values of this culture. The following list was prepared by the National Academy, Gallaudet University, (1990):

1. Membership is based on deafness. Members have little or no hearing and define themselves as deaf.
2. There is a heavy emphasis on vision. American Sign Language, a visual mode of communication, is the language used within the deaf community. Members gain the vast majority of their information through their eyes and make a point of observing closely what is happening around them.
3. There is a specific set of social norms. Members follow certain social customs that are somewhat different from the general society. Among these are the following:

a. Members do not generally use their voices with deaf friends, but will with hearing friends. In fact, many members of the deaf community dissociate themselves from speech.
b. Members will wave, tap, or throw a small piece of paper to attract a person's attention.
c. Members use a variety of devices to replace ordinary alarm clocks, door bells, telephones, fire alarms, and so on.
d. Members place a strong emphasis on fostering and maintaining social ties within the community.

Social etiquette within the deaf community can be slightly different from that of the hearing community. For example, although the hearing culture generally considers staring to be rude, the deaf culture has no prohibition against this as staring is necessary for effective sign communication.

The two most common descriptors related to individuals who have a hearing loss are: **deaf** (cannot make use of residual hearing for the purposes of communication) and **hard of hearing** (can use residual hearing to assist in communication). The term *hearing impaired* is often avoided for two reasons. First, as with many other contemporary issues, deafness is influenced by its own political agendas and for some deaf individuals the term hearing impaired suggests that something is "broken." This descriptor therefore is viewed as inaccurate and undesirable by many in the deaf community. Second, this terminology does not usefully distinguish between "deaf" and "hard of hearing" and so has limited practical use. Keeping up with terms that are constantly changing is not easy, particularly when individual health educators live outside many of the cultures in which they are asked to work. However, educators should make every possible attempt to remain current in order to prevent offending individuals and to maintain crucial credibility.

Deafness can then be divided into two types: **congenital** (deaf from birth) and **acquired** (hearing at birth and becoming deaf later due to illness or accident). Acquired deafness can then also be divided into two subgroups: **prelingual** (becoming deaf before spoken language skills have been developed) and **postlingual** (becoming deaf after spoken language has been developed). See Figure 7-10.

Although at first glance these distinctions might seem subtle, they carry important implications for health educators as they approach program and material development. Those individuals who are congenitally or prelingually deaf will not have been exposed to the more typical methods of language development—repetition of the spoken word, constantly hearing words and sounds, and learning to read by hearing written words spoken aloud. As a result, congenitally

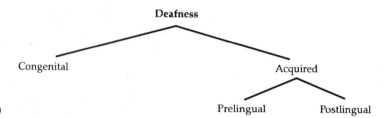

FIGURE 7-10

or prelingually deaf individuals may struggle with written and spoken English. Studies have shown that many deaf and hard-of-hearing students read at lower than normal grade levels for their age. One study estimated that approximately half of those individuals with hearing loss aged 18 and below read on less than a fourth grade reading level, while only 10 percent of 18-year-olds with hearing loss could read at above an eighth-grade level (Trybus and Karchmer, 1977). Unfortunately, many individuals mistakenly equate reading levels with intelligence, and health educators must be careful not to make this assumption. Although deaf and hard-of-hearing individuals might indeed read at lower grade levels, their IQ scores do not differ greatly from the hearing population. However, because of this lack of comprehension of both written and spoken language, communication can become a major barrier between deaf and hearing people . . . a barrier of which the health educator must be aware. Consideration must then be given as to how to overcome the barrier and effectively educate the deaf and hard-of-hearing communities about important health issues.

Look at the following examples of questions addressed to the health educator of a college for the deaf, via the computer/mail system (Morrone-Joseph, 1992). Take note of the wide range of linguistic ability between students.

Example 1

Hi . . . I want to know and curious. Suppose I did period on the end of the month at Feb . . . later in the two weeks and the sperm did in the vagina. But the period will come on the end of march . . . is it possible to be pregnant or not . . . please let me know this week so I can aware that . . .

Example 2

There are two questions I need to know . . . I am 20 years old female. Am I suppose to take pap-smear and breast check up? Or is it too early for me to test? Can you tell me the difference between the pap-smear and breast check up?

Example 3

Which days are safe to have sex without getting pregnant, without using any method of birth control? I was told that the time before ovulation is safe.

The three preceding examples clearly represent a cross section of written English levels. Although the writing levels are very different, it is interesting to note that these excerpts do effectively communicate their questions. It is often necessary to read for content and not be put off by "strange" English. The health educator must be aware that all deaf individuals are *not* the same, nor do they operate at identical levels of communication. This factor must be taken into account when developing and planning programs.

Once the health educator has become cogniscent of potential communication difficulties, he/she must also become aware of just how deaf individuals do communicate. Consider the following examples.

• If I speak in a clear manner, can deaf people read my lips?

In the previous case study, Jill made the common error of assuming that by speaking in a loud voice with clear enunciation everyone would understand her. The notion that a good way to communicate with the deaf is for them to read lips is a myth. There are many reasons why reading lips is fraught with problems, not the least of which is that the English language has many words that are pronounced the same but have very different meanings. One estimate places the proportion of words in the English language that are considered homophonous (pronounced the same) to be from 40 to 60 percent (Fitzgerald and Fitzgerald, 1980). In addition, factors such as distance from the speaker, people in between, poor lighting, head movements, and poor speech patterns all contribute to making lip reading an ineffective mode of communication. It is perhaps ironic to note that because they have developed speech and language through hearing, the best lip readers are in fact hearing individuals (Lowell, 1958).

Here are some examples of words with very different meanings but identical pronunciations:

MAIL	MALE
BAIL	BALE
PAIL	PALE
SAIL	SALE

• What if I were to take a quick course in sign language?

The idea that a hearing person could take a brief course in sign language and then effectively communicate with a deaf person is, unfortunately, as common as it is absurd! Imagine that in one month you will be expected to present a one-hour workshop on stress management to a group of 30 Russian immigrants who speak no English. In preparation for this, you will polish your presentation material and then take a short course in Russian! As absurd as this example might appear, the comparison is not inaccurate. Many people believe that deaf individuals communicate in a language that is essentially English which is simply signed. This is not the case. *American Sign Language (ASL) which is the native language of most culturally deaf Americans is not English.* ASL is a visually based language which bears little relationship to English, particularly in grammar and syntax. An interpreter who is signing for a deaf person is not always signing what is being said word for word. Rather, concepts and ideas are signed. Most cultures have a colloquial element to their language which all of us outside that specific culture find difficult to follow. People from the northern regions of the United States often find expressions unique to the South impossible to understand and vice versa. Also, many of us who have taken French in school or college have experienced the horrors of visiting Paris or other French cities only to be left wondering just what language those people were speaking! This problem with understanding colloqualisms is no less important for the deaf. Here are just a few examples of idioms that hearing health educators would probably not hesitate to use under normal circumstances, but might prove to be dysfunctional in the communication process with the deaf:

"pulling my leg"   "check it out"
"really hits home"   "sink or swim"
"cut the light"   "hooking up"

Health educators must be aware that many deaf individuals are in an almost identical situation to foreigners. English is a *second* language to them. This does not mean that they are less intelligent or able. It simply means that efforts to communicate will be compromised unless this factor is understood, taken into account, and measures are implemented that can alleviate this situation.

Sources of Information

As with health and deafness in general, very little data exist to assist the health educator in comprehending the world of deaf people. Do deaf individuals gain most of their health information in the same manner as their hearing peers, or do they follow an alternative route? One of the few studies that even considers this issue seems to suggest that deaf individuals do indeed tend to gather information and learn about health in a manner that is different from the typical hearing individual. Fitzgerald and Fitzgerald (1980) postulate that at least in the area of sexuality, deaf individuals, because of their lack of hearing, are denied access to all the usual agents that contribute to sexual knowledge and awareness. For example, young people in the hearing world gain information in a multitude of ways: talking with others, watching television, going to the movies, listening to the radio, attending classes, reading, listening to others, and, personal experience. The authors suggest that deaf individuals are denied the "incidental learning" opportunities which hearing individuals take for granted. Very few films are captioned, radio is not an option, limited language skills often make reading difficult, and even observations can lead to mistaken impressions. Fitzgerald and Fitzgerald (1980) relate the story of the 11-year-old deaf boy who on entering the classroom began to share his packet of Certs with the girls in the class. It quickly became obvious that the young man was expecting to be kissed by the girls in return for the Certs! The boy had seen the televised Certs commercial without the benefit of sound, had missed the verbal communication related to breath freshness, and had come to the very reasonable conclusion that anyone who was given a Cert was expected to respond with a kiss.

It is the contention of Fitzgerald and Fitzgerald (1980) that without the benefit of "incidental learning" deaf individuals might rely on personal experience more than their hearing counterparts. The pitfalls and dangers of learning through experience are obvious for most areas of health, but are particularly acute given the presence of AIDS, sexually transmitted diseases, and unintended pregnancy in the arena of contemporary sexuality. One of the few studies ever to compare the sexual knowledge, attitudes, and beliefs of deaf and hearing college students was performed by Grossman in 1972. This study reported that deaf individuals had less sexual knowledge, were more accepting of myths, and were more sexually active than their hearing peers. In addition to missing the benefits of "incidental learning," deaf individuals were also less likely to have the opportunity to attend formal sex education courses. Sexual knowledge for many deaf individuals therefore might often be derived from personal experience. A more recent study comparing the sexual knowledge, behavior, and sources of health information between hearing and deaf students reported some interesting significant differences between the populations (Sawyer, Desmond, and Joseph, 1994). Hearing students scored higher than deaf students on sexual knowledge items, although both groups of students demonstrated poor knowledge levels. Deaf students had received significantly less sex education at middle school, high school, and college levels and reported lower levels of sexual activity than their hearing counterparts. With regard to contraception, hearing students were much more likely to use the pill and condom, while deaf students reported a significantly higher incidence of withdrawal. There were no significant differences between the populations with respect to sexual activity (having had sexual intercourse at least once) and number of sexual partners. However, one particularly alarming difference between the populations was the greater reported incidence of forced sexual intercourse among deaf students than hearing students, 23 percent versus 14 percent. The authors comment on the obvious need for awareness and education around the issues of contraception, sexuality and communication, date rape, and sexual assault. They conjecture that the forced-intercourse data suggest evidence that hearing loss might sufficiently compromise sexual communication to the extent that date rape might occur. Finally, this study described differences in sources of health information between deaf and hearing students. Deaf and hard-of-hearing students were more likely than their hearing peers to use friends, workshops, and posters as sources of health information, while hearing students reported a significantly greater reliance on physicians.

There is insufficient research to demonstrate whether or not these types of findings could be generalized to other populations or even other areas of health. However, the limited research that is available does seem to suggest that the health education approach, which assumes that deaf individuals have the identical health interests, concerns, and behaviors as hearing people, might be a dangerously oversimplified perspective.

Teaching Methods and Strategies

Research into the effectiveness of health education teaching methodology for the deaf is scant. Tomasetti, Beck, and Clearwater (1983) compared the effectiveness of three different types of teaching methods used in cardiopulmonary resuscitation (CPR) education for both the hearing and deaf populations. Three deaf groups each received a different teaching method: standard course through signed instruction, standard instruction with a captioned videotape; and standard instruction with an uncaptioned videotape, signed by an interpreter. The hearing group which received a standard course, performed the best of all groups on psychomotor skills in an immediate posttest. However, in a four-month retest, the deaf group that had received a signed videotape performed better on psychomotor skills than any of the other groups, including the hearing group. It is not clear why the signed film may have been more effective than the captioned. One possibility might have been that poor reading levels compromised the ability to comprehend the captions, or perhaps the presence of an interpreter might have caused the students to identify with the instructor, thus influencing retention levels. An interesting addition to this study would have been a group that was instructed by a deaf health educator who was able to sign. Whether or not levels of learning are enhanced by having an educator from the same community as the group receiving the education is a subject worthy of further research. Yet this concept would seem no less important to the deaf community as it would in the African American or Hispanic populations. However, the limited number of minority health educators underlines the necessity for nonminority health educators to be educated about other cultures.

Beck and Tomasetti (1984) make an important contribution to health education teaching methodology and the deaf in their description of a safety training program. The authors describe the preparation for teaching a special population and the adaptations they made to successfully complete the workshop. Many of their recommendations are included in the following methods summary.

The almost complete absence of research related to the health education needs, knowledge, attitudes, and behavior of the deaf ensures that health educators working with this population must really give a great deal of thought to method selection. Hopefully, this section of the text will have helped the reader understand that not all deaf or hard-of-hearing individuals are alike, and some effort by the educator should be made to discover specific information about individuals and their needs. Here are some suggestions that might facilitate working with the deaf:

- Make no assumptions! Obtain as much information as you can about the individual(s)—hearing levels, reading levels, and so on.
- Come to terms with the idea that most presentations will require an interpreter. Forget about reading lips or speaking clearly . . . get an interpreter.[1] Some organizations will provide them, some deaf individuals will bring their own . . . make some inquiries! Often the expense or shortage of interpreters continues to limit deaf people's access to health education.
- Do not expect a deaf person to look at printed information and the interpreter at the same time. Allow time for the participants to look over any printed information before resuming the discussion.
- If you are using an overhead or slide projector or any method where the lights are dimmed, give some thought to the interpreter. Provide the interpreter with a side light or turn the lights back on between slides or transparencies to discuss information.
- Take a hands-on approach to learning. This move away from the lecture format necessitates less translation and, in addition, may be a more effective means to facilitate comprehension.
- Practical demonstrations rather than descriptions and handouts can facilitate learning when poor reading comprehension levels exist. Use models and pictures.

---

[1]The Americans with Disabilities Act (ADA) was initiated in 1988 and provides civil rights protections to persons with disabilities. It is comparable to legislation in force to protect women and minorities. The act protects individuals with disabilities from discrimination and states that physical and communication barriers must be removed. Reasonable accommodation must be made for all persons with disabilities (West, 1991). To that end, presentations performed by public agencies (e.g., state, local, and community) must provide and pay for interpreters if requested. In addition, private agencies (e.g. a health maintenance organization) must also provide and fund any reasonable accommodation, including an interpreter, if requested.

Myths About Deafness

Like all minority groups, deaf people suffer from stereotyping by many who do not know and understand them. A number of myths about deaf people circulate widely in our society and get in the way of understanding between hearing and deaf people.

MYTH: All hearing losses are the same.
FACT: The single term deafness covers a wide range of hearing losses that have very different effects on a person's ability to process sound and thus to understand speech.

MYTH: All deaf people are mute.
FACT: Some deaf people speak very well and clearly; others do not because their hearing loss prevented them from learning spoken language. Deafness usually has little effect on the vocal chords, and very few deaf people are truly mute.

MYTH: People with impaired hearing are "deaf and dumb."
FACT: The inability to hear affects neither native intelligence nor the physical ability to produce sounds. Deafness does not make people dumb in the sense of being either stupid or mute. Deaf people, understandably, find this stereotype particularly offensive.

MYTH: All deaf people use hearing aids.
FACT: Many deaf people benefit considerably from hearing aids. Many others do not; indeed, they find hearing aids to be annoying and choose not to use them.

MYTH: Hearing aids restore hearing.
FACT: Hearing aids amplify sound. They have no effect on a person's ability to process that sound. In cases where a hearing loss distorts incoming sounds, a hearing aid can do nothing to correct this and may even make the distortion worse.

MYTH: All deaf people can read lips.
FACT: Some deaf people are very skilled lip readers, but many are not. This is because many speech sounds have identical mouth movements. For example, *p* and *b* look exactly alike on the lips.

MYTH: Deaf people are not sensitive to noise.
FACT: Some types of hearing loss actually accentuate sensitivity to noise. Loud sounds become garbled and uncomfortable. Hearing-aid users often find loud sounds, which are greatly magnified by their hearing aids, very unpleasant.

MYTH: Deaf people are less intelligent.
FACT: Hearing ability is unrelated to intelligence. Lack of knowledge about deafness has often limited educational and occupational opportunities for deaf people.

MYTH: Deaf people are alike in abilities, tastes, ideas, and outlooks.
FACT: Deaf people are as diverse in their abilities, tastes, ideas, habits, and outlooks as any other large group of people.

- Films should be captioned or an interpreter used. Here again, the absence of good, captioned materials continues to be a major problem in program delivery.
- The use of games as a teaching method can be an effective way to involve participants in an interactive manner.
- Be aware that programs might take more time with a deaf audience and allow for this difference. This allows individuals to feel less pressure and permits the educator to reiterate and consolidate important points and to go over issues requiring more complex levels of comprehension.
- Never ask "Do you understand?" The likely response will be an affirmative nod of the head. Always use the "check back" technique, asking for a review of information understood.

Helpful Tips for Speaking[2]
- Face the deaf person.
- Maintain eye contact with the deaf person.
- Be sure that there is a light source in front of you.
- Speak slowly and clearly.
- Do not exaggerate your mouth movements.
- Keep objects/hands away from your mouth.
- Isolate or emphasize key words when appropriate.
- Give the deaf person as many visual cues as possible.
- Consider your choice of words carefully.

[2]These tips were developed for use by health professionals by The National Academy, Gallaudet University, 1991. Reprinted with permission.

Helpful Tips for Communicating through Writing/ Drawing[2]

- Keep your writing brief and to the point.
- Look for meaning in the deaf person's message; ignore any grammatical errors.
- When appropriate, use a drawing in addition to your written message.
- Use open-ended questions.
- Face the deaf person after you have written your messages and ask for a communication check.
- Often, requesting that the deaf person rephrase what he/she has understood is the best way to identify and prevent potential misunderstandings.

Helpful Tips for Working with an Interpreter

- Stand or sit close to the interpreter.
- Place graphics or models near you and the interpreter.
- Speak at a reasonable pace.
- Look at deaf person(s).
- Address deaf person(s) directly. Do not say to the interpreter, "Tell her . . ."
- Leave time for the interpreter to finish.
- Adjust lighting appropriately.
- Allow time for the deaf person(s) to ask and respond to questions.
- Say only what you want interpreted; remember that it is the interpreter's job to interpret everything you say and everything the deaf person signs.

EXERCISES

1. Consider the previous case study where Monica's presentation to the Mexican American women went so poorly. You have been asked to perform the same one-hour workshop for middle-aged Mexican American women on the importance of having a regular pelvic exam. Take into account the features of this population and design a presentation plan (including behavioral objectives) that you think would be appropriate.

2. You have been asked to present a program on HIV/ AIDS to an African American youth group (approximately 20 boys and girls aged 14 to 16 years). Make a list of strategies/methods that you feel might be successful with this group (keeping in mind what your objectives might be). Then select *two* of the possible methods and justify their inclusion in your program.

3. A group of deaf college students (approximately 15 male and female students aged 19 to 23 years) has requested a speaker on birth control. You have been

given the assignment. With your new-found knowledge of people who are hearing impaired or deaf, describe the steps you would take to plan for this presentation. Then list some presentation methods related to contraception education that might be appropriate with this group.

4. You are teaching a combination ninth- and tenth-grade high school health education course. You have been informed that 3 of the 25 students are special education students. Describe the steps you would take to accommodate these students in your course, both in preparation for teaching and during individual classes. (You can either respond in general terms or select specific learning disabilities.)

5. Jennifer, one of the students in your seventh-grade health education class, is visually impaired. Describe the steps you would take to discover the extent of the impairment and then make some suggestions as to how you would accommodate Jennifer in your class.

SUMMARY

1. Health educators need to have a good working knowledge of non-majority populations, including important information such as basic demographics and health problems unique to specific populations.
2. All individuals within minority populations are not the same. Appropriate methods of presentation must be considered to optimize the effectiveness of the program. Health educators can consult the minority individuals themselves or ask people within the community to suggest some effective methods of presentation.
3. There is very little available research data on the health needs and ways of addressing special populations. Optimally, health educators who themselves are members of the minority population are likely to be more effective than "outsiders." However, the availability of such educators is not a reality, and nonminority health educators will need to adequately prepare themselves to work with minority populations.
4. Health educators will need to familiarize themselves with the laws relating to the provision of services for the disabled.
5. As the trend to mainstream disabled individuals continues, the health educator is more likely to have to be prepared to devise presentation methods which will optimally include these individuals in the learning process.
6. Health educators will need to familiarize themselves with available resources specifically designed to meet the needs of minority populations.

REFERENCES

Aukerman, R. 1972. *Reading in the Secondary Classroom.* New York: McGraw-Hill.

Beck, K. H., and J. A. Tomasetti. 1984. Safety training for the deaf. *Professional Safety* (May):20–23.

CDC. 1992. *HIV/AIDS Surveillance.* Atlanta: Public Health Service.

Clements, S. D. 1966. Minimal brain dysfunction in children: Terminology and Identification, phase 1 of a three phase project. Public Health Service Bulletin no. 1415. Washington, DC: U.S. Department of Health, Education, and Welfare.

Cratty, B. J. 1971. *Movement and Spatial Awareness in Blind Children and Youth.* Springfield, IL: Charles Thomas.

Ellerbrock, J. V., T. J. Bush, Me. E. Chamberland, and M. J. Oxtoby. 1991. The epidemiology of women with AIDS in the U.S. 1980–90. *Journal of the American Medical Association* 265(22):2971–2975.

Federal Register (Part III). Washington, DC: Department of Health, Education, and Welfare, December 29, 1977, 42 (65083).

Federal Register (Part IV). Washington, DC: Department of Health, Education, and Welfare, August 23, 1977, 42 (163).

Fitzgerald, D., and M. Fitzgerald. 1980. Sexuality and deafness—An American overview. *British Journal of Sexual Medicine* (September):30–34.

Galludet University. 1990. *Deaf Culture.* Handout prepared by College for Continuing Education, National Academy. Washington, DC.

Goldstein, H., C. Arkell, S. C. Ashcroft, O. L. Hurley, and M. S. Lilly. 1975. In *Issues in the Classification of Children,* edited by N. Hobbs. San Francisco: Jossey-Bass.

Gordon, S. 1973. *The Sexual Adolescent,* North Scituate, MA: Duxbury.

Grossman, S. 1972. Sexual knowledge, attitudes and experiences of deaf college students. Unpublished Master's Thesis. George Washington University.

Haight, S. L., and D. D. Fachting. 1986. Materials for teaching sexuality, love and maturity to high school students with learning disabilities. *Journal of Learning Disabilities* 19(6):344–350.

Hammill, D. D., and N. R. Bartel. 1978. *Teaching Children with Learning Disabilities and Behavior Problems.* Boston: Allyn and Bacon.

Harlan, L. C., A. B. Bernstein, and L. G. Kessler. 1991. Cervical cancer screening: Who is not screened and why? *American Journal of Public Health* 81(7):885–890.

Jones, J. 1981. *Bad Blood: The Tuskegee Syphilis Experiment—A Tragedy of Race and Medicine.* New York: Free Press.

Lowell, E. L. 1958. *John Tracey Clinic Research Papers III–VII.* Los Angeles: John Tracey Clinic.

Lowenfeld, B. 1962. Psychological foundations of special methods of teaching blind children. In *Blindness,* edited by P.A. Zahl. New York: Hafner.

Mandell, C. J., and E. Fiscus. 1981. *Understanding Exceptional People.* St. Paul: West Publishing.

Meyen, E. L. 1978. *Exceptional Children and Youth.* Denver: Love Publishing.

Morrone-Joseph, J. 1992. Personal files. Gallaudet University, Washington, DC.

Myers, E., D. Ethington, and S. Ashcroft. 1958. Readability of Braille as a function of three spacing variables. *Journal of Applied Psychology* 42:163–165.

National Commission on AIDS. 1990. Hearings on HIV disease in the African American communities.

Parran, T. 1937. *Shadow on the Land: Syphilis.* New York: Reynal and Hitchcock.

Report of the Secretary's Task Force on Black and Minority Health. 1985. U.S. Department of Health and Human Services, Washington, DC.

Sawyer, R. G., S. M. Desmond, and J. Joseph. 1994. A comparison of sexual knowledge, behavior and sources of health information between hearing and deaf university students. *Journal of Health Education* (in press).

Sharon, L. M. 1992. Assessing the AIDS education needs of black women in an urban epicenter for HIV infection: A descriptive analysis. Unpublished Master's Thesis. University of Maryland.

Thomas, S. B. and S. C. Quinn. 1991. The Tuskegee syphilis study, 1932–1972: Implications for HIV education and AIDS risk education programs in the black community. *American Journal of Public Health* 81(11):1498–1505.

Tomasetti, J. A., K. H. Beck, and H. E. Clearwater. 1983. An analysis of selected instructional methods on CPR retention competency of deaf and non-deaf college students. *American Annals of the Deaf.* (August):474–478.

Trybus, R. J., and M. A. Karchmer. 1977. School achievement scores of hearing impaired children: National data on achievement status and growth patterns. *American Annals of the Deaf Directory of Programmes and Services* 122:62–69.

U.S. Census. 1990. U.S. Department of Commerce News Release, June 12, 1991, CB 91-215, Washington, DC.

West, J. 1991. *The Americans with Disabilities Act: From Policy to Practice.* New York: Milbank Memorial Fund.

Controversial Topics

Entry-Level Health Educator Competencies Addressed in This Chapter

Responsibility I: Assessing Individual and Community Needs for Health Education

Competency A: Obtain health-related data about social and cultural environments, growth and development factors, needs, and interests.

Competency C: Infer needs for health education on the basis of obtained data.

Responsibility III: Implementing Health Education Programs

Competency B: Infer enabling objectives as needed to implement instructional program in specified settings.

Competency C: Select methods and media best suited to implement program plans for specific learners.

Responsibility IV: Evaluating Effectiveness of Health Education Programs

Competency C: Interpret results of program evaluation.

Competency D: Infer implications from findings for future program planning.

Responsibility VII: Communicating Health and Health Education Needs, Concerns, and Resources

Competency A: Interpret concepts, purposes, and theories of health education.

Method Selection in Health Education

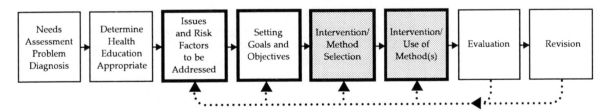

Needs Assessment Problem Diagnosis → Determine Health Education Appropriate → Issues and Risk Factors to be Addressed → Setting Goals and Objectives → Intervention/ Method Selection → Intervention/ Use of Method(s) → Evaluation → Revision

Heavy-bordered boxes indicate subjects addressed in this text; shaded boxes indicate subject(s) of current chapter.

Competency B: Predict the impact of societal value systems on health education programs.

Competency C: Select a variety of communication methods and techniques in providing health information.

Taken from *A Framework for the Development of Competency-Based Curricula for Entry Level Health Educators,* National Task Force on the Preparation and Practice of Health Educators, Inc., 1985. Reprinted by permission.

Case Study

Todd is a recently appointed health educator who has been asked to attend an upcoming PTA meeting to discuss the proposed implementation of a new sex education component in the school system's curriculum. Todd is a fervent believer in the necessity of sex education and puts together an impressive set of overhead transparencies which explains the curriculum. He intends to strengthen his presentation by citing national data on the prevalence rates of adolescent STDs, HIV infection, and unintended pregnancy. Todd's initial enthusiasm as he sees large numbers of parents at the meeting quickly turns to dismay as his presentation is largely ignored and some very vocal parents barrage him with questions and comments that he is not adequately prepared to answer: "Why do we need sex education in our town . . . our community doesnt have these problems," "These programs only increase sexual activity, don't they?" "Can you say that your program will reduce pregnancy rates?" "Why don't you teach some type of moral values?" "Why don't you stay out of this . . . this type of education should happen in the home, not the school." The meeting deteriorates into a shouting match, Todd is unable to make any progress, and the evening ends without any type of resolution.

Todd had allowed his own belief and enthusiasm in sex education to blind himself to the realization that many individuals are extremely opposed to the inclusion of sex education in the school curriculum. Setting up new programs is one of the most difficult facets of sex education, and health educators who are involved in any controversial programming should be as prepared as possible to defend against a sometimes vociferous opposition. As health educators we sometimes forget that, although responses to health concerns appear obvious to us, many individuals will greet our propositions with great skepticism. To that end, an ever-increasing role played by the health educator is that of politician, who must carefully prepare the ground for innovative ideas which might be met by strong public opposition. Support for programming must be carefully but consistently developed with influential community individuals, and opposition arguments must be anticipated and appropriate responses prepared.

After studying the chapter the reader will be able to:

- describe the potential problems inherent in planning, implementing, and evaluating programs concerning controversial topics
- provide a justification and rationale for implementing human sexuality and drug abuse prevention programs

- develop meaningful, realistic goals and objectives in human sexuality and drug abuse prevention programs
- describe the major concerns of sexuality education opponents
- list the most common mistakes that occur when presenting programs on sexuality education
- describe a diversity of approaches to sex and drug education

Key Issues

Goals and Objectives
Educational Philosophy
Educational Approaches
Opposition Concerns

Defending a Program
Effects of Programming
Resources

Health education today deals with many topics and issues that are sometimes construed as controversial. Obviously, sex education/human sexuality/family living comes immediately to mind when controversy is mentioned. A second major topic that has drawn criticism is that of alcohol and other drug education, and in fact almost any health topic can become controversial!

Because of the focus of this text, this chapter will concentrate mainly on sex education as an example of how to anticipate and minimize potential controversy. However, the health educator should be aware that even the areas within health education that appear at first glance to be benign are sometimes fraught with problems. Nutrition, particularly when concerned with dieting, has become an area that can stir emotions, and achieving a concensus about weight management is often very difficult. Also, the topic of death and dying is considered by many to be sufficiently sensitive that the home is the only place to deal with the issue.

BRIEF HISTORY

Although an in-depth historical analysis is beyond the scope of this text, it is interesting to note that drug education and sex education seem to have followed a very similar evolutionary direction when considering the development of strategies and methods of education. In the 1960s when many of the first sexuality and drug education programs were being implemented, the focus was clearly on disseminating factual information. The rational but simplistic triad of knowlege, attitude, and behavior was being routinely utilized . . . the hypothesis being that if we give individuals the "facts" (knowledge), then their attitudes will change for the better, and ultimately the individuals will cease their risky and dangerous health behaviors. This type of approach then dictated that the methods of educating about these subjects would take a biological/physiological direction. It is interesting to note that as long ago as 1919 the U.S. Government

Printing Office published a text entitled *A High School Course in Physiology in Which the Facts of Life Are Taught* (Means, 1962). There is no need to guess the method utilized in this approach to sexuality! In the drug area nearly 20 years later, the element of fear was added to the educator's arsenal in the form of a new film intended to depict the evils of marijuana use. The now classic 1936 film entitled *Reefer Madness* showed how paragons of normalcy could be transformed into crazed perpetrators of rape and murder after a single exposure to marijuana (Anderson, 1973). Although this type of hysterical approach can be viewed as ridiculous by today's more sophisticated youth, elements of this method still survive today as health educators struggle to stimulate just the right amount of anxiety (Taqi, 1972)!

In more contemporary times, health educators began to realize that facts alone would not change human behavior. Sex education in the form of "plumbing" which stressed biology and drug education which focused on pharmacology seemed to have little relevance and effect on the lives of young people. The trend that seems to characterize contemporary methods in both drug and sex education is that of decision making. Most of the newer curricula, although still including factual information, tend to focus on the more abstract practice of decision making. For example, in drug education a plethora of school-based programs have been developed which stress the skills of saying "No" to drugs, and where students actively learn how to resist the

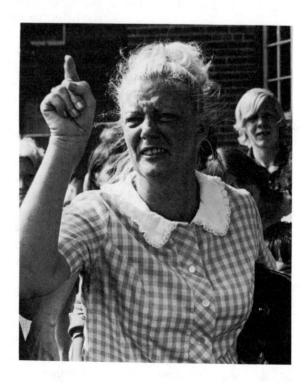

pressures to use drugs (Botvin, 1983; Battjes, 1985). One example of a much utilized school-based drug education program is the DARE program. This program, adopted now in as many as 49 states, relies on the cooperation of specially trained uniformed police officers and combines factual information with a major emphasis on the resistance of societal and peer pressures to use drugs (Ringwalt, Ennett, and Holt, 1991). Students are actively encouraged to participate in the development and practice of measures of resistance. Methods and strategies with this type of program necessitate more innovative learning opportunities than the simple exchange of facts. However, there are studies of such programming that seem to suggest that this educational approach might hold at least some promise of a favorable outcome (Gersick, Grady, and Snow, 1988).

Sexuality education has traveled a similar road to drug education in its diversion from straight facts to individual and group process, incorporating decision making. The whole field of sexuality education has taken on a broader perspective, with more organizations involved in the process, more children being exposed to education at an earlier age, and the development of programs that address the emotional as well as the physical components of the issue (Greenberg and Bruess, 1981). Statistically, there does appear to have been an increase in the prevalence of sex education. In 1980 only 3 states mandated sex education, compared to 47 states in 1993 which require or *recommend* sex education (*Time*, 1993). Of course, these statistics cannot report how much of the recommended sexuality education actually occurs or describe the quality or amount of the teaching in this area. This increase in exposure to sexuality education remains well below the levels that most sexuality experts believe are needed to achieve minimally effective educational levels. For example, Popham (1993) suggests that for an AIDS education unit to have the slightest possible chance of influencing behavior, it must consist of a number of 3- to 5-hour instructional activities in the early grades, 10 to 15 hours of education in grades 9 or 10, followed by one or more 3- to 5-hour booster sessions after the main AIDS unit has been concluded . . . all, by the way, taught by the most talented, first-rate teachers. How do these minimal standards compare with common AIDS education practices in our public schools?

The AIDS epidemic is undoubtedly responsible for allowing sexuality educators to gain access to hitherto unreachable audiences, and most states and regions have mandated some compulsory AIDS education programming. Despite this temporary acceptance of the need for increased awareness, sexuality education continues to meet much opposition from individuals and groups who either oppose the approach taken by educators or feel that such education should not even exist. Health educators involved with human sexuality should at least acknowledge the strong possibility of individual and community opposition to such programming.

JUSTIFICATION OF PROGRAM DEVELOPMENT

Justifying and developing a rationale for program development is a crucial factor in gaining support and acceptance for new or continuing programs. When one takes a cursory glance at the scope of the problems related to sexuality and drug abuse, there would seem to be little argument against the necessity for program development. During the past decade, although there is evidence of a reduction in the use of illicit drugs, the following data from the 1991 High School Senior Survey (National Institute of Drug Abuse, 1991) should still be of major concern:

> 54 percent of high school seniors used alcohol in the past month.
>
> 75 percent of college students used alcohol in the past month.
>
> 30 percent of high school seniors reported at least one occasion of heavy drinking (five or more drinks in a row) in the past two months.
>
> 13.8 percent of high school seniors used marijuana in the past month.
>
> 14.1 percent of college students used marijuana in the past month.

Earlier surveys reported similar widespread use of the most popular drugs by this nation's youth:

> 70 percent of 12- to 17-year-olds in the United States have ever used alcohol.
>
> 37 percent of 12- to 17-year-olds have used alcohol in the past 30 days (National Institute of Drug Abuse, 1986).
>
> 12 percent of 12- to 17-year-olds have used marijuana in the past 30 days.
>
> 27 percent of 18- to 25-year-olds have used marijuana in the past 30 days (U.S. Department of Health and Human Services, 1984).

Despite a slowly moderating trend in adolescent drug usage, data describing the use of both legal and illegal substances would clearly indicate levels higher than most parents and educators would like.

Data chronicling the sexual behavior of young people is also difficult to ignore. The Youth Risk Behavior Survey of 1990 (Centers for Disease Control, 1991) paints an all too graphic picture of the sexual behavior of high school students:

> 54 percent of all students in grades 9 through 12 have had sexual intercourse.

39 percent of all students in grades 9 through 12 reported
having had sexual intercourse during the three months
preceding the survey.

The percentage of students ever having had sexual intercourse
increased steadily by grade level:

9th Grade	40 percent have had sex
10th Grade	48 percent have had sex
11th Grade	57 percent have had sex
12th Grade	72 percent have had sex

Obviously, a substantial number of young people who are sexually active translates into a significant potential for increased health
problems. Again, there is an abundance of available data which reflects
the problems inherent in widespread, often unsafe sexual activity.

Unintended Pregnancy

The United States leads the Western world in unintended pregnancy
rates. Compare the following pregnancy rates for women under 20
years of age (Jones, et al., 1986):

United States	96 per 1,000
Great Britain	45 per 1,000
Canada	44 per 1,000
France	43 per 1,000
Sweden	35 per 1,000
Holland	14 per 1,000

1 out of every 12 unmarried American teenagers becomes
pregnant every year; half of them carry the pregnancy to
term. (Trussell, 1988)

Sexually active American youth is at high risk for many sexually
transmitted diseases and in fact:

Nearly 86% of all cases of sexually transmitted diseases and
AIDS occur among persons aged 15–29 years. (Centers for
Disease Control, 1992)

Despite any amount of persuasive information that clearly points
to the fact that American youth has a problem with both alcohol, and
drugs and sexuality issues, the health educator should not be surprised when individuals and groups do not share his/her vision of
the situation. Opponents of education around these issues may acknowledge that a national problem exists, but they tend to see the
problem in a vacuum . . . one that does not involve their particular
family. To that end, when beginning a program, the cooperation of
local experts and respected community leaders who can speak force-

fully in favor of programming is absolutely essential. Also, in addition to national statistics, the health educator should make a concerted effort to obtain local data which can be used more effectively to personalize an issue to specific communities.

DEVELOPING GOALS AND OBJECTIVES FOR SEXUALITY EDUCATION

One of the most difficult and sometimes dangerous components of sexuality education is developing meaningful, useful, and attainable objectives. Just what will the program accomplish? What will happen to the students after they experience such a program? Developing objectives in this area can be dangerous because the opponents of sexuality programming are often looking for possible ammunition with which to challenge the legitimacy of sex education. Reasonable, achievable objectives must be formulated; otherwise the health educator will be literally ensuring failure. For example, at first glance the following behavioral objective for a high school sexuality class does not seem unreasonable:

> As a result of a recently developed sex education class, there will be fewer pregnancies at All American High School.

In the community setting an objective for HIV education might look like:

> Following a two-hour presentation on safer sex, the participants will report higher levels of condom usage.

In both cases the objectives developed are almost certainly doomed to failure.

School   In isolation, very few human sexuality courses have ever been effective enough to significantly reduce the rates of unintended pregnancy. Therefore, if an objective is written to reduce such rates and no decrease occurs, then the objective has not been reached and many will judge the class to be ineffective . . . a failure. Reducing overall pregnancy rates might be a sound *goal* of any sexuality class and as such should be included. Decreased pregnancy rates is not a reasonable, attainable objective under these conditions.

Community   The possibility that condom usage will increase significantly after a two-hour presentation is almost nonexistent! As with most behaviors related to sexuality, condom usage is a complex psychosexual dynamic which is unlikely to be influenced in such a short period of time. If increased condom usage is written as an objective, then the likelihood of failure, or not achieving the objective, is almost certain. Again, increased condom usage might be a realistic *goal* to set, but under the present conditions a very unrealistic behavioral objective.

So what are some reasonable objectives that can be developed in sexuality education? Some educators have made a definite attempt to avoid the pitfalls outlined previously by purposely designing objectives that are *not* easily measurable. For example, Kirby, Alter, and Scales (1979a) suggest the following objectives:

> to provide accurate information about sexuality
> to facilitate insights into personal sexual behavior
> to reduce fears and anxieties about personal sexual developments and feelings
> to encourage more informed, responsible, and successful decision making
> to encourage students to question, explore, and assess their sexual attitudes
> to develop more tolerant attitudes toward the sexual behavior of others
> to facilitate communication about sexuality with parents and others
> to develop skills for the management of sexual problems
> to facilitate rewarding sexual expression
> to integrate sex into a balanced and purposeful pattern of living
> to create satisfying interpersonal relationships
> to reduce sex-related problems such as venereal disease and unwanted pregnancies (Kirby, Alter, and Scales, 1979a, pp. 3–4)

The authors of these objectives have cast their net very wide in order to include most of the major facets they consider germane to sexuality education. Under the terminology used in this text, these "objectives" would be better characterized as "goals." These goals are obviously a far cry from objectives/goals that might have been generated for the "plumbing" sexuality course. The major advantage to this type of objective/goal is that the educator can promote very generalized aims, without being restricted to more narrow, specific, and quantifiable projections. This certainly facilitates the avoidance of developing objectives that are unreasonable and likely to remain unattainable. However, this same strength is often viewed by opponents as a definite weakness. If objectives/goals are developed without an eye to some type of evaluation, how is program effectiveness then determined? In times of economic difficulty, particularly in education, accountability has become a crucial factor in funding. As thorough and appropriate as the objectives/goals developed by Kirby, Alter, and Scales might be, most program developers would make an attempt to include objectives that relate to specific sexuality issues and that are quantifiable.

To that end, as in most disciplines, quantifiable behavioral objectives can be confidently written in the cognitive domain. A significant increase in knowledge is often the criteria for evaluating any classroom performance, and human sexuality is no exception.

Some examples of cognitive domain objective might include the following:

> The students will be able to list in order of effectiveness four methods of contraception, as described in class.

> The students will be able to describe three factors that might precipitate date rape, according to the film viewed in class.

These types of objectives are valid, easily measurable, and attainable. A sound, well-taught class/workshop should be able to achieve objectives like these without much difficulty.

Objectives in the affective domain are more difficult to achieve than their cognitive counterparts described previously. Nevertheless, affective domain objectives should be a reasonable inclusion when planning programs in sexuality. Given that the field of human sexuality has now expanded to be considered more than mere "plumbing," an attempt to consider affective concerns is crucial. One of the simplest ways to evaluate attitudinal changes is by using a pretest/posttest. Give the students/participants a short questionnaire before the workshop or unit and then have the individuals complete a similar questionnaire at the conclusion of the unit. This procedure, however, raises two important concerns: How valid is the instrument you are using? Will any changes in attitude that arise be only short term in nature? The first concern is of prime importance, but one remedy would be to use an already developed instrument with proven levels of reliability and validity. This is not always possible, but there is an increasing number of available instruments as more evaluation is performed in this field (Davis, Davis, and Yarber,1988). The second concern about short-lived effects on attitude change is also valid, and yet it would be unrealistic to assume that, as a result of a single unit or workshop, any changes would be long term. Only consistent follow-up programming would be likely to maintain attitude change, and that is not always possible. Health educators have to be prepared to take small gains where they can, and there is nothing wrong with the idea of "planting a seed." To that end, writing behavioral objectives that would address only immediate attitude change is not so unreasonable.

Some examples of affective domain objectives might include the following:

> As a result of the unit on AIDS, the students will demonstrate higher levels of perceived susceptibility to HIV infection.

As a result of the workshop on safer sex, participants will report a higher level of acceptance of using a condom.

Both of these examples reflect affective objectives, which are reasonable and attainable. AIDS education should include components that are intended to personalize the issue to students who fail to see themselves at risk, and one of the most important factors in attempting to increase condom usage is having individuals feel comfortable in accepting condom use. Both of these objectives are also measurable, and by using a pretest/posttest questionnaire educators can gain a sense of what might have been accomplished.

As discussed earlier, addressing specific behavioral objectives related to behavior change is a potentially dangerous undertaking, and this type of objective might be better written as a less specific program/unit goal. Given the extremely limited time students spend in a sexuality education classroom, or individuals spend in community workshops, it would not be fair or reasonable to expect changes in sexual behavior such that pregnancy rates or sexually transmitted disease rates dramatically declined. Should a student who has studied French once a week for 50 minutes during one semester be able to pass fluency tests? Incidentally, the French class was taught by the physical education teacher who had, after all, taken a two-day course in preparation for this teaching assignment! Sexuality educators should try to ensure that their programs are not evaluated by criteria not used to measure other courses. One way to avoid such unfair scrutiny, however, is not to write unreasonable behavioral objectives that could guarantee failure. One study investigating the goals of various school districts found the following:

- promoting rational and informed decision making about sexuality—94%
- increasing students' knowledge of reproduction—77%
- reducing the sexual activity of teenagers—25%
- reducing teenage childbearing—21% (Hofferth, 1981)

It is interesting to note that in this particular study, "plumbing" has been superseded by a decision-making focus and that much smaller percentages of school districts make mention of behavior change, even as goals.

OPPOSITION TO SEXUALITY EDUCATION

Since the inception of widespread sexuality education, opposition groups have attempted to discredit and, in many cases, remove existing programs. A long history of such opposition is beyond the scope of this chapter, and yet a knowledge of some of the major complaints

Even the rivers of ignorance contain clever crocodiles.
—Mohan Singh

might prove useful to those planning or maintaining programs. The same principles apply to any area of study.

Majority or Minority?

Many opponents of sexuality education would have us believe that they are in the majority . . . that most Americans oppose sexuality education. Objective barometers of this issue, various national polls, clearly demonstrate that the majority of Americans favor some form of organized sexuality education. One poll carried out in 1986 (Louis Harris and Associates, 1988) found that 85 percent of U.S. adults favored sexuality instruction in schools, up from 76 percent in 1975 (National Opinion Research Center, 1982) and 69 percent in 1965 (Gallup Poll, 1976). In addition, studies have demonstrated that a large majority of teachers are also in favor of sexuality education in schools (Forrest and Silverman, 1989). Evidently, opponents of some form of sexuality education have never been in the majority! Unfortunately, as with many other issues, the "squeaky wheel" gathers all the attention, disproportionate to the size of the group. The lesson is clear. Those people in favor of sexuality education should be proactive in order to maintain the gains made over the past 20 years and should not take for granted what has been achieved.

Sex Education Increases Sexual Activity

Perhaps the most common claim made by opponents of sexuality education is that such education will result in and encourage increased sexual behavior. Professional educators or even those of us whose memories stretch back to those halcyon days of our adolescence might

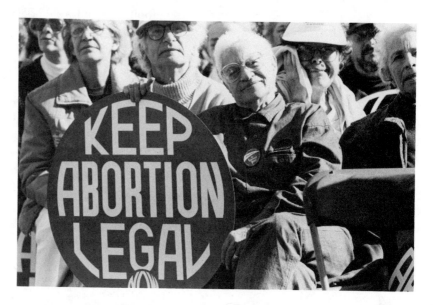

perhaps marvel at the notion that without sex education teenagers would not think about sex at all! As facile as that idea might seem, many opponents view sex educators as their child's first contact or thought about sex. Opponents view high rates of teen pregnancy, pandemic levels of sexually transmitted diseases (STDs), and, of course, the AIDS epidemic as clear evidence that sex educators have corrupted today's youth. Contrary to these subjective and sometimes hysterical beliefs, objective evaluation of sexuality programs does not point to increased sexual activity. Studies on the effects of sex education demonstrate that it increases knowledge levels of young people, increases the likelihood of contraceptive usage, and in some cases delays the onset of initial sexual intercourse. There is absolutely no empirical evidence that sexuality education encourages young people to initiate or increase sexual activity (Marsiglio and Mott, 1986; Dawson, 1986; Zelnik and Kim, 1982; Louis Harris and Associates, 1986). In addition, how many American teens actually receive regular, consistent dosages of sex education, sufficient to ruin their souls? A large, national study performed in the late 1970s placed that figure at no more than 10 percent (Kirby, Alter, and Scales, 1979b), and a more recent study showed a modest increase to a maximum of 15 percent (Sonenstein and Pittman, 1984). Pregnancies and pandemic levels of STDs can hardly be blamed on comprehensive sexuality education when only a small percentage of American youth are receiving such education! Figure 8-1 depicts the many influences related to sexuality experienced by young people today, and formalized sex education plays only one small part. Given that all schooling takes up only 8 percent of an individual's life, and that sex education is just one tiny fraction of that amount, the idea that sex education is responsible for a mountain of social ills is not grounded in reality (Finn, 1986).

FIGURE 8-1
Factors Influencing the
Lives of Young People

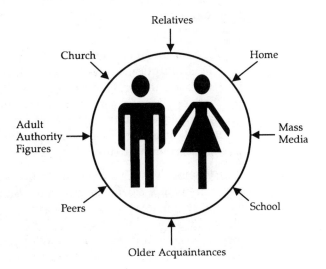

Sex Education Does Not Work

A major criticism leveled at sex education is that it simply does not work. Since sex education has become more common in schools in the United States, there has been little reduction in teenage pregnancy and rates of STD transmission. As discussed earlier, blaming sex education for exacerbating sexual problems is simply not logical when so few children receive any meaningful sex education. However, sex educators need to be able to defend against this type of criticism as programs come under closer scrutiny. Sex educators can help prevent some of this criticism by not promising more than can be realistically delivered. Be extremely cautious about writing behavioral objectives promising to reduce the rates of pregnancy and STDs . . . sex education on its own will not achieve these objectives. Individuals who claim that sex education does not work need to be "educated" to the reality that little or no meaningful sex education exists in our schools today and so it is unfair to expect a minimalistic approach to have any meaningful effects. Also, other subjects in school are not held to the same levels of outcome accountability as sex education. The most used example is social studies. Should schools abandon teaching about civics because fewer than 50 percent of the population votes in presidential elections and vast numbers of adolescents cannot name the vice president? Another study found that nearly one-half of the nation's 17-year-olds did not know that each state has two senators (National Assessment of Educational Progress, 1976)! Obviously, very few people would suggest that American schools discontinue teaching social studies because of these dismal findings, but the unfairness and disparity in how programs are evaluated need to be noted.

A more tangential but valid response to this criticism would be that the objectives of sexuality education are about more than just pregnancy, STD, and AIDS prevention. For example, the Sex Information and Education Council of the United States (SIECUS) defines sexuality as follows:

> Human sexuality encompasses the sexual knowledge, beliefs, attitudes, values and behaviors of individuals. It deals with the anatomy, physiology, and biochemistry of the sexual response system; with roles, identity and personality; with individual thoughts, feelings, behaviors, and relationships. It addresses ethical, spiritual, and moral concerns, and group and cultural variations.

Obviously, such a broad definition suggests an educational experience in which sexual health plays only one particular role. Even a cursory glance at the following position statement formulated by SIECUS to address sex education affords a good example of how education in this area is not simply concerned with sexual health.

There is something I don't know
that I am supposed to know
I don't know what it is I don't know,
and yet I am supposed to know.
and I feel I look stupid
if I seem both not to know it
and not know what it is I don't know.
Therefore I pretend I know it.
This is nerve-racking
since I don't know what I must pretend to know.
Therefore I pretend to know everything.
I feel you know what I am supposed to know
but you can't tell me what it is
because you don't know that I don't know what it is.
You may know what I don't know, but not
that I don't know it,
and I can't tell you. So you will have to tell me
everything.

—R.D. Laing

From: Knots (1972) Laing, R.D., Random House Inc., New York, NY. Reprinted by permission.

Sex Education Should Be Done in the Home

Many opponents of sex education vehemently state that sex is a private matter and children should be educated in the home by the parents. A sex educator would be foolish to deny such a claim, and indeed the previous statement prepared by SIECUS clearly endorses parental responsibility in this area. However, the fact remains that, although many parents do a wonderful job of educating their children about sexuality, some parents pass on harmful myths and partial truths, and some parents do nothing. The ideal sex education is one that begins at home and is then augmented by many individuals and agencies, one of which is the school. The reality of the situation is that for some children the *only* sexuality education they receive is performed by the school.

People Who Teach Sex Education Are Not Qualified

Unfortunately, this is one area where sexuality education does seem vulnerable to criticism. Although there are numerous well-trained, qualified individuals currently teaching human sexuality, there are also too many others who have unwillingly accepted responsibility for this area, lacking both enthusiasm and expertise. There is little or no consistency nationally in the type of preparation individuals receive to teach human sexuality. One of the few examples of an attempt to standardize sexuality education training is the American Association of Sex Educators, Counselors, and Therapists (AASECT) who developed standards for granting certification to sex educators. The Guttmacher Institute performed a large survey to identify who is teaching sex education in our schools (Guttmacher Institute, 1989). It is interesting to note that this study identified the greatest proportion of sex education teachers as primarily physical education specialists. Figure 8-2 indicates the breakdown by responsibility area. This study revealed that about 60 percent of sex education teachers are women, half are over 40 years old, and nearly half have been teaching sex education for at least eight years. The majority of these individuals have received some type of preparation to teach sex education, although any type of state or local certification in human sexuality education is rare. Thus a good proportion of sex education teachers are mature and experienced individuals who have received professional preparation. However, given that there is little quality control in the types of preparation available, school districts and individual schools would be very wise to ensure that any individuals who are asked to teach sex education have adequate training in this field and that they teach within the accepted curricular framework. To do any less than this would make a school and/or school district extremely vulnerable to complaint and criticism, ultimately jeopardizing an entire program.

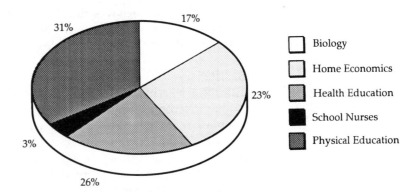

FIGURE 8-2
Sex Education Teachers
by Specialty

OBSTACLES TO TEACHING SEX EDUCATION

Although sexuality education has now existed for quite some time, and despite the fact that the AIDS epidemic has legitimized the need for sex education for at least some people, many obstacles still exist that impede the development and implementation of comprehensive programming. More than one in five sex education teachers report that they face curriculum limitations; a similar proportion report that they experience negative pressure from parents and community groups; one in three feel that their school administration is nervous about negative community reactions; and one in five believe that their school administrators do not support them (Guttmacher Institute, 1989). On the surface, with more states mandating AIDS education, it would seem that sexuality is now an accepted part of educational programming and that obstacles are diminishing. However, the concerns of the teachers mentioned previously clearly paint a different picture—a picture of an uneasy and potentially volatile truce between school administrators, who have to do *something* because of the new mandates, and the opponents of sexuality education, who are ever vigilant for mistakes that could provide ammunition for their cause. Often the result of such a situation is that the administrator, in an attempt not to offend anyone, restricts and dilutes the sexuality curriculum to the degree that it becomes ineffectual. Another way to effectively "lose" sex education is to have small segments taught in various classes by regular classroom teachers. This way state requirements are met and yet no one actually realizes that sex education took place . . . and given the level of expertise by many teachers unprepared in this area, sex education did not take place!

Peter Scales believes that there are five major barriers that sex educators must overcome now or in the future in order to make sexuality education flourish (Scales, 1989, pp. 172–176).

Barrier 1.
Taking a Narrow View of Sexuality Education

Within this context Scales describes how sex educators must avoid the temptation to "oversell" the impact of sexuality education. As described earlier, sex education in isolation cannot achieve major behavioral changes, and these changes should not be expected.

Sexuality education should not be evaluated solely on the basis of its short-term *measurable* impact. Instead, included in an assessment of the value of sexuality education should be a component of sex education's intrinsic value to the development of the total human being. This would necessitate an acceptance that sex education plays a fundamental role in defining a holistic viewpoint of "being educated."

Instead of a "back to basics" approach, Scales believes educators need to move forward in order to prepare children for a different and complex world. Children will need to develop critical thinking skills to cope with a new and challenging world environment.

Barrier 2.
Failure to Understand the Importance of Self-Efficacy

Although sex educators have historically held the opinion that self-esteem is pivotal in sexual decision making, Scales argues that perhaps a more relevant component for behavioral change is self-efficacy. However, Scales would argue that neither self-esteem nor self-efficacy can really be taught, so educators and policymakers should attempt through social action to create conditions in which self-efficacy can flourish.

Barrier 3.
Failure to Resolve the Role of Public
Schools as "Surrogate Parents"

Schools today are asked to do much more than the "three R's" of education. As we adapt to new demands and pressures, sexuality education must also change to contribute more to the students' broader education. Scales describes how sexuality education must go beyond mere pregnancy prevention and tackle issues of sexism, racism, homophobia and social action.

Barrier 4.
AIDS and the Decline of Pluralism

AIDS prevention of late has included a rather antisex message, which Scales argues is causing a decrease in a national acceptance of pluralism and diversity. Acceptance of different ideas and values is seen as a central premise to modern sexuality education, and Scales suggests that all sex educators, whether conservative or liberal, should strive to maintain a flexible and pluralistic approach to the field.

Barrier 5.
Inadequate Political Skills
Although the political savvy of sex educators has improved over the years, Scales sees much room for improvement in the three following areas: translating beliefs into budgets, setting the right agenda, and speaking for ourselves. These areas underline the importance of realizing that political battles are about resource allocation and that educators must translate ideas and beliefs into funding, that the "right agenda" is much more than just having greater numbers of better trained sex educators, and, finally, that sexuality education advocates must be proactive and not just allow others to say what they think advocates believe.

The observations of Scales are a far cry from the early concerns of sexuality educators and certainly reflect a wider and more visionary perspective of sexuality education. There is no doubt, however, that the politicization of issues such as abortion, contraception, AIDS, and sexual orientation will necessitate that teachers of human sexuality be continuously aware that their educational efforts will receive a unique form of public scrutiny. To that end, political awareness should now be considered a prerequisite for teachers involved in sexuality education.

There is no doubt that making mistakes while implementing a sexuality curriculum can have far more severe consequences than making errors in other subject areas. Even minor examples of poor judgment could compromise an entire program, particularly when administrators might exhibit little or no support for sexuality education.

AVOIDING TROUBLE

Gilbert (1979) believes there are 10 easy ways of getting into trouble when teaching sex education.*

1. Inadequate Knowledge and Background
Just as with any subject, an ill-prepared teacher or presenter will inevitably experience great difficulty in providing solid, correct information in a meaningful way. However, the implications of poor preparation in human sexuality are potentially disastrous for the recipients of the program, the teacher/facilitator, and the program itself. In the

---

*From "Easy Ways of Getting Into Trouble When Teaching Sex Education," *Health Education*, Sept/Oct 1979. Reprinted by permission.

school setting where the students are often immature and impressionable, being given incorrect information could lead to disasterous consequences for the students. Then the entire program is judged in the light of this obvious misinformation, the program very quickly loses credibility, and the next step is the abandonment of the program. Ideally, individuals teaching in this area should have the utmost preparation and strive to keep "current" in a field that is always changing. Pragmatically, particularly in the school setting, it is unlikely that this ideal situation will occur. Teachers are often coerced into teaching sex education and/or they have an interest in the area but have very little professional background. If programs are to survive, administrators must ensure that they select individuals who at least have an interest in the subject and that these individuals receive sufficient training to enable them to be effective. Teachers need to be able to attend continuing education workshops and courses that will keep them up to date on new information and teaching methods. Community health sexuality educators need to be no less qualified and prepared. The organizations they represent, whether they are private or public agencies, will be judged by the response to their presentations, and community groups can be every bit as critical and volatile as parent groups in the school setting. Whenever possible, school and community sex educators should not accept assignments for which they know they are unprepared . . . the damage could be irreparable.

2. Unrealistic Curriculum Goals and Objectives

As mentioned earlier, a major criticism by sex education opponents is that sex education simply does not work. To minimize such attacks, sexuality educators must be very prudent when designing course goals and objectives. Do not write behavioral objectives that are unrealistic. Most sex educators would laugh if a fellow educator wrote as an objective for a 10-week course that his students would discover a cure for AIDS! And yet some of these same sex educators will happily promise to miraculously reduce unintended pregnancy as the result of a once-a-week, 10-week sex education course. By all means write broad, generalized goals that might include pregnancy reduction or higher rates of condom usage. However, specific behavioral objectives, which must all be *measurable*, should be far more realistic and attainable. Objectives that promise knowledge gains, for example, are entirely appropriate. Sexuality educators should not promise what they have no hope of delivering.

3. Not Being Prepared to Defend the Program

Unlike other areas of school curriculum or community health topics, sexuality education is consistently placed under the microscope of scrutiny. Despite the publicity and awareness surrounding the AIDS epidemic, sexuality education remains in many communities a commodity to be either grudgingly tolerated or viewed with intense suspicion. Although studies mentioned earlier in this chapter clearly demonstrate that opponents of sexuality education are in the minority, these groups continue to be a voluble and persistent nuisance. Therefore both sex educators and administrators of such programs should be prepared to defend programming in the face of intense criticism. Preparation should include a knowledge of the major opposition arguments (these have not changed greatly over the years), a rebuttal to these arguments, a developed support system within the community to help bolster acceptance of the program, and a major effort to ensure that the sex educators are well trained and teaching within the accepted curriculum guidelines. Of course, not all criticism of programming will be irrational and unreasonable. Administrators should be honest enough to accept valid criticism and be prepared to alter program guidelines in an attempt to improve programming standards and overall quality.

4. Inappropriate Materials or Assignments

More ammunition for opponents of sexuality education and a very quick way to lose program credibility is for the sex educator to use inappropriate materials. The difficulty here is with the definition of "inappropriate." There may be nothing intrinsically wrong with the materials themselves, but it is the setting in which they are to be used that will determine their appropriateness. The school setting allows for less discussion than the community setting as most school districts have fairly strict policies about "sensitive" materials. A committee will preview a film or videotape and determine its acceptability. Of course, frustration occurs when the teacher feels that the material is acceptable and useful, but the committee in its infinite wisdom thinks otherwise! The teacher has little choice but to accept the committee's decision, other than perhaps approaching the committee members individually to lobby for their support and a possible re-review. Most school districts have a catalog or list of accepted materials which are well publicized and to which the area teachers must conform. The community health situation is much less regulated and if the sex educator is at all uncertain about the acceptability of his/her materials, then people living in, or familiar with, the targeted community should preview the materials and provide feedback before any presentations are made. If the community health educator is actually working as a guest speaker in a classroom, it is most important to ensure that materials and content are acceptable in that particular school.

Inappropriate assignments are obviously more relevant to school health, but could also occur in a community health environment. Asking students to visit a drug store to purchase condoms is one example of an assignment that would likely cause an uproar with many parents and school administrators. Giving the same assignment to a youth or church group in a community setting would also inspire a similar negative reaction. The point is that the assignment itself is perhaps not a bad one, but simply inappropriate in many settings. Problems like this can be minimized if the sexuality educator consults administrators or community leaders *before* the damage is done. Also, many of these problems would not arise if all or even most sexuality educators were professionally trained and adequately prepared (see item 1).

5. Using Materials Without Preview

Using materials without previewing them is never a good idea in school or community health. At least in the school situation, if the educator is using materials from the approved catalog the worst that could happen is the students will not understand the material or, more likely, will become incredibly bored! Of course, using nonapproved sexuality materials in the school with or without preview is grounds for dismissal so such an action could have severe implications. In the community setting, again where few regulations exist, the sexuality educator certainly needs to preview the materials to evaluate their appropriateness and usefulness. The sexuality educator needs to thoroughly evaluate the materials him/herself (see Chapter 5) and not fall into the trap of using something recommended by a friend or colleague. Once the sex educator has previewed the materials, having students or any intended audience also preview the materials can provide useful feedback. Educators can easily fall into the trap of assuming because we think materials are great that our audiences will feel the same way. Obviously, this is not always the case.

6. Inappropriate Guest Speakers

Just as certain materials will be deemed by communities and organizations to be "inappropriate," using guest speakers can potentially raise the same concerns. For example, if a school sex educator is fortunate enough to be able to explore sexual orientation as a topic, how will the school and community react if the teacher invites a homosexual or lesbian to speak to the class? How will the community church group react when the sex educator schedules a panel on AIDS which will include a bisexual, a prostitute, and a drug abuser who are all HIV positive? As valuable and educational as both these examples might be, are they worth potentially placing the programs in jeopardy? As stated before, experience in this field usually prevents this type of problem from occurring, but there are some simple safeguards the sex educator can take. In the school setting the teacher can check to see if there is a list of approved guest speakers already in existence. If not, or the desired speaker is not on the list, the teacher should consult a school administrator to seek official approval. In this way, if there is any fall-out following the guest speaker's presentation, the teacher has protected him/herself and the administrator will handle the conflict. In the community setting there will be few, if any, formal regulations. As with materials discussed previously, the community sex educator should consult a few community leaders in an attempt to solicit their opinions regarding the guest speaker. Individuals within the community setting will have a much more accurate reading on how their peers will react to certain types of speakers than will the health educator.

Regardless of the setting, the educator should always discuss with the speaker beforehand just what material the speaker is going to cover. Similarly to previewing audiovisual materials, ideally the educator should have heard the guest speaker present before extending an invitation. An important concern should not only be *what* the individual is going to say but *how well* he or she is going to say it! There are many health experts or other individuals who have important messages to send but who are such poor speakers that the value of their presence is minimized. In the school setting where attention spans are often very short, a stunningly boring speaker will quickly be "tuned out" regardless of the quality of the information.

7. Personal Bias in Teaching

All teachers and communicators have some types of biases, no matter how subtle. This is a crucial issue for sexuality educators to consider as biases related to so many sensitive issues could potentially cause major problems for the educator and overall program. For example, the sex educator who is "pro choice" on the volatile abortion issue and provides a one-sided and very subjective view of the issue can cause many problems. Obviously, those participants who would describe themselves as "pro life" will be greatly offended as perhaps would those individuals who are undecided. Many school sexuality education programs do not allow any discussion about abortion, but, for those that do, if the sex educator merely promotes his/her own subjective views, the school will quickly hear about it! Once again, sexuality educators must take great care not to do anything that might place the entire program at risk. There is nothing wrong with having personal biases, and there are very few human beings who have none! The important point, however, is that the well-prepared sexuality educator should be aware of and sensitive to his/her own biases and ensure that they do not influence how material is presented. At the risk of being redundant, the well-prepared and experienced sexuality educator should have achieved these higher levels of self-awareness.

8. Using Slang

For many students and participants in both the school and community settings, using correct clinical terms to describe reproductive anatomy and sexual behavior will be a new experience. The sexuality educator will play an important role in modeling and normalizing the use of correct terminology, particularly in the school setting. Because there are so many different cultures in the United States, slang terminology will be extremely varied; therefore if slang is used communication becomes very complicated. There is nothing wrong with addressing the slang issue early in the class or presentation, where "translations" can be made and the correct terminology established. But, for the sake of accuracy and consistency, correct terminology should be used whenever possible. Community health educators, when dealing with specific subcultures, might argue that correct terminology is only an unnecessary diversion, and to some extent that might be true. For example, when attempting to encourage condom usage among inner-city, minority intravenous drug abusers, to insist on using the correct terminology would seem overzealous and could quite possibly be dysfunctional. Community sexuality educators must therefore use their best judgment, attempting to use correct terminology whenever possible, but being sensitive to the possibility of exceptions.

9. Sharing Personal Sexual Experience

A more generalized term for this issue might be self-disclosure. How much of his/her own experiences does the sexuality educator share? At first glance this would appear to be a simple issue—the sexuality educator should *never* self-disclose any information. But perhaps we are defining *sexual experience* in too narrow a fashion. Look at the following examples and consider whether or not the disclosures are appropriate:

> A female sex educator while teaching about menstruation to a class of sixth-grade girls relates how she had felt about her own period beginning.

> A male sex educator while discussing relationships in a coed senior high school class describes how he had felt when his "first love" had ended the relationship.

> A female sex educator presenting a workshop for community youth on becoming sexually active describes her own fears of having sex for the first time when she was a teenager.

> A female sex educator describes her own experience with inorgasmia (inability to orgasm) to an adult community group interested in sexual dysfunction.

> A male peer sexuality educator during a workshop on date rape explains how he had previously had sex with a women after she had said "No."

Clearly, the gratuitous use of graphic depictions of personal sexual experiences has no place in sexuality education. However, as you consider the preceding examples, you might gain a sense that not all personal revelation in the area of sexuality needs to be viewed as negative and forbidden. There is no doubt that in many instances self-revelation by the educator places the participants at greater ease, thus encouraging more meaningful contributions. Self-disclosure allows the participants to perceive that the "expert" or educator is not so different from them and that the environment for participant disclosure is safe. Again, experience and training will help the educator avoid trouble, and a good rule of thumb, particularly in the school setting, is that if there is any doubt as to the appropriateness of the disclosure . . . then do not do it! Do not feel duty bound to answer every question that you are asked.

For example, while discussing decision-making skills related to becoming sexually active a student asks, "How old were you when you had sex for the first time?" How should you respond? This is probably not an appropriate question, nor an appropriate issue about which to self-disclose. A possible reply might be:

> That is a personal issue which I would prefer to remain private. I will respect your privacy about such issues and I won't ask you personal questions, and I'd be grateful if you would respect me in the same way.

In the school setting students will always ask inappropriate questions . . . that is their job! The sexuality educator therefore must always be alert to possible problems that might arise from impulsive self-disclosure and be prepared to politely, but firmly, decline to answer certain questions.

10. Behind Closed Doors

All individuals who work with youth are placed in a position of trust—a trust that they will not abuse their positions of power to take advantage, in any way, of the young person. To many individuals sexuality educators are a little "suspect" anyway, as a result of the sensitive nature of the material that they teach. Ironically, to students, in particular, the sexuality educator is often viewed as a warm, caring individual and certainly one of very few adult figures with whom they could discuss personal concerns and problems. There is no question that in the school setting good, effective sexuality educators will frequently be consulted by students on many diverse issues. Some of the issues may involve simple clarification of fact; others may include student disclosure of unintended pregnancies, STDs, and even sexual abuse. There is no simple formula or recipe for dealing with these issues, but the sexuality educator must balance an honest and genuine concern for the student with an awareness of the dangers to his/her professional reputation and the integrity of the entire program. To minimize the potential for problems, do not meet students in "private places" outside class. There is nothing wrong with having a private conversation, but have it in an office or classroom, where the wrong assumptions are less likely to be made. If a student wants to relate something in confidence, explain that there are certain issues that the law requires an educator to report, child sexual abuse, for example. Many sexuality educators, because of the types of individuals they are, can provide an incredibly important outlet for student concerns and this invaluable service should not be compromised. However, the educator needs to be aware of the potential dangers and misinterpretations that may develop, and take preventive measures to avoid such problems.

Mary Krueger (1993) provides an interesting and thought-provoking list of *assumptions to avoid* when discussing sex education, particularly in the classroom. Some of the following ideas may seem obvious, but they are definitely worthy of our attention:

1. **All students come from traditional families.** With divorce rates of over 50 percent, the "traditional" family is not necessarily the norm. Do not make any assumptions about home situations.
2. **All students are heterosexual.** Whatever the rate of homosexuality/bisexuality in our society, alternate sexual orientations certainly exist. Include all segments of society in the educative process.
3. **All students are sexually involved.** Not all young people are sexually active, so do not present information as if being a virgin is somehow abnormal and undesirable.
4. **No students are sexually involved.** Alternately, do not make an assumption that *no one* is sexually active, which often leads to an emphasis on abstinence . . . a concept to which some individuals might have some difficulty relating.
5. **All students' sexual involvements are consensual.** Given the prevalence of sex abuse in our society, particularly with school-aged children, an educator should assume that some students/participants are experiencing or have experienced sexual exploitation. Sexuality educators can expect to be approached about this type of issue and will hopefully be receptive and helpful in giving aid and advice.
6. **Students who are "sexually active" are having intercourse.** There are many different forms of sexual behaviors that do not include penis/vagina intercourse. Therefore discussion should not be confined to preventing pregnancy and STD/HIV transmission, but should incorporate other behaviors such as masturbation, mutual masturbation, oral sex, petting, and kissing and hugging.

CURRENT ISSUE: ABSTINENCE VERSUS RESPONSIBILITY

Like all topics in health education, particularly controversial issues such as human sexuality or drug education, nothing remains static and different approaches to education come and go. One of the current dilemmas in approaching sexuality education in both the school and community can be categorized as abstinence versus responsibility. Should we teach young people from the perspective that if only they would remain or become sexually abstinent, then they would not have to be concerned with sexual problems? Or should we take a more pragmatic approach and acknowledge that, whether adults like it or not, young people are sexually active and therefore we need to talk about sexual responsibility. There is no question that much of education is politically motivated and that, during the past 12 years of conservatism, the message has clearly been one of abstinence, beautifully depicted in the slogan, Just Say No! Nearly 10 years ago, Congress appropriated money for the development of abstinence education programs, and since then abstinence-based programs like *Sex Respect* have been adopted in several states (*Wall Street Journal, 1992*). Many school districts have adopted such programs in the belief that traditional types of programming have not been effective. Students are schooled in the virtues of chastity and are taught that premarital sex can lead to emotional turmoil, disease, pregnancy, and guilt. The *Sex Respect* curriculum includes a chart which marks a prolonged kiss as "the beginning of danger" and the course uses the slogan, No Petting if You Want to be Free (*Wall Street Journal, 1992*). Students are encouraged to create bumper stickers which read, Control Your Urgin'/Be A Virgin, and suggest alternative activities to sex, such as bicycling, dinner parties, and playing Monopoly (*Time 1993*). Opponents of abstinence curricula argue that such an approach does little but cause extremely negative ideas about sex. In addition, because such curricula do not include information about preventing pregnancy, HIV infection, and STDs, they may have disasterous effects on sexual behavior.

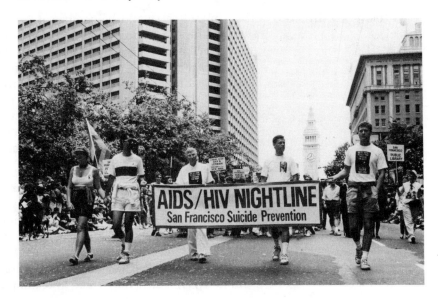

In 1993 Planned Parenthood of Northeast Florida, and local citizens in Duval County, Florida sued the local school board for rejecting a broad-based sex education curriculum in favor of an abstinence-only program from Teen-Aid, of Spokane, Washington. Also, in Shreveport, Louisiana, a district judge ruled that the abstinence-only text of *Sex Respect* was biased and inaccurate, ordering its removal from the Caddo Parish junior high schools (*Time* 1993). Most sexuality educators take a middle position on this issue and believe that abstinence should certainly be included in comprehensive sexuality programs. However, to omit information to assist those students who will not remain abstinent might be viewed as foolhardy and dangerous. Recently trained health educators who will be teaching sexuality education in schools should take a long and careful look at the curriculum to be sure just what it is they are being asked to teach!

ESTABLISHING A CURRICULUM OR PROGRAM IN A CONTROVERSIAL AREA

Whether you are establishing a potentially controversial program in sexuality, drug education, nutrition, or whatever subject matter, it is important to follow procedures that will minimize complaints and address the standards of the environment in which you are working. Following procedures previously discussed in conducting a needs assessment will be very important. Another step that should be considered is the two-committee (writing and advisory) structure. The use of two such committees is an important tool in dealing with diverse points of view.

Writing Committee

This committee should be composed of professionals in the area of study. If this is a school curriculum, this committee should be made up of employees of the school district only. The size is very important since the charge of this committee is to write or adapt materials for use. Therefore it is recommended that the committee never exceed eight members with the optimal size being six members. The writing committee has final say on what is submitted to the supervising board for approval. School districts generally have a school board and health agencies have some type of board of directors.

Advisory Committee

This committee is to be composed of citizens from the community who have an interest in the subject matter to be addressed. The charge is to react to materials developed by the writing committee and to make suggestions. This can be a large committee since it is advisory in nature and reacts to the work of the professional committee. Care should be taken in membership to ensure proportionate representation of the community. It is generally a good idea to place a representative of the opposition on the committee. This will demonstrate there is nothing secret and there is a willingness to listen to all sides. However, it is important not to let this person or group dominate the discussions. Care should be taken to appoint a strong chair and representative membership so the opposition voices are not dominating. This is a lay advisory group and might include ministers or other religious leaders, physicians and other appropriate members of the medical community, parents, community leaders, police, and community and organization leaders.

EXERCISES

1. You have been asked by your rather reluctant high school principal to design a one-semester human sexuality course which may become mandatory for all tenth-grade students. Consider what you think is feasible, then construct relevant goals and objectives that you will present to the principal.

2. You have been given the onerous task of speaking for the development of a human sexuality program in the local school system. The public meeting is expected to be volatile and opposition to the proposed program very vocal. Describe the steps you will take in preparing your presentation and on which points you will focus your discussion.

3. Anystate University, where you are employed as a health educator, has an obvious alcohol problem. You have been asked by your supervisor to design a workshop for incoming freshmen about alcohol use and abuse. Consider your own philosophy, likely university administration philosophy, and the current political climate before briefly describing your approach to such a workshop. Which goals and objectives would you choose? What types of strategies/methods would you utilize?

4. You are a community health educator responsible for designing and implementing a sexuality program for a local youth group (ages 14 to 16 years). While describing the program to the parents of the prospective participants, one parent becomes extremely antagonistic and demands to know why "responsible sex" is even mentioned as abstinence is the only message that should be given. Briefly describe how you would respond to such an attack and justify your reasoning.

5. You are a community health educator working in an inner-city clinic which deals mostly with unintended pregnancy, sexually transmitted disease treatment, and HIV testing. A 13-year-old girl tells you that she has been having sexual intercourse regularly during her period and cannot understand why she has not become pregnant. She explains that she "needs" to get pregnant in order to keep her boyfriend who has threatened to leave her unless she has his baby. You try the predictable counseling route discussing the difficulties of a 13-year-old's raising a baby, not finishing school, the boyfriend's leaving anyway . . . all the rational reasons why she should not get pregnant. None of these arguments makes a difference, and the girl demands to know what she is doing wrong. How will you respond? Will you help her to become pregnant? Is it ethical to suggest that she keep having sex during her period? Does the end truly justify the means? Respond briefly to this situation and justify your answers.

6. One of your tenth-grade students comes to you after class, visibly upset. She confides in you that she is pregnant and needs information about having an abortion but is uncertain where to go for help. Despite your encouragement to discuss this with her parents, the girl is adamant that she cannot involve them. You are the only person she felt comfortable enough to approach and she needs your help. What are you going to do? Carefully think through the issue and then briefly describe and justify your actions.

Responding to these last two exercises will not be easy. Health education students must realize that, because they deal with sensitive issues, they will invariably become involved in real-life, personal problems, not just the more abstract design of objectives or workshop protocols. Thinking through your own ideas and listening to the philosophies of others will prepare you, at least in some small way, to handle extremely difficult situations.

SUMMARY

1. There are many issues within the discipline of health education that might be considered controversial.
2. Sexuality education and drug education have traced parallel paths with regard to the evolution of teaching strategies.
3. There is an ever-increasing number of "canned" or commercially prepared programs being utilized in both the drug and sexuality areas.
4. Health educators must be prepared to defend the existence of programming in controversial areas.
5. The accurate development of feasible, attainable objectives is of crucial importance when developing programs in controversial areas.
6. Health educators must be knowledgeable about the existence and tactics of opposition groups.
7. Health educators must be aware of the major obstacles to developing a sexuality education program.
8. Health educators must be aware of and avoid some of the more common pitfalls in teaching/presenting sex education.
9. The current struggle in sex education, particularly in the schools, is the adoption of abstinence versus responsibility curricula.
10. Developers of potentially controversial programs should consider the two-committee strategy of development.

REFERENCES

Anderson, P. 1973. The pot lobby. *New York Times Magazine* (January 21):8–9.

Battjes, R. J. 1985. Prevention of adolescent drug abuse. *International Journal of Addiction* 20:1113–1134.

Botvin, G. J. 1983. Prevention of adolescent substance abuse through the development of personal and social competence. In *Preventing Adolescent Drug Abuse: Intervention Strategies*, edited by T. Glynn, C. Leukefeld, and J. P. Ludford. Rockville, MD: NIDA.

Centers for Disease Control. 1991. Youth Risk Behavior Survey of 1990. Atlanta.

Centers for Disease Control. 1992. *HIV/AIDS Prevention Newsletter* 3(1):4.

Davis, C. M., S. L. Davis, and W. L. Yarber, eds. 1988. *Sexuality Related Measures: A Compendium*. Lake Mills, IA: Graphic Publishing.

Dawson, D. A. 1986. The effects of sex education on adolescent behavior. *Family Planning Perspectives* 18 (July/August).

Finn, C. 1986. Educational excellence: Eight elements. *Foundations News* 27(2):40–45.

Forrest, J. D. and J. Silverman. 1989. What public

school teachers teach about pregnancy prevention and AIDS, *Family Planning Perspectives* 21 (March/April).

Gallup Poll. 1976. Growing number of Americans favor discussion of sex in the classroom. News Release. Princeton, NJ.

Gersick, K. E., K. Grady, and D. Snow. 1988. Social-cognitive skill development with 6th graders and its initial impact on substance use. *Journal of Drug Education* 18:55–69.

Gilbert, G. G. 1979. Easy ways of getting into trouble when teaching sex education. *Health Education* (September/October).

Greenberg, J. S., and C. E. Bruess. 1981. *Sex Education: Theory and Practice*. Belmont, CA: Wadsworth.

Guttmacher Institute. 1989. *Risk and Responsibility*, p.7. 111 Fifth Avenue, New York.

Hofferth, S. L. 1981. Effects of number and timing of births on family well-being over the life cycle. Final Report to National Institute of Child Health and Human Development (Contract 1-HD-82850).

Jones, E. F., et al. 1986. *Teenage Pregnancy in Industrialized Countries*. New Haven: Yale University Press.

Kirby, D., J. Alter, and P. Scales. 1979a. An analysis of U.S. sex education programs and evaluation methods. Springfield, VA: National Technical Information Service.

Kirby, D., J. Alter, and P. Scales. 1979b. Executive summary. In *An Analysis of U.S. Education Programs and Evaluation Methods*. Atlanta: U.S. Department of Health, Education, and Welfare.

Kreuger, M. 1993. Sexuality education. *Phi Delta Kappan* (March):550–553.

Laing, R. D. 1972. *Knots*. New York: Random House.

Louis Harris and Associates. 1986. American teens speak: Sex, myth, T.V. and birth control. New York.

Louis Harris and Associates. 1988. Public attitudes toward teenage pregnancy, sex education and birth control. New York, p. 24. H. Quinley of Yankelovich Clancy Shulman, memorandum to all data users regarding *Time*/Yankelovich Clancy Shulman Poll Findings on Sex Education, November 17, 1986.

Marsiglio, W. and F. L. Mott. 1986. The impact of sex education on sexual activity, contraceptive use and premarital pregnancy among American teenagers. *Family Planning Perspectives* 18 (July/August).

Means, R. K. 1962. *A History of Health Education in the U.S.* Philadelphia: Lea and Febiger.

National Assessment of Educational Progress. 1976. Bicentennial Citizenship Survey. Denver.

National Institute of Drug Abuse. 1986. National Survey on Drug Abuse. DHHS Publication (ADM) 84-1356. Washington, DC.

National Institute of Drug Abuse. 1991. High School Senior Survey. Washington, DC.

National Opinion Research Center. 1982. General Social Surveys, 1972–1978: Cumulative Code Book. Chicago.

Popham, W. J. 1993. Wanted: AIDS education that works. *Phi Delta Kappan* (March):559–562.

Ringwalt, C., S. T. Ennett, and K. D. Holt. 1991. An outcome evaluation of project DARE. *Health Education Research*, 3(6):327–337.

Scales, P. 1989. Overcoming future barriers to sexuality education, theory into practice. *Health Education* 28(3):172–176.

SIECUS Report. December 1989/January 1991.

Sonenstein, F. L., and K. J. Pittman. 1984. The availability of sex education in large school districts. *Family Planning Perspectives* 16:19–25.

Taqi, S. 1972. The drug cinema. *Bulletin on Narcotics* 24:19–24.

Time. 1993. How should we teach our children about sex? (May):60–66.

Trussell, J. 1988. Teenage pregnancy in the U.S. *Family Planning Perspectives*, 20(6):262–272.

U.S. Department of Health and Human Services. 1984. Highlights from the National Survey on Drug Abuse. DHHS Publication (ADM) 83-1277. Washington, DC.

Wall Street Journal. 1992. Schools teach the virtues of virginity. (February 20):B1.

Zelnik, M., and Y. J. Kim. 1982. Sex education and its association with teenage sexual activity, pregnancy and contraceptive use. *Family Planning Perspectives* 14 (May/June).

Resources

Entry-Level Health Educator Competencies Addressed in These Appendixes

Responsibility VI: Acting as a Resource Person in Health Education

Competency A: Utilize computerized health information retrieval systems effectively.

Competency B: Establish effective consultative relationships with those requesting assistance in solving health-related problems.

Competency C: Interpret and respond to requests for health information.

Competency D: Select effective resource materials for dissemination.

Responsibility VII: Communicating Health and Health Education Needs, Concerns, and Resources

Competency C: Select a variety of communication methods and techniques in providing health information.

Taken from *A Framework for the Development of Competency-Based Curricula for Entry Level Health Educators,* National Task Force on the Preparation and Practice of Health Educators, Inc., 1985. Reprinted by permission.

Method Selection in Health Education

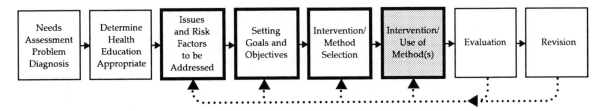

Heavy-bordered boxes indicate subjects addressed in this text; shaded boxes indicate subject(s) of current chapter.

Key Issues   Entry-Level Health Educator   Sources of Materials
                Competencies   National Hotlines
             SOPHE Code of Ethics   Year 2000 Health Objectives
             Professional Organizations   Additional Readings

ENTRY-LEVEL HEALTH EDUCATOR COMPETENCIES

Responsibility I: Assessing Individual and Community Needs for Health Education

Competency A: Obtain health-related data about social and cultural environments, growth and development factors, needs, and interests.

Competency B: Distinguish between behaviors that foster and those that hinder well-being.

Competency C: Infer needs for health education on the basis of obtained data.

Responsibility II: Planning Effective Health Education Programs

Competency A: Recruit community organizations, resource people, and potential participants for support and assistance in program planning.

Competency B: Develop a logical scope and sequence plan for a health education program.

Competency C: Formulate appropriate and measurable program objectives.

Responsibility III: Implementing Health Education Programs

Competency A: Exhibit competence in carrying out planned educational programs.

Competency B: Infer enabling objectives as needed to implement instructional program in specified settings.

Competency C: Select methods and media best suited to implement program plans for specific learners.

Competency D: Monitor educational programs, adjusting objectives and activities as necessary.

Responsibility IV: Evaluating Effectiveness of Health Education Programs

Competency A: Develop plans to assess achievement of program objectives.

Competency B: Carry out evaluation plans.

Competency C: Interpret results of program evaluation.

Competency D: Infer implications from findings for future program planning.

Responsibility V: Coordinating Provision of Health Education Services

Competency A: Develop a plan for coordinating health education services.

Competency B: Facilitate cooperation between and among levels of program personnel.

Competency C: Formulate practical modes of collaboration among health agencies and organizations.

Competency D: Organize in-service training programs for teachers, volunteers, and other interested personnel.

Responsibility VI: Acting as a Resource Person in Health Education

Competency A: Utilize computerized health information retrieval systems effectively.

Competency B: Establish effective consultative relationships with those requesting assistance in solving health-related problems.

Competency C: Interpret and respond to requests for health information.

Competency D: Select effective resource materials for dissemination.

Responsibility VII: Communicating Health and Health Education Needs, Concerns, and Resources

Competency A: Interpret concepts, purposes, and theories of health education.

Competency B: Predict the impact of societal value systems on health education programs.

Competency C: Select a variety of communication methods and techniques in providing health information.

Taken from *A Framework for the Development of Competency-Based Curricula for Entry Level Health Educators,* National Task Force on the Preparation and Practice of Health Educators, Inc., 1985. Reprinted by permission.

SOCIETY FOR PUBLIC HEALTH EDUCATION CODE OF ETHICS[1]

PREAMBLE

Health educators, in using educational processes to influence human well-being, take on profound responsibilities. Their professional situation is varied and complex, they work with people of different backgrounds, in diverse settings, and have varying responsibilities in this country as well as overseas. Health educators are involved with their discipline, their colleagues, their employees, their constituents, their government's position, other interest groups, and processes and issues affecting the general welfare of people, locally, nationally and internationally.

In a field of complex involvements, value conflicts generate ethical dilemmas. It is a prime responsibility of health educators to anticipate and to resolve them in such way as not to do damage either to the constituency with whom they work or their profession. Where these conditions cannot be met, the health educator would be well advised not to be involved.

The health educator must be committed to the principles of self-determination and liberty. Ethical precepts which guide the design of strategies and methods

continued

---

[1]Society for Public Health Education. 1987. SOPHE code of ethics. *Health Education Quarterly* 14:79–90.

must ultimately reflect a respect for the right of individuals and communities to form their own ways of living.

The following principles are deemed fundamental to health educators' responsible ethical pursuit of their profession:

ARTICLE I
RELATIONS WITH THE PUBLIC

Health educators' ultimate responsibility is to the general public. When there is a conflict of interest among individuals, groups, agencies, or institutions, health educators must consider all issues and give priority to those whose goals are closest to the principles of self-determination and enhancement of freedom of choice.

Section 1
Health educators must protect the right of individuals to make their own decisions regarding health as long as such decisions pose no threat to the health of others.

Section 2
Health educators should be candid and truthful in their dealings with the public.

Section 3
Health educators should not exploit the public by misrepresenting or exaggerating the potential benefits of services or programs with which they are associated.

Section 4
As people who devote their professional lives to improving people's well-being, health educators bear a responsibility to speak out on issues which would have a deleterious effect upon the public's health.

Section 5
In all dealings health educators should be honest about their qualifications and the limitations of their expertise.

Section 6
In a world where privacy is frequently threatened, health educators should protect the physical, social and psychological welfare of the public, and ensure their privacy and dignity.

Section 7
Health educators should involve clients actively in the entire educational change process so that all aspects are clearly understood by clients.

Section 8
Health educators affirm an egalitarian ethic. Believing that health is a basic human right, they act to ensure that neither the benefits nor the quality of their professional services are denied or impaired to all people to whom they are responsible.

ARTICLE II
RESPONSIBILITY TO THE PROFESSION

Health educators are responsible for the good reputation of their discipline.

Section 1
They should maintain their competence at the highest level through continuing study and training, for example:

- Active membership in professional organizations
- Review of professional, technical, and lay journals
- Previewing of new products and media materials
- Creation and distribution of new programs and materials including the publication of professional and lay papers
- Involvement in economic and legislative issues related to public health
- Assumption of a leadership or participative role in cooperative endeavors

Section 2
When they participate in actions related to hiring, promotion, or advancement, they should ensure that no exclusionary practices be enacted against individuals on the basis of sex, marital status, color, age, social class, religion, sexual preference, ethnic background, national origin, or older non-professional attributes.

Section 3
Health educators should protect and enhance the integrity of the profession by responsible discussion and criticism of the profession.

ARTICLE III
RESPONSIBILITY TO COLLEAGUES

Section 1
Health educators should maintain high standards of professional conduct as recommended by the Code of Ethics, and should encourage health education colleagues to do likewise.

Section 2

Health educators should make no critical remarks about colleagues in situations where possible conflicts of interest exist, especially where their own personal gain is involved or the personal gain of close friends.

Section 3

Health educators should take action through appropriate channels against unethical conduct by any other member of the profession.

ARTICLE IV
RESPONSIBILITY IN EMPLOYING EDUCATIONAL STRATEGIES AND METHODS

In designing strategies and methods, health educators must not compromise their professional standards, nor reduce the trust in health education held by the general public. They should be sensitive to the prevailing community standard and existing cultural or social norms. Health educators should also be aware of the possible impact of their strategies and methods upon the community and other health professionals.

The strategies and methods must not place the burden of change solely on the targeted population but must involve other appropriate groups to bring effective change.

In the design/implementation of strategies and methods, health educators have an obligation to two principles. First, that the people do have a right to make decisions affecting their lives. Second, there is a moral imperative to provide them all relevant information and resources possible to make their choice freely and intelligently.

Section 1

To protect public confidence in the profession, health educators should avoid strategies and methods that are clearly in violation of accepted moral and legal standards.

Section 2

In conducting programs the health educator's responsibility is not only to the participants, but also to the community at large.

Section 3

The selection of strategies and methods should include the active involvement of the people to be affected.

Section 4

The potential outcomes, both positive and negative, that can result from the proposed strategies should be communicated to all the appropriate individuals who will be affected.

Section 5

Health educators should implement strategies and methods which direct change whenever possible by choice, rather than by coercion. However, where a community is being harmed, or would be harmed by others, actions which limit the freedom of the harm-producing agents are justified. Where voluntary action has not succeeded in producing a desired outcome, coercive strategies and methods may be necessary but should be employed most cautiously.

ARTICLE V
RESPONSIBILITIES TO EMPLOYERS

In their relations with employers, health educators should

Section 1

Be honest about their qualifications (education, experience, training), capabilities, and aims.

Section 2

Reflect seriously upon the goals of the organization for which they are to work and consider with great care their employer's stated aims and their past behaviors, prior to entering any commitment.

Section 3

Act within the boundaries of their professional competence.

Section 4

Accept responsibility and accountability for their areas of practice, including responsibility for maintenance of optimum standards.

Section 5

Exercise informed judgment and use professional standards and guidelines as criteria in seeking consultation, accepting responsibilities, and delegating health education activities to others.

Section 6

Maintain competence in their areas of professional practice.

Section 7

Be careful not to promise outcomes or to imply acceptance of conditions contrary to their professional ethics.

Continued

Section 8

Avoid competing commitments, conflict of interest situations, secret agreements and endorsement of products.

ARTICLE VI
RESPONSIBILITY TO STUDENTS

The preparation and training of prospective health educators entails serious responsibilities affecting the well-being of the profession, the public, and the students. All those involved in such preparation and training, including teachers, administrators, and practicum supervisors, have an obligation to accord students the same respect and treatment accorded all other client groups, and to provide the highest quality education possible.

Educators should be receptive and seriously responsive to students' interests, opinions, and desires in all aspects of their academic work and relationships. The principles and methods of health education that are taught should be practiced in the education of future professionals. Teachers and educators should share their passions, convictions, commitments, and visions as well as their knowledge and skills with their students. Personal and professional honesty and integrity are the essential qualities of a good teacher.

Section 1

Selection of students for professional preparation programs should preclude discrimination on any grounds other than ability and potential contribution to the profession and the public health.

Section 2

The ethical dimensions of the practice of health education should be stressed at all levels of professional preparation.

Section 3

The education environment–physical, social, and emotional–should to the greatest degree possible be conducive to the health of all involved.

Section 4

The responsibilities of all teachers to their students include careful preparation; presentation of material that is accurate, up-to-date, and timely; providing reasonable and timely feed-back; having and stating clear and reasonable expectations; and fairness in grading and evaluation.

Section 5

Faculty owe students a reasonable degree of accessibility. Other demands such as research and administration must be kept in balance with responsibilities to students.

Section 6

Students should receive counseling regarding career opportunities and assistance in securing professional employment upon completion of their studies.

Section 7

Field work and internships should be based upon the professional interests and needs of the student and should provide meaningful opportunities to gain useful experience and adequate supervision.

ARTICLE VII
RESPONSIBILITY IN RESEARCH AND EVALUATION

The health educator engaged in research and evaluation studies should

Section 1

Consider carefully its possible consequences for human beings.

Section 2

Ascertain that the consent of participants in research is voluntary and informed, without any implied deprivation or penalty for refusal to participate, and with due regard for the participant's privacy and dignity.

Section 3

Protect participants from unwarranted physical or mental discomfort, distress, harm, danger, or deprivation.

Section 4

Treat all information secured from participants as confidential.

Section 5

Take credit only for work actually done and credit contributions made by others.

Section 6

Provide no reports to sponsors that are not also available to the general public and, where practicable, to the populations studied.

Section 7

Discuss the results of evaluation of services only with the person directly and professionally concerned with them.

SOPHE'S CODE OF ETHICS (BRIEF EDITION)

To guide professional behaviors of its members toward highest standards; SOPHE adopted a Code of Ethics in

1976 and acknowledged the need for periodic review and improvement of the Code.

- I will accurately represent my capability, education, training, and experience, and will act within the boundaries of my professional competence.

- I will maintain my competence at the highest level through continuing study, training, and research.

- I will report research findings and practice activities honestly and without distortion.

- I will not discriminate because of race, color, national origin, religion, age, or socioeconomic status in rendering service, employing, training, or promoting others.

- I value the privacy, dignity, and worth of the individual, and will use skills consistent with these values.

- I will observe the principle of informed consent with respect to individuals and groups served.

- I will support change by choice, not by coercion.

- I will foster an educational environment that nurtures individual growth and development.

- If I become aware of unethical practices, I am accountable for taking appropriate action concerning these practices.

PROFESSIONAL ORGANIZATIONS

Organization	Publication	Address	Abbreviation	Approximate Membership
American School Health Association	*Journal of School Health*	P.O. Box 708 Kent, OH 44240 216-678-1601	ASHA	4,500
American Public Health Association	*American Journal of Public Health Umbrella organizations include PHES and SHES*	1015 15th St. NW Washington, DC 20005 (202) 789-5600	APHA	32,000
APHA–Public Health Education Section	Newsletter	1015 15th St. NW Washington, DC 20005 202-789-5600	PHES	
APHA–School Health Education Section	Newsletter	1015 15th St. NW Washington, DC 20005	SHES	
American College Health Association	*Journal of American College Health*	15879 Crabbs Branch Way Rockville, MD 20852 301-963-1100	ACHA	
American Alliance for Health, Physical Education, Recreation, and Dance	Umbrella organization includes AAHE	1900 Association Dr. Reston, VA 22091 703-476-3400	AAHPERD	30,000
Association for the Advancement of Health Education	*Journal of Health Education*	1900 Association Dr. Reston, VA 22091 703-476-3441	AAHE	10,000

Continued

Organization	Publication	Address	Abbreviation	Approximate Membership
Council of Health Education Programs in Higher Education	No Journal	c/o Department of Health Education University of Maryland College Park, MD 20742-2611 301-405-2467	The Council	100 Institutions
Eta Sigma Gamma	*The Gamman*	2000 University Ave. Ball State University Muncie, IN 47306 317-285-5961		2,600
National Commission for Health Education Credentialing, Inc.	Newsletter	475 Riverside Dr., 8th Floor New York, NY 10115 212-870-2047	The Commission	Membership through examination
Society for Public Health Education	*Health Education Quarterly*	2001 Addison St. Suite 220 Berkeley, CA 94704 510-644-9242	SOPHE	1,000
Society of State Directors of Health, Physical Education, and Recreation	No Journal		SSDHPER	55

SELECTED SOURCES OF HEALTH EDUCATION MATERIALS

There are numerous sources of health education materials in the United States and a comprehensive list would be unwieldy. The following source list represents a compilation of the larger, established distributors that provide a variety of materials in varying formats. The authors are certainly not endorsing these companies or all their materials. However, this list will provide the health educator with a starting point in the search for interesting health education materials.

American Health Foundation
320 E. 43rd St.
New York, NY 10017
(800) 953-1900

The Know Your Body Curriculum and other related materials.

Comprehensive Health Education Foundation
22323 Pacific Hgwy. S.
Seattle, WA 98198
(206) 824–2907

Curriculum materials and supporting materials.

Coronet/MTI
108 Wilmot Rd.
Deerfield, IL 60015
(800) 621–2131

Films and videotapes on a number of health issues. Particularly good selection on rape, sexual assault, and violence.

DINE System, Inc.
586 N. French Rd.,
  Suite 2
Amherst, NY 14228
(716) 688–2492

Nutrition analysis software and other related products.

Education Development Center, Inc.
55 Chapel St.
Newton, MA 02160
(617) 969–7100

Curriculum materials, Comprehensive School Health Network newsletter, and other materials.

Education Programs Associates
1 W. Campbell Ave., Bldg. D
Campbell, CA 95008
(408) 374–3720

Books and pamphlets on many health issues. Emphasis on patient education.

ETR Associates
P.O. Box 1830
Santa Cruz, CA 95061–4407
(800) 321–4407

Videos, books, and pamphlets on many topics. Particularly aimed at children and adolescents.

Filmakers Library
124 E. 40th St.
New York, NY 10016
(212) 808–4980

Films and videos on sexuality, aging, death education, disabilities, alcoholism, suicide, violence, child development, and the environment.

Films for the Humanities and Sciences
P.O. Box 2053
Princeton, NJ 08543–2053
(800) 257–5126

Films, videos, and videodiscs on a wide-ranging area of health and medical topics.

Fisher–EMD
4901 W. LeMoyne St.
Chicago, IL 60651
(800) 955–1177

Anatomical models, displays, and skeletons.

Focus International
14 Oregon Dr.
Huntington Station
New York, NY 11746
(800) 843–0305

Numerous films and videotapes on human sexuality, from childhood to adult.

Health Edco
P.O. Box 21207
Waco, TX 76702–1207
(800) 299–3366, Ext. 295

Health Visions
10930 Little Sparrow Pl.
Columbia, MD 21044
(410) 997–9419

Films specifically related to sexuality at the college and high school levels.

Intermedia
1300 Dexter N.
Seattle, WA 98109
(800) 553–8336

Films and videotapes with particular emphasis on teen and young adult issues.

Krames Communications
1100 Grundy Ln.
San Bruno, CA 94066–3030
(800) 333–3032

Booklets, pamphlets, and brochures on many health topics. These products are extremely colorful and of very high quality, but tend to be expensive.

NASCO
901 Janesville Ave.
Fort Atkinson, WI 53538–0901
(414) 563–2446

Anatomical models, charts, displays, CPR mannequins, and videotapes.

National School Products
101 E. Broadway
Maryville, TN 37801–2498

Books, pamphlets, posters, displays, models, software, and videotapes. Emphasis on the school setting, particularly the teenager.

Positive Promotions
222 Ashland Pl.
Brooklyn, NY 11217
(800) 635–2666

Interesting health-related promotion materials on various topics intended for children and adults. Many materials in Spanish.

Select Media
74 Varick St., 3rd Floor
New York, NY 10013
(212) 431–8923

Films, videotapes, and interactive videodiscs. Some materials in Spanish. Many materials related to sexuality.

Sunburst
39 Washington Ave.
P.O. Box 40
Pleasantville, NY 10570–0040
(800) 431–1934

Curriculum modules, videotapes, posters, teacher's guides, and games. Some videotapes are open captioned or in Spanish. Emphasis is grades 2 through 12.

Wisconsin Clearinghouse
P.O. Box 1468
Madison, WI 53701–1468
(800) 322–1468

Videotapes, posters, software, pamphlets, and complete projects/programs on many health topics, ranging from the elementary school level through college and adulthood.

HEALTH HOTLINES/800 NUMBERS

Note the following is the federal clearinghouse on clearinghouses. If in doubt call them for advice.

National Health Information Center
(800) 336–4797
P.O. Box 1133
Washington, DC 20013–1133

IDS Clinical Trials Information
   Service (ACTIS)
(800) TRIALS–A (874–2572)
(800) 243–7012 (TTY)
P.O. Box 6421
Rockville, MD 20859-6421

Al-Anon, Alateen Family Group
   Hotline
(800) 344–2666
(800) 245–4656 (within New York)
(800) 443–4525 (within Canada)
P.O. Box 862 Midtown Station

New York, NY 10018-0862

Alcohol Rehab for the Elderly
(800) 354–7089
(800) 344–0824 (within Illinois)
P.O. Box 267
Hopedale, IL 61747

Alliance of Genetic Support
   Groups
(800) 336–GENE (4363)
1001 22nd St. NW, Suite 800
Washington, DC 20037

Alzheimer's Association
(800) 272–3900
919 N. Michigan Ave., Suite 1000
Chicago, IL 60611–1676

American Association of Retired
 Persons
(800) 424–2277
601 E St. NW
Washington, DC 20049

American Cancer Society
National Office
(800) ACS–2345 (within each state
 with a divisional office)
1599 Clifton Rd. NE
Atlanta, GA 30329

American Council on Alcoholism
(800) 527–5344
5024 Campbell Blvd., Suite H
Baltimore, MD 21236

American Diabetes Association
(800) 232–3472
1660 Duke St.
Alexandria, VA 22314

American Foundation for the Blind
(800) 232–5463
15 W. 16th St.
New York, NY 10011

American Kidney Fund
(800) 638–8299
(800) 492-8361 (within Maryland)
6110 Executive Blvd., Suite 1010
Rockville, MD 20852

American Liver Foundation
Hepatitis Hotline
(800) 223–0179
1425 Pompton Ave.
Cedar Grove, NJ 07009

American Lupus Society
(800) 331–1802
3914 Del Arno Blvd., Suite 922
Torrance, CA 90503

American Narcolepsy Association
(800) 222–6085
425 California Ave., Suite 201
San Francisco, CA 94104

American Paralysis Association
(800) 225–0292
500 Morris Ave.
Springfield, NJ 07081

American Parkinson's Disease
 Association
(800) 223–2732
60 Bay St., Suite 401
Staten Island, NY 10301

American Schizophrenia
 Association
(800) 847–3802
900 N. Federal Hgwy.
Boca Raton, FL 33432

American School Health
 Association
(800) 227–8922 (National STD
 Hotline)
(800) 342–AIDS (National AIDS
 Hotline)
(800) 344–SIDA (Spanish)
(800) AIDS–TTY (Hearing
 Impaired)
P.O. Box 13827
Research Triangle Park, NC 27709

Ankylosing Spondylitis
 Association
(800) 777–8189
511 N. La Cienega, Suite 216
Los Angeles, CA 90048

Arthritis Foundation
(800) 283–7800
1314 Spring St. NW
Atlanta, GA 30309

Bulemia Anorexia Self-Help
 (BASH)
(800) BASH–STL (227–4785)
6125 Clayton Ave., Suite 215
St. Louis, MO 63139–3295

Cancer Information Service
(800) 4–CANCER (in various states
 and regions)

Office of Cancer Communications,
    NCI/NIH
Bldg. 31, Room 10A24
9000 Rockville Pike
Bethesda, MD 20892

Children's Craniofacial Association
(800) 535–3643
10210 N. Central Expwy, L.B. 37
Dallas, TX 75231

Cleft Palate Foundation
(800) 242–5338
1218 Grandview Ave.
Pittsburgh, PA 15211

Cocaine Anonymous
(800) 347–8998
3740 Overland Ave., Suite G
Los Angeles, CA 90034

Consumer Product Safety
    Commission (CPSC)
(800) 638–2772 (Product Safety
    Line)
(800) 638–8270 (TTY National)
(800) 492–8104 (TTY Maryland)
Washington, DC 20207

Cooley's Anemia Foundation
(800) 221–3571
(800) 522–7222 (within New York)
105 E. 22nd St.
New York, NY 10010

Cornelia de Lange Syndrome
    Foundation
(800) 223–8355
(800) 735–2357 (Connecticut and
    Canada only)
(Birth defects information)
60 Dyer Ave.
Collinsville, CT 06022

Crohn's and Colitis Foundation of
    America
(800) 343–3637
444 Park Ave. S., 11th Floor
New York, NY 10018

Cystic Fibrosis Foundation
(800) 344–4823
6931 Arlington Rd.
Bethesda, MD 20814

Device Experience Network
Division of Product Surveillance
Office of Compliance and
    Surveillance
Center for Devices and
    Radiological Health (FDA)
(800) 638–6725
FDA-HFZ-343
8757 Georgia Ave.
Silver Spring, MD 20910

Endometriosis Association
(800) 992–ENDO (3636)
P.O. Box 92187
Milwaukee, WI 53202

Epilepsy Foundation of America
(800) EFA–1000 (outside Maryland)
4351 Garden City Dr., Suite 406
Landover, MD 20785

Health Resources and Services
    Administration
Office of Health Facilities
(800) 492–0359 (English and
    Spanish, within Maryland)
(800) 638–0742 (English and
    Spanish, outside Maryland)
Department of Health and Human
    Services
Public Health Service
5600 Fishers Ln.
Rockville, MD 20857

Healthy Mothers, Healthy Babies
    Coalition
(800) 673–8444, Ext. 2458
409 12th St. SW
Washington, DC 20024–2188

Huntington's Disease Society of
    America
(800) 345–4372
140 W. 22nd St., 6th Floor
New York, NY 10011–2420

Juvenile Diabetes Foundation (JDF)
(800) 223–1138
432 Park Ave. S., 16th Floor
New York, NY 10016

La Leche League International
(800) 525–3243
P.O. Box 1209
Franklin Park, IL 60131–8209

Little People of America
(800) 243–9273
P.O. Box 9897
Washington, DC 20016

Living Bank
(800) 528–297
(Organ donation)
P.O. Box 6725
Houston, TX 77265

Lupus Foundation of America
(800) 558–0121
1717 Massachusetts Ave. NW,
   Suite 203
Washington, DC 20036

Medic Alert Foundation
   International
(800) ID–ALERT (432–5378)
(800) 344–3226 (within California)
2323 Colorado
Turlock, CA 95381-1009

Missing Children Help Center
(800) USA–KIDS (872–5437)
410 Ware Blvd., Suite 400
Tampa, FL 33619

Mothers Against Drunk Drivers
(800) 438–6233 (Victim hotline)
P.O. Box 541688
Dallas, TX 75354–1688

Myasthenia Gravis Foundation
(800) 541–5454
53 W. Jackson Blvd., Suite 660
Chicago, IL 60604

National AIDS Hotline
Centers for Disease Control
(800) 342–AIDS
(800) 344–SIDA (Spanish)
(800) AIDS–TTY (Hearing
   Impaired)
Atlanta, GA 30333

National AIDS Information
   Clearinghouse
(800) 458–5231
P.O. Box 6003
Rockville, MD 20850

National Association for Parents of
   the Visually Impaired
(800) 562–6265
2180 Linway Dr.
Beloit, WI 53511

National Association for Sickle
   Cell Disease, Inc.
(800) 421–8453
3345 Wilshire Blvd., Suite 1106
Los Angeles, CA 90010–1880

National Association of People
   with AIDS (NAPWA)
(800) 673–8538
P.O. Box 18345
Washington, DC 20036

National Center for Missing and
   Exploited Children
(800) 843–5678
2101 Wilson Blvd., Suite 550
Arlington, VA 22201

National Center for Stuttering
(800) 221–2483
200 E. 33rd St.
New York, NY 10016

National Child Abuse Hotline
(800) 422–4453
Box 630
Hollywood, CA 90028

National Child Safety Council
Childwatch
(800) 222–1464
P.O. Box 1368
Jackson, MI 49204

National Clearinghouse for
    Alcohol and Drug Information
(800) SAY–NOTO (729–6686)
P.O. Box 2345
Rockville, MD 20852

National Cocaine Hotline
(800) 262–2463
P.O. Box 100
Summit, NJ 07902–0100

National Council in Alcoholism
    and Drug Dependent Hopeline
(800) NCA–CALL (622–2255)
12 W. 21st St., Suite 700
New York, NY 10010

National Council on Child Abuse
    and Family Violence
(800) 222–2000
1155 Connecticut Ave. NW, Suite
    300
Washington, DC 20036

National Council on the Aging
(800) 424–9046
409 3rd St. SW, 2nd Floor
Washington, DC 20024

National Domestic Violence
    Hotline
Michigan Coalition Against
    Domestic Violence
(800) 333–SAFE (7233)
P.O. Box 463100
Mt. Clemens, MI 48043

National Down Syndrome
    Congress
(800) 232–NDSC (6372)
1800 Dempster St.
Park Ridge, IL 60068–1146

National Down Syndrome Society
(800) 221–4602
666 Broadway
New York, NY 10012

National Drug Information and
    Referral Line
National Institute on Drug Abuse
(800) 662–HELP (4357)
5635 Fishers Ln.
Rockville, MD 20852

National Easter Seal Society
(800) 221–6827
70 E. Lake St.
Chicago, IL 60601

National Eye Care Project
(800) 222–EYES (3937)
(Medical and surgical care for the
    elderly at no out-of-pocket
    expense)
P.O. Box 9688
San Francisco, CA 94101–9688

National Eye Research Foundation
(800) 621–2258
910 Skokie Blvd., #207A
Northbrook, IL 60062

National Fire Protection
    Association
(800) 344–3555
Batterymarch Park
Quincy, MA 02269

National Foundation for
    Depressive Illness
(800) 248–4344
P.O. Box 2257
New York, NY 10116

National Headache Foundation
(800) 843–2256
5252 N. Western Ave.
Chicago, IL 60625

National Head Injury Foundation
(800) 444–6443
1140 Connecticut Ave. NW, Suite
    812
Washington, DC 20036

National Health Information
    Center
(800) 336–4797
P.O. Box 1133
Washington, DC 20013–1133

National Hearing Aid Society
Hearing Aid Helpline
(800) 521–5247
20361 Middlebelt Rd.
Livonia, MI 48152

National Highway Traffic Safety
    Administration
Auto Safety Hotline
(800) 424–9393
400 7th St. SW, Room 5319
Washington, DC 20590

National Hospice Organization
(800) 658–8898
1901 N. Moore St., Suite 901
Arlington, VA 22209

National Information Center for
    Children and Youth with
    Handicaps
(800) 999–5599
P.O. Box 1492
Washington, DC 20013

National Information Center for
    Orphan Drugs and Rare
    Diseases
(800) 456–3505
P.O. Box 1133
Washington, DC 20013–1133

National Information
    Clearinghouse for Infants with
    Disabilities and Life-
    Threatening Conditions
Center for Developmental
    Disabilities

(800) 922–9234
University of South Carolina
Benson Bldg., 1st Floor
Columbia, SC 29208

National Institute for Occupational
    Safety and Health (NIOSH)
(800) 356–4674
4676 Columbia Pkwy.
Cincinnati, OH 45226

National Resource Center on
    Homelessness and Mental
    Illness
(800) 444–7415
262 Delaware Ave.
Delmar, NY 12054

National Reye's Syndrome
    Foundation, Inc.
(800) 233–7393
(800) 231–7393 (within Ohio)
P.O. Box 829
Bryan, OH 43506

National Runaway Switchboard
(800) 621–4000
3080 N. Lincoln
Chicago, IL 60657

National Safety Council
(800) 621–7619
444 N. Michigan Ave.
Chicago, IL 60611

National Second Surgical Opinion
    Program
(800) 638–6833
200 Independence Ave. SW
Washington, DC 20201

National Society to Prevent
    Blindness
(800) 221–3004
500 E. Remington Rd.
Schaumberg, IL 60173

National Spinal Cord Injury
  Association
(800) 962–9629
600 W. Cummings Park, Suite
  2000
Woburn, MA 01801

National STD Hotline
(800) 227–8922
(Sexually transmitted diseases)
Centers for Disease Control
Atlanta, GA 30333

National Stroke Association
(800) 787–6537
300 E. Hampden Ave., Suite 240
Englewood, CO 80110

National Sudden Infant Death
  Syndrome Foundation
(800) 221–SIDS (outside Maryland)
10500 Little Patuxent Pkwy., Suite
  420
Columbia, MD 21044

Office of Minority Health Resource
  Center
(800) 444–6472
P.O. Box 37337
Washington, DC 20013–7337

Planned Parenthood Federation of
  America
(800) 829–7732
810 7th Ave.
New York, NY 10019

PMS Access
(800) 222–4PMS
(Information on premenstrual
  syndrome)
P.O. Box 9326
Madison, WI 53715

Runaway Hotline
(800) 231–6946
(800) 392–3552 (within Texas)
P.O. Box 12428
Austin, TX 78711

Spina Bifida Association of
  America
(800) 621–3141
1700 Rockville Pike, Suite 250
Rockville, MD 20852

Spinal Cord Injury Hotline
(800) 526–3456
2201 Argonne Drive
Baltimore, MD 21218

Tourette Syndrome Association
  (TSA)
(800) 237–0717
42-40 Bell Blvd.
Bayside, NY 11361

Y-Me Breast Cancer Support
  Program
(800) 221–2141 (9–5 central time)
18220 Harwood Ave.
Homewood, IL 60430

Year 2000 Objectives

Duplicate objectives, which appear in two or more priority areas, are marked with an asterisk (*).

Except as otherwise noted, all rates in the following objectives are annual. Where the baseline rate is age adjusted, it is age adjusted to the 1940 U.S. population, and the target is age adjusted also.

1. Physical Activity and Fitness
Health Status Objectives

1.1* Reduce coronary heart disease deaths to no more than 100 per 100,000 people. (Age-adjusted baseline: 135 per 100,000 in 1987)

Special Population Target

Coronary Deaths (per 100,000)	1987 Baseline	2000 Target
1.1a Blacks	163	115

1.2* Reduce overweight to a prevalence of no more than 20 percent among people aged 20 and older and no more than 15 percent among adolescents aged 12 through 19. (Baseline: 26 percent for people aged 20 through 74 in 1976–80, 24 percent for men and 27 percent for women; 15 percent for adolescents aged 12 through 19 in 1976–80)

Special Population Targets

Overweight Prevalence	1976–80 Baseline†	2000 Target
1.2a Low-income women aged 20 and older	37%	25%
1.2b Black women aged 20 and older	44%	30%
1.2c Hispanic women aged 20 and older		
Mexican American women	39%‡	
Cuban women	34%‡	
Puerto Rican women	37%‡	

1.2d American Indians/Alaska Natives	29–75%§	30%
1.2e People with disabilities	36%+	25%
1.2f Women with high blood pressure	50%	41%
1.2g Men with high blood pressure	39%	35%

†1976–80 baseline for people aged 20–74
‡1982–84 baseline for Hispanics aged 20–74.
§1984–88 estimates for different tribes.
+1985 baseline for people aged 20–74 who report any limitation in activity due to chronic conditions.

Note: For people aged 20 and older, overweight is defined as body mass index (BMI) equal to or greater than 27.8 for men and 27.3 for women. For adolescents, overweight is defined as BMI equal to or greater than 23.0 for males aged 12 through 14, 24.3 for males aged 15 through 17, 25.8 for males aged 18 through 19, 23.4 for females aged 12 through 14, 24.8 for females aged 15 through 17, and 25.7 for females aged 18 through 19. The values for adolescents are the age- and gender-specific 85th percentile values of the 1976–80 National Health and Nutrition Examination Survey (NHANES II), corrected for sample variation. BMI is calculated by dividing weight in kilograms by the square of height in meters. The cut points used to define overweight approximate the 120 percent of desirable body weight definition used in the 1990 objectives.

Risk Reduction Objectives

1.3* Increase to at least 30 percent the proportion of people aged 6 and older who engage regularly, preferably daily, in light to moderate physical activity for at least 30 minutes per day. (Baseline: 22 percent of people aged 18 and older were active for at least 30 minutes 5 or more times per week and 12 percent were active 7 or more times per week in 1985)

Note: Light to moderate physical activity requires sustained, rhythmic muscular movements, is at least equivalent to sustained walking, and is performed at less that 60 percent of maximum heart rate for age. Maximum heart rate equals roughly 220 beats per minute minus age. Examples may include walking, swimming, cycling, dancing, gardening and yardwork, various domestic and occupational activities, and games and other childhood pursuits.

1.4 Increase to at least 20 percent the proportion of people aged 18 and older and to at least 75 percent the proportion of children and adolescents aged 6 through 17 who engage in vigorous physical activity that promotes the development and maintenance of cardiorespiratory fitness 3 or more days per week for 20 or more minutes per occasion. (Baseline: 12 percent for people aged 18 and older in 1985; 66 percent for youth aged 10 through 17 in 1984)

	Special Population Target		
	Vigorous Physical Activity	*1985 Baseline*	*2000 Target*
1.4a	Lower-income people aged 18 and older (annual family income < $20,000)	7%	12%

Note: Vigorous physical activities are rhythmic, repetitive physical activities that use large muscle groups at 60 percent or more of maximum heart rate for age. An exercise heart rate of 60 percent of maximum heart rate for age is about 50 percent of maximal cardiorespiratory capacity and is sufficient for cardiorespiratory conditioning. Maximum heart rate equals roughly 220 beats per minute minus age.

1.5 Reduce to no more than 15 percent the proportion of people aged 6 and older who engage in no leisure-time physical activity. (Baseline: 24 percent for people aged 18 and older in 1985)

	Special Population Targets		
	No Leisure-Time Physical Activity	*1985 Baseline*	*2000 Target*
1.5a	People aged 65 and older	43%	22%
1.5b	People with disabilities	35%	20%
1.5c	Lower-income people (annual family income < $20,000)	32%†	17%

†*Baseline for people aged 18 and older.*

Note: For this objective, people with disabilities are people who report any limitation in activity due to chronic conditions.

1.6 Increase to at least 40 percent the proportion of people aged 6 and older who regularly perform physical activities that enhance and maintain muscular strength, muscular endurance, and flexibility. (Baseline data available in 1991)

1.7* Increase to at least 50 percent the proportion of overweight people aged 12 and older who have adopted sound dietary practices combined with regular physical activity to attain an appropriate body weight. (Baseline: 30 percent of overweight women and 25 percent of overweight men for people aged 18 and older in 1985)

Services and Protection Objectives

1.8 Increase to at least 50 percent the proportion of children and adolescents in 1st through 12th grade who participate in daily school physical education. (Baseline: 36 percent in 1984–86)

1.9 Increase to at least 50 percent the proportion of school physical education class time that students spend being physically active, preferably engaged in lifetime physical activities. (Baseline: Students spent an estimated 27 percent of class time being physically active in 1983)

Note: Lifetime activities are activities that may be readily carried into adulthood because they generally need only one or two people. Examples include swimming, bicycling, jogging, and racquet sports. Also counted as lifetime activities are vigorous social activities such as dancing. Competitive group sports and activities typically played only by young children such as group games are excluded.

1.10 Increase the proportion of worksites offering employer-sponsored physical activity and fitness programs as follows:

Worksite Size	1985 Baseline	2000 Target
50–99 employees	14%	20%
100–249 employees	23%	35%
250–749 employees	32%	50%
≥ 750 employees	54%	80%

1.11 Increase community availability and accessibility of physical activity and fitness facilities as follows:

Facility	1986 Baseline	2000 Target
Hiking, biking, and fitness trail miles	1 per 71,000 people	1 per 10,000 people
Public swimming pools	1 per 53,000 people	1 per 25,000 people
Acres of park and recreation open space	1.8 per 1.000 people (553 people per managed acre)	4 per 1,000 people (250 people per managed acre)

1.12 Increase to at least 50 percent the proportion of primary care providers who routinely assess and counsel their patients regarding the frequency, duration, type, and intensity of each patient's physical activity practices. (Baseline: Physicians provided exercise counseling for about 30 percent of sedentary patients in 1988)

2. Nutrition
Health Status Objectives
2.1* Reduce coronary heart disease deaths to no more than 100 per 100,000 people. (Age-adjusted baseline: 135 per 100,000 in 1987)

	Special Population Target	
Coronary Deaths (per 100,000)	1987 Baseline	2000 Target
2.1a Blacks	163	115

2.2* Reverse the rise in cancer deaths to achieve a rate of no more than 130 per 100,000 people. (Age-adjusted baseline: 133 per 100,000 in 1987)

Note: In its publications, the National Cancer Institute age-adjusts cancer death rates to the 1970 U.S. population. Using the 1970 standard, the equivalent baseline and target values for this objective would be 171 and 175 per 100,000, respectively.

2.3* Reduce overweight to a prevalence of no more than 20 percent among people aged 20 and older and no more than 15 percent among adolescents aged 12 through 19. (Baseline: 26 percent for people aged 20 through 74 in 1976–80, 24 percent for men and 27 percent for women; 15 percent for adolescents aged 12 through 19 in 1976–80)

Special Population Targets

Overweight Prevalence	1976–80 Baseline†	2000 Target
2.3a Low-income women aged 20 and older	37%	25%
2.3b Black women aged 20 and older	44%	30%
2.3c Hispanic women aged 20 and older		
Mexican American women	39%‡	
Cuban women	34%‡	
Puerto Rican women	37%‡	
2.3d American Indians/Alaska Natives	29–75%§	30%
2.3e People with disabilities	36%+	25%
2.3f Women with high blood pressure	50%	41%
2.3g Men with high blood pressure	39%	35%

†1976–80 baseline for people aged 20–74
‡1982–84 baseline for Hispanics aged 20–74.
§1984–88 estimates for different tribes.
+ 1985 baseline for people aged 20–74 who report
any limitation in activity due to chronic conditions.

Note: For people aged 20 and older, overweight is defined as body mass index (BMI) equal to or greater than 27.8 for men and 27.3 for women. For adolescents, overweight is defined as BMI equal to or greater than 23.0 for males aged 12 through 14, 24.3 for males aged 15 through 17, 25.8 for males aged 18 through 19, 23.4 for females aged 12 through 14, 24.8 for females aged 15 through 17, and 25.7 for females aged 18 through 19. The values for adolescents are the age- and gender-specific 85th percentile values of the 1976–80 National Health and Nutrition Examination Survey (NHANES II), corrected for sample variation. BMI is calculated by dividing weight in kilograms by the square of height in meters. The cut points used to define overweight approximate the 120 percent of desirable body weight definition used in the 1990 objectives.

2.4 Reduce growth retardation among low-income children aged 5 and younger to less than 10 percent. (Baseline: Up to 16 percent among low-income children in 1988, depending on age and race/ ethnicity)

	Special Population Target	
Prevalence of Short Stature	*1988 Baseline*	*2000 Target*
2.4a Low-income black children < age 1	15%	10%
2.4b Low-income Hispanic children < age 1	13%	10%
2.4c Low-income Hispanic children aged 1	16%	10%
2.4d Low-income Asian/Pacific Islander children aged 1	14%	10%
2.4e Low-income Asian/Pacific Islander children aged 2–4	16%	10%

Note: Growth retardation is defined as height-for-age below the fifth percentile of children in the National Center for Health Statistics'reference population.

Risk Reduction Objectives

2.5* Reduce dietary fat intake to an average of 30 percent of calories or less and average saturated fat intake to less than 10 percent of calories among people aged 2 and older. (Baseline: 36 percent of calories from total fat and 13 percent from saturated fat for people aged 20 through 74 in 1976–80; 36 percent and 13 percent for women aged 19 through 50 in 1985)

2.6* Increase complex carbohydrate and fiber-containing foods in the diets of adults to 5 or more daily servings for vegetables (including legumes) and fruits, and to 6 or more daily servings for grain products. (Baseline: 2½ servings of vegetables and fruits and 3 servings of grain products for women aged 19 through 50 in 1985)

2.7* Increase to at least 50 percent the proportion of overweight people aged 12 and older who have adopted sound dietary practices combined with regular physical activity to attain an appropriate body weight. (Baseline: 30 percent of overweight women and 25 percent of overweight men for people aged 18 and older in 1985)

2.8 Increase calcium intake so at least 50 percent of youth aged 12 through 24 and 50 percent of pregnant and lactating women consume 3 or more servings daily of foods rich in calcium, and at least 50 percent of people aged 25 and older consume 2 or more servings daily. (Baseline: 7 percent of women and 14 percent of men aged 19 through 24 and 24 percent of pregnant and lactating women consumed 3 or more servings, and 15 percent of women and 23 percent of men aged 25 through 50 consumed 2 or more servings in 1985–86)

Note: The number of servings of foods rich in calcium is based on milk and milk products. A serving is considered to be 1 cup of skim milk or its equivalent in calcium (302 mg). The number of servings in this objective will generally provide approximately three-fourths of the 1989 Recommended Dietary Allowance (RDA) of calcium. The RDA is 1200 mg for people aged 12 through 24, 800 mg for people aged 25 and older, and 1200 mg for pregnant and lactating women.

2.9 Decrease salt and sodium intake so at least 65 percent of home meal preparers prepare foods without adding salt, at least 80 percent of people avoid using salt at the table, and at least 40 percent of adults regularly purchase foods modified or lower in sodium. (Baseline: 54 percent of women aged 19 through 50 who served as the main meal preparer did not use salt in food preparation, and 68 percent of women aged 19 through 50 did not use salt at the table in 1985; 20 percent of all people aged 18 and older regularly purchased foods with reduced salt and sodium content in 1988)

2.10 Reduce iron deficiency to less that 3 percent among children aged 1 through 4 and among women of childbearing age. (Baseline: 9 percent for children aged 1 through 2, 4 percent for children aged 3 through 4, and 5 percent for women aged 20 through 44 in 1976-80)

	Special Population Target	
	1976-80	
Iron Deficiency Prevalence	*Baseline*	*2000 Target*
2.10a Low-income children aged 1–2	21%	10%
2.10b Low-income children aged 3–4	10%	5%
2.10c Low-income women of childbearing age	8%†	4%
	1983–85	
Anemia Prevalence	*Baseline*	*2000 Target*
2.10d Alaska Native children aged 1–5	22–28%	10%

2.10e Black, low-income pregnant
   women (third trimester)   41%‡   20%
†*Baseline for women aged 20–44.*
‡*1988 baseline for women aged 15–44.*

Note: Iron deficiency is defined as having abnormal results for 2 or more of the following tests: mean corpuscular volume, erythrocyte protoporphyrin, and transferrin saturation. Anemia is used as an index of iron deficiency. Anemia among Alaska Native children was defined as hemoglobin < 11 mg/dL or hematocrit < 34 percent. For pregnant women in the third trimester, anemia was defined according to CDC criteria. The preceding prevalences of iron deficiency and anemia may be due to inadequate dietary iron intakes or to inflammatory conditions and infections. For anemia, genetics may also be a factor.

2.11* Increase to at least 75 percent the proportion of mothers who breastfeed their babies in the early postpartum period and to at least 50 percent the proportion who continue breastfeeding until their babies are 5 to 6 months old. (Baseline: 54 percent at discharge from birth site and 21 percent at 5 to 6 months in 1988)

Special Population Targets

Mothers Breastfeeding Their Babies During Early Postpartum Period	1988 Baseline	2000 Target
2.11a Low-income mothers	32%	75%
2.11b Black mothers	25%	75%
2.11c Hispanic mothers	51%	75%
2.11d American Indian/Alaska Native mothers	46%	75%
At Age 5–6 Months		
2.11e Low-income mothers	9%	50%
2.11f Black mothers	8%	50%
2.11g Hispanic mothers	16%	50%
2.11h American Indian/Alaska Native mothers	28%	50%

2.12* Increase to at least 75 percent the proportion of parents and caregivers who use feeding practices that prevent baby bottle tooth decay. (Baseline data available in 1991)

Special Population Targets

Appropriate Feeding Practices	Baseline	2000 Target
2.12a Parents and caregivers with less than high school education	—	65%

    2.12b American Indian/Alaska
           Native parents and care-
           givers   —   65%

2.13 Increase to at least 85 percent the proportion of people aged 18 and older who use food labels to make nutritious food selections. (Baseline: 74 percent used labels to make food selections in 1988)

Services and Protection Objectives

2.14 Achieve useful and informative nutrition labeling for virtually all processed foods and at least 40 percent of fresh meats, poultry, fish, fruits, vegetables, baked goods, and ready-to-eat carry-away foods. (Baseline: 90 percent of sales of processed foods regulated by FDA had nutrition labeling in 1988; baseline data on fresh and carry-away foods unavailable)

2.15 Increase to at least 5,000 brand items the availability of processed food products that are reduced in fat and saturated fat. (Baseline: 2,500 items reduced in fat in 1986)

2.16 Increase to at least 90 percent the proportion of restaurants and institutional food service operations that offer identifiable low-fat, low-calorie food choices, consistent with the *Dietary Guidelines for Americans.* (Baseline: About 70 percent of fast-food and family restaurant chains with 350 or more units had at least one low-fat, low-calorie item on their menu in 1989)

2.17 Increase to at least 90 percent the proportion of school lunch and breakfast services and child care food services with menus that are consistent with the nutrition principles in the *Dietary Guidelines for Americans.* (Baseline data available in 1993)

2.18 Increase to at least 80 percent the receipt of home food services by people aged 65 and older who have difficulty in preparing their own meals or are otherwise in need of home-delivered meals. (Baseline data available in 1991)

2.19 Increase to at least 75 percent the proportion of the nation's schools that provide nutrition education from preschool through 12th grade, preferably as part of quality school health education. (Baseline data available in 1991)

2.20 Increase to at least 50 percent the proportion of worksites with 50 or more employees that offer nutrition education and/or weight management programs for employees. (Baseline: 17 percent offered nutrition education activities and 15 percent offered weight control activities in 1985)

2.21 Increase to at least 75 percent the proportion of primary care providers who provide nutrition assessment and counseling and/or referral to qualified nutritionists or dietitians. (Baseline: Physicians provided diet counseling for an estimated 40 to 50 percent of patients in 1988)

3. Tobacco
Health Status Objectives

3.1* Reduce coronary heart disease deaths to no more that 100 per 100,000 people. (Age-adjusted baseline: 135 per 100,000 in 1987)

Special Population Target

	Coronary Deaths (per 100,000)	1987 Baseline	2000 Target
3.1a	Blacks	163	115

3.2* Slow the rise in lung cancer deaths to achieve a rate of no more that 42 per 100,000 people. (Age-adjusted baseline: 37.9 per 100,000 in 1987)

Note: In its publications, the National Cancer Institute age-adjusts cancer death rates to the 1970 U.S. population. Using the 1970 standard, the equivalent baseline and target values for this objective would by 47.9 and 53 per 100,000, respectively.

3.3 Slow the rise in deaths from chronic obstructive pulmonary disease to achieve a rate of no more than 25 per 100,000 people. (Age-adjusted baseline: 18.7 per 100,000 in 1987)

Note: Deaths from chronic obstructive pulmonary disease include deaths due to chronic bronchitis, emphysema, asthma, and other chronic obstructive pulmonary diseases and allied conditions.

Risk Reduction Objectives

3.4* Reduce cigarette smoking to a prevalence of no more than 15 percent among people aged 20 and older. (Baseline: 29 percent in 1987, 32 percent for men and 27 percent for women)

Special Population Targets

	Cigarette Smoking Prevalence	1987 Baseline	2000 Target
3.4a	People with a high school education or less aged 20 and older	34%	20%
3.4b	Blue-collar workers aged 20 and older	36%	20%
3.4c	Military personnel	42%†	20%
3.4d	Blacks aged 20 and older	34%	18%
3.4e	Hispanics aged 20 and older	33%‡	18%
3.4f	American Indians/Alaska Natives	42–70%§	20%
3.4g	Southeast Asian men	55%+	20%
3.4h	Women of reproductive age	29%††	12%
3.4i	Pregnant women	25%‡‡	10%
3.4j	Women who use oral contraceptives	36%§§	10%

†1988 baseline.

‡1982–84 baseline for Hispanics aged 20–74.

§1979–87 estimates for different tribes.

+1984–88 baseline.

††Baseline for women aged 18–44.

‡‡1985 baseline.

§§1983 baseline.

Note: A cigarette smoker is a person who has smoked at least 100 cigarettes and currently smokes cigarettes.

3.5 Reduce the initiation of cigarette smoking by children and youth so that no more than 15 percent have become regular cigarette smokers by aged 20. (Baseline: 30 percent of youth had become regular cigarette smokers by ages 20 through 24 in 1987)

Special Population Target

		2000 Target
Initiation of Smoking	1987 Baseline	
3.5a Lower socioeconomic status youth†	40%	18%

†As measured by people aged 20–24 with a high school education or less.

3.6 Increase to at least 50 percent the proportion of cigarette smokers aged 18 and older who stopped smoking cigarettes for a least one day during the preceding year. (Baseline: In 1986, 34 percent of people who smoked in the preceding year stopped for at least one day during the year)

3.7 Increase smoking cessation during pregnancy so that at least 60 percent of women who are cigarette smokers at the time they become pregnant quit smoking early in pregnancy and maintain abstinence for the remainder of their pregnancy. (Baseline: 39 percent of white women aged 20 through 44 quit at any time during pregnancy in 1985)

Special Population Target

Cessation and Abstinence During Pregnancy	1985 Baseline	2000 Target
3.7a Women with less than a high school education	28%†	45%

†Baseline for white women aged 20–44.

3.8 Reduce to no more than 20 percent the proportion of children aged 6 and younger who are regularly exposed to tobacco smoke at home. (Baseline: More than 39 percent in 1986, as 39 percent of households with one or more children aged 6 or younger had a cigarette smoker in the household)

Note: Regular exposure to tobacco smoke at home is defined as the occurrence of tobacco smoking anywhere in the home on more than 3 days each week.

3.9   Reduce smokeless tobacco use by males aged 12 through 24 to a prevalence of no more than 4 percent. (Baseline: 6.6 percent among males aged 12 through 17 in 1988; 8.9 percent among males aged 18 through 24 in 1987)

	Special Population Target	
	1986–87	2000
Smokeless Tobacco Use	*Baseline*	Target
3.9a American Indian/Alaska Native youth	18–64%	10%

Note: For males aged 12 through 17, a smokeless tobacco user is someone who has used snuff or chewing tobacco in the preceding month. For males aged 18 through 24, a smokeless tobacco user is someone who has used either snuff or chewing tobacco at least 20 times and who currently uses snuff or chewing tobacco.

Services and Protection Objectives

3.10 Establish tobacco-free environments and include tobacco use prevention in the curricula of all elementary, middle, and secondary schools, preferably as part of quality school health education. (Baseline: 17 percent of school districts totally banned smoking on school premises or at school functions in 1988; antismoking education was provided by 78 percent of school districts at the high school level, 81 percent at the middle school level, and 75 percent at the elementary school level in 1988)

3.11 Increase to at least 75 percent the proportion of worksites with a formal smoking policy that prohibits or severely restricts smoking at the workplace. (Baseline: 27 percent of worksites with 50 or more employees in 1985; 54 percent of medium and large companies in 1987)

3.12 Enact in 50 states comprehensive laws on clean indoor air that prohibit or strictly limit smoking in the workplace and enclosed public places (including health care facilities, schools, and public transportation). (Baseline: 42 states and the District of Columbia had laws restricting smoking in public places; 31 states restricted smoking in public workplaces; but only 13 states had comprehensive laws regulating smoking in private as well as public worksites and at least 4 public places, including restaurants, as of 1988)

3.13 Enact and enforce in 50 states laws prohibiting the sale and distribution of tobacco products to youth younger than age 19. (Baseline: 44 states and the District of Columbia had, but rarely enforced, laws regulating the sale and/or distribution of cigarettes or tobacco products to minors in 1990; only 3 set the age of majority at 19 and only 6 prohibited cigarette vending machines accessible to minors)

Note: Model legislation proposed by DHHS recommends licensure of tobacco vendors, civil money penalties and license suspension or revocation for violations, and a ban on cigarette vending machines.

3.14 Increase to 50 the number of states with plans to reduce tobacco use, especially among youth. (Baseline: 12 states in 1989)

3.15 Eliminate or severely restrict all forms of tobacco product advertising and promotion to which youth younger than age 18 are likely to be exposed. (Baseline: Radio and television advertising of tobacco products were prohibited, but other restrictions on advertising and promotion to which youth may be exposed were minimal in 1990)

3.16 Increase to at least 75 percent the proportion of primary care and oral health care providers who routinely advise cessation and provide assistance and follow-up for all of their tobacco-using patients. (Baseline: About 52 percent of internists reported counseling more than 75 percent of their smoking patients about smoking cessation in 1986; about 35 percent of dentists reported counseling at least 75 percent of their smoking patients about smoking in 1986)

4. Alcohol and Other Drugs
Health Status Objectives

4.1 Reduce deaths caused by alcohol-related motor vehicle crashes to no more than 8.5 per 100,000 people. (Age-adjusted baseline: 9.8 per 100,000 in 1987)

Special Population Targets		
Alcohol-Related Motor Vehicle Crash Deaths (per 100,000)	*1987 Baseline*	*2000 Target*
4.1a American Indian/Alaska Native men	52.2	44.8
4.1b People aged 15–24	21.5	18

4.2 Reduce cirrhosis deaths to no more than 6 per 100,000 people. (Age-adjusted baseline: 9.1 per 100,000 in 1987)

Special Population Targets		
Cirrhosis Deaths (per 100,000)	*1987 Baseline*	*2000 Target*
4.2a Black men	22	12
4.2b American Indians/Alaska Natives	25.9	13

4.3 Reduce drug-related deaths to no more than 3 per 100,000 people. (Age-adjusted baseline: 3.8 per 100,000 in 1987)

4.4   Reduce drug-abuse-related hospital emergency department visits by at least 20 percent. (Baseline data available in 1991)

Risk Reduction Objectives

4.5   Increase by at least 1 year the average age of first use of cigarettes, alcohol, and marijuana by adolescents aged 12 through 17. (Baseline: Age 11.6 for cigarettes, age 13.1 for alcohol, and age 13.4 for marijuana in 1988)

4.6   Reduce the proportion of young people who have used alcohol, marijuana, and cocaine in the past month, as follows:

Substance/Age	1988 Baseline	2000 Target
Alcohol/aged 12–17	25.2%	12.6%
Alcohol/aged 18–20	57.9%	29%
Marijuana/aged 12–17	6.4%	3.2%
Marijuana/aged 18–25	15.5%	7.8%
Cocaine/aged 12–17	1.1%	0.6%
Cocaine/aged 18–25	4.5%	2.3%

Note: The targets of this objective are consistent with the goals established by the Office of National Drug Control Policy, Executive Office of the President.

4.7   Reduce the proportion of high school seniors and college students engaging in recent occasions of heavy drinking of alcoholic beverages to no more than 28 percent of high school seniors and 32 percent of college students. (Baseline: 33 percent of high school seniors and 41.7 percent of college students in 1989)

Note: Recent heavy drinking is defined as having 5 or more drinks on one occasion in the previous 2-week period as monitored by self-reports.

4.8   Reduce alcohol consumption by people aged 14 and older to an annual average of no more than 2 gallons of ethanol per person. (Baseline: 2.54 gallons of ethanol in 1987)

4.9   Increase the proportion of high school seniors who perceive social disapproval associated with the heavy use of alcohol, occasional use of marijuana, and experimentation with cocaine, as follows:

Behavior	1989 Baseline	2000 Target
Heavy use of alchol	56.4%	70%
Occasional use of marijuana	71.1%	85%
Trying cocaine once or twice	88.9%	95%

Note: Heavy drinking is defined as having 5 or more drinks once or twice each weekend.

4.10   Increase the proportion of high school seniors who associate risk of physical or psychological harm with the heavy use of alcohol, regular use of marijuana, and experimentation with cocaine, as follows:

Behavior	1989 Baseline	2000 Target
Heavy use of alcohol	44%	70%
Occasional use of marijuana	77.4%	90%
Trying cocaine once or twice	54.9%	80%

Note: Heavy drinking is defined as having 5 or more drinks once or twice each weekend.

4.11 Reduce to no more than 3 percent the proportion of male high school seniors who use anabolic steroids. (Baseline: 4.7 percent in 1989)

Services and Protection Objectives

4.12 Establish and monitor in 50 states comprehensive plans to ensure access to alcohol and drug treatment programs for traditionally underserved people. (Baseline data available in 1991)

4.13 Provide to children in all school districts and private schools primary and secondary school educational programs on alcohol and other drugs, preferably as part of quality school health education. (Baseline: 63 percent provided some instruction, 39 percent provided counseling, and 23 percent referred students for clinical assessments in 1987)

4.14 Extend adoption of alcohol and drug policies for the work environment to at least 60 percent of worksites with 50 or more employees. (Baseline data available in 1991)

4.15 Extend to 50 states administrative driver's license suspension/ revocation laws or programs of equal effectiveness for people determined to have been driving under the influence of intoxicants. (Baseline: 28 states and the District of Columbia in 1990)

4.16 Increase to 50 the number of states that have enacted and enforce policies, beyond those in existence in 1989, to reduce access to alcoholic beverages by minors.

Note: Policies to reduce access to alcoholic beverages by minors may include those that address restriction of the sale of alcoholic beverages at recreational and entertainment events at which youth make up a majority of participants/consumers, product pricing, penalties and license revocation for sale of alcoholic beverages to minors, and other approaches designed to discourage and restrict purchase of alcoholic beverages by minors.

4.17 Increase to at least 20 the number of states that have enacted statutes to restrict promotion of alcoholic beverages that is focused principally on young audiences. (Baseline data available in 1992)

4.18 Extend to 50 states legal blood alcohol concentration tolerance levels of .04 percent for motor vehicle drivers aged 21 and older and .00 percent for those younger than age 21. (Baseline: 0 states in 1990)

4.19 Increase to at least 75 percent the proportion of primary care providers who screen for alcohol and other drug use problems and provide counseling and referral as needed. (Baseline data available in 1992)

5. Family Planning
Health Status Objectives

5.1 Reduce pregnancies among girls aged 17 and younger to no more than 50 per 1,000 adolescents. (Baseline: 71.1 pregnancies per 1,000 girls aged 15 through 17 in 1985)

	Special Population Targets		
	Pregnancies (per 1,000)	*1985 Baseline*	*2000 Target*
5.1a	Black adolescent girls aged 15–19	186†	120
5.1b	Hispanic adolescent girls aged 15–19	158	105
	†Non-white adolescents.		

Note: For black and Hispanic adolescent girls, baseline data are unavailable for those aged 15 through 17. The targets for these two populations are based on data for women aged 15 through 19. If more complete data become available, a 35 percent reduction from baseline figures should be used as the target.

5.2 Reduce to no more than 30 percent the proportion of all pregnancies that are unintended. (Baseline: 56 percent of pregnancies in the previous 5 years were unintended, either unwanted or earlier than desired, in 1988)

	Special Population Target		
	Unintended Pregnancies	*1988 Baseline*	*2000 Target*
5.2a	Black women	78%	40%

5.3 Reduce the prevalence of infertility to no more than 6.5 percent. (Baseline: 7.9 percent of married couples with wives aged 15 through 44 in 1988)

	Special Population Targets		
	Prevalence of Infertility	*1988 Baseline*	*2000 Target*
5.3a	Black couples	12.1%	9%
5.3b	Hispanic couples	12.4%	9%

Note: Infertility is the failure of couples to conceive after 12 months of intercourse without contraception.

Risk Reduction Objectives

5.4* Reduce the proportion of adolescents who have engaged in sexual intercourse to no more than 15 percent by age 15 and no more than 40 percent by age 17. (Baseline: 27 percent of girls and 33 percent of boys by age 15; 50 percent of girls and 66 percent of boys by age 17; reported in 1988)

5.5 Increase to at least 40 percent the proportion of ever sexually active adolescents aged 17 and younger who have abstained from sexual activity for the previous 3 months. (Baseline: 26 percent of sexually active girls aged 15 through 17 in 1988)

5.6 Increase to at least 90 percent the proportion of sexually active, unmarried people aged 19 and younger who use contraception, especially combined method contraception that both effectively prevents pregnancy and provides barrier protection against disease. (Baseline: 78 percent at most recent intercourse and 63 percent at first intercourse; 2 percent used oral contraceptives and the condom at most recent intercourse; among young women aged 15 through 19 reporting in 1988)

Note: Strategies to achieve this objective must be undertaken sensitively to avoid indirectly encouraging or condoning sexual activity among teens who are not yet sexually active.

5.7 Increase the effectiveness with which family planning methods are used, as measured by a decrease to no more than 5 percent in the proportion of couples experiencing pregnancy despite use of a contraceptive method. (Baseline: Approximately 10 percent of women using reversible contraceptive methods experienced an unintended pregnancy in 1982)

Services and Protection Objectives

5.8 Increase to at least 85 percent the proportion of people aged 10 through 18 who have discussed human sexuality, including values surrounding sexuality, with their parents and/or have received information through another parentally endorsed source, such as youth, school, or religious programs. (Baseline: 66 percent of people aged 13 through 18 have discussed sexuality with their parents; reported in 1986)

Note: This objective, which supports family communication on a range of vital personal health issues, will be tracked using the National Health Interview Survey, a continuing, voluntary, national sample survey of adults who report on household characteristics including such items as illnesses, injuries, use of health services, and demographic characteristics.

5.9 Increase to at least 90 percent the proportion of pregnancy counselors who offer positive, accurate information about adoption to their unmarried patients with unintended pregnancies. (Baseline: 60 percent of pregnancy counselors in 1984)

Note: Pregnancy counselors are any providers of health or social services who discuss the management or outcome of pregnancy with a woman after she has received a diagnosis of pregnancy.

5.10* Increase to at least 60 percent the proportion of primary care providers who provide age-appropriate preconception care and counseling. (Baseline data available in 1992)

5.11* Increase to at least 50 percent the proportion of family planning clinics, maternal and child health clinics, sexually transmitted disease clinics, tuberculosis clinics, drug treatment centers, and primary care clinics that screen, diagnose, treat, counsel, and provide (or refer for) partner notification services for HIV infection and bacterial sexually transmitted diseases (gonorrhea, syphilis, and chlamydia). (Baseline: 40 percent of family planning clinics for bacterial sexually transmitted diseases in 1989)

6. Mental Health and Mental Disorders
Health Status Objectives

6.1* Reduce suicides to no more than 10.5 per 100,000 people. (Age-adjusted baseline: 11.7 per 100,000 in 1987)

Special Population Targets

Suicides (per 100,000)	1987 Baseline	2000 Target
6.1a Youth aged 15–19	10.3	8.2
6.1b Men aged 20–34	25.2	21.4
6.1c White men aged 65 and older	46.1	39.2
6.1d American Indian/Alaska Native men in reservation states	15	12.8

6.2* Reduce by 15 percent the incidence of injurious suicide attempts among adolescents aged 14 through 17. (Baseline data available in 1991)

6.3 Reduce to less than 10 percent the prevalence of mental disorders among children and adolescents. (Baseline: An estimated 12 percent among youth younger than aged 18 in 1989)

6.4 Reduce the prevalence of mental disorders (exclusive of substance abuse) among adults living in the community to less than 10.7 percent. (Baseline: One-month point prevalence of 12.6 percent in 1984)

6.5 Reduce to less than 35 percent the proportion of people aged 18 and older who experienced adverse health effects from stress within the past year. (Baseline: 42.6 percent in 1985)

Special Population Target

	1985 Baseline	2000 Target
6.5a People with disabilities	53.5%	40%

Note: For this objective, people with disabilities are people who report any limitation in activity due to chronic conditions.

Risk Reduction Objectives

6.6 Increase to at least 30 percent the proportion of people aged 18 and older with severe, persistent mental disorders who use community support programs. (Baseline: 15 percent in 1986)

6.7 Increase to at least 45 percent the proportion of people with major depressive disorders who obtain treatment. (Baseline: 31 percent in 1982)

6.8 Increase to at least 20 percent the proportion of people aged 18 and older who seek help in coping with personal and emotional problems. (Baseline: 11.1 percent in 1985)

Special Population Target

		1985 Baseline	2000 Target
6.8a	People with disabilities	14.7%	30%

6.9 Decrease to no more than 5 percent the proportion of people aged 18 and older who report experiencing significant levels of stress who do not take steps to reduce or control their stress. (Baseline: 21 percent in 1985)

Services and Protection Objectives

6.10* Increase to 50 the number of states with officially established protocols that engage mental health, alcohol and drug, and public health authorities with corrections authorities to facilitate identification and appropriate intervention to prevent suicide by jail inmates. (Baseline data available in 1992)

6.11 Increase to at least 40 percent the proportion of worksites employing 50 or more people that provide programs to reduce employee stress. (Baseline: 26.6 percent in 1985)

6.12 Establish mutual help clearinghouses in at least 25 states. (Baseline: 9 states in 1989)

6.13 Increase to at least 50 percent the proportion of primary care providers who routinely review with patients their patients' cognitive, emotional, and behavioral functioning and the resources available to deal with any problems that are identified. (Baseline data available in 1992)

6.14 Increase to at least 75 percent the proportion of providers of primary care for children who include assessment of cognitive, emotional, and parent-child functioning, with appropriate counseling, referral, and follow-up, in their clinical practices. (Baseline data available in 1992)

7. Violent and Abusive Behavior
Health Status Objectives

7.1 Reduce homicides to no more than 7.2 per 100,000 people. (Age-adjusted baseline: 8.5 per 100,000 in 1987)

Special Population Target

Homicide Rate (per 100,000)	1987 Baseline	2000 Target
7.1a Children aged 3 and younger	3.9	3.1
7.1b Spouses aged 15–34	1.7	1.4
7.1c Black men aged 15–34	90.5	72.4
7.1d Hispanic men aged 15–34	53.1	42.5
7.1e Black women aged 15–34	20.0	16.0
7.1f American Indians/Alaska Natives in reservation states	14.1	11.3

7.2* Reduce suicides to no more than 10.5 per 100,000 people. (Age-adjusted baseline: 11.7 per 100,000 in 1987)

Special Population Targets

Suicides (per 100,000)	1987 Baseline	2000 Target
7.2a Youth aged 15–19	10.3	8.2
7.2b Men aged 20–34	25.2	21.4
7.2c White men aged 65 and older	46.1	39.2
7.2d American Indian/Alaska Native men in reservation states	15	12.8

7.3 Reduce weapon-related violent deaths to no more than 12.6 per 100,000 people from major causes. (Age-adjusted baseline: 12.9 per 100,000 by firearms, 1.9 per 100,000 by knives, in 1987)

7.4 Reverse to less than 25.2 per 1,000 children the rising incidence of maltreatment of children younger than age 18. (Baseline: 25.2 per 1,000 in 1986)

Type-Specific Targets

Incidence of Types of Maltreatment (per 1,000)	1986 Baseline	2000 Target
7.4a Physical abuse	5.7	<5.7
7.4b Sexual abuse	2.5	<2.5
7.4c Emotional abuse	3.4	<3.4
7.4d Neglect	15.9	<15.9

7.5 Reduce physical abuse directed at women by male partners to no more than 27 per 1,000 couples. (Baseline: 30 per 1,000 in 1985)

7.6 Reduce assault injuries among people aged 12 and older to no more than 10 per 1,000 people. (Baseline: 11.1 per 1,000 in 1986)

7.7 Reduce rape and attempted rape of women aged 12 and older to no more than 108 per 100,000 women (Baseline: 120 per 100,000 in 1986)

Special Population Target

Incidence of Rape and Attempted Rape (per 100,000)	1986 Baseline	2000 Target
7.7a Women aged 12–34	250	225

7.8* Reduce by 15 percent the incidence of injurious suicide attempts among adolescents aged 14 through 17. (Baseline data available in 1991)

Risk Reduction Objectives

7.9 Reduce by 20 percent the incidence of physical fighting among adolescents aged 14 through 17. (Baseline data available in 1991)

7.10 Reduce by 20 percent the incidence of weapon carrying by adolescents aged 14 through 17. (Baseline data available in 1991)

7.11 Reduce by 20 percent the proportion of people who possess weapons that are inappropriately stored and therefore dangerously available. (Baseline data available in 1992)

Services and Protection Objectives

7.12 Extend protocols for routinely identifying, treating, and properly referring suicide attempters, victims of sexual assault, and victims of spouse, elder, and child abuse to at least 90 percent of hospital emergency departments. (Baseline data available in 1992)

7.13 Extend to at least 45 states implementation of unexplained child death review systems. (Baseline data available in 1991)

7.14 Increase to at least 30 the number of states in which at least 50 percent of children identified as neglected or physically or sexually abused receive physical and mental evaluation with appropriate follow-up as a means of breaking the intergenerational cycle of abuse. (Baseline data available in 1993)

7.15 Reduce to less than 10 percent the proportion of battered women and their children turned away from emergency housing due to lack of space. (Baseline: 40 percent in 1987)

7.16 Increase to at least 50 percent the proportion of elementary and secondary schools that teach nonviolent conflict resolution skills, preferably as a part of quality school health education. (Baseline data available in 1991)

7.17 Extend coordinated, comprehensive violence prevention programs to at least 80 percent of local jurisdictions with populations over 100,000. (Baseline data available in 1993)

7.18* Increase to 50 the number of states with officially established protocols that engage mental health, alcohol and drug, and public health authorities with corrections authorities to facilitate identification and appropriate intervention to prevent suicide by jail inmates. (Baseline data available in 1992)

8. Educational and Community-Based Programs
Health Status Objective

8.1* Increase years of healthy life to at least 65 years. (Baseline: An estimated 62 years in 1980)

Special Population Targets

	Years of Healthy Life	1980 Baseline	2000 Target
8.1a	Blacks	56	60
8.1b	Hispanics	62	65
8.1c	People aged 65 and older	12†	14†

†*Years of healthy life remaining at age 65.*

Note: Years of healthy life (also referred to as quality-adjusted life years) is a summary measure of health that combines mortality (quantity of life) and morbidity and disability (quality of life) into a single measure. For people aged 65 and older, active life expectancy, a related summary measure, also will be tracked.

Risk Reduction Objective

8.2 Increase the high school graduation rate to at least 90 percent, thereby reducing risks for multiple problem behaviors and poor mental and physical health. (Baseline: 79 percent of people aged 20 through 21 had graduated from high school with a regular diploma in 1989)

Note: This objective and its target are consistent with the National Education Goal to increase high school graduation rates. The baseline estimate is a proxy. When a measure is chosen to monitor this National Education Goal, the same measure and data source will be used to track this objective.

Services and Protection Objectives

8.3 Achieve for all disadvantaged children and children with disabilities access to high-quality and developmentally appropriate preschool programs that help prepare children for school, thereby improving their prospects with regard to school performance, problem behaviors, and mental and physical health. (Baseline: 47 percent of eligible children aged 4 were afforded the opportunity to enroll in Head Start in 1990)

Note: This objective and its target are consistent with the National Education Goal to increase school readiness and its objective to increase access to preschool programs for disadvantaged and disabled children. The baseline estimate is an available, but partial, proxy. When a measure is chosen to monitor this National Education Goal, the same measure and data source will be used to track this objective.

8.4 Increase to at least 75 percent the proportion of the nation's elementary schools that provide planned and sequential kindergarten through 12th grade quality school health education. (Baseline data available in 1991)

8.5 Increase to at least 50 percent the proportion of postsecondary institutions with institutionwide health promotion programs for students, faculty, and staff. (Baseline: At least 20 percent of higher education institutions offered health promotion activities for students in 1989–90)

8.6 Increase to at least 85 percent the proportion of workplaces with 50 or more employees that offer health promotion activities for their employees, preferably as part of a comprehensive employee health promotion program. (Baseline: 65 percent of worksites with 50 or more employees offered at least one health promotion activity in 1985; 63 percent of medium and large companies had a wellness program in 1987)

8.7 Increase to at least 20 percent the proportion of hourly workers who participate regularly in employer-sponsored health promotion activities. (Baseline data available in 1992)

8.8 Increase to at least 90 percent the proportion of people aged 65 and older who had the opportunity to participate during the preceding year in at least one organized health promotion program through a senior center, lifecare facility, or other community-based setting that serves older adults. (Baseline data available in 1992)

8.9 Increase to at least 75 percent the proportion of people aged 10 and older who have discussed issues related to nutrition, physical activity, sexual behavior, tobacco, alcohol, other drugs, or safety with family members on at least one occasion during the preceding month. (Baseline data available in 1992)

Note: This objective, which supports family communication on a range of vital personal health issues, will be tracked using the National Health Interview Survey, a continuing, voluntary, national sample survey of adults who report on household characteristics including such items as illnesses, injuries, use of health services, and demographic characteristics.

8.10 Establish community health promotion programs that separately or together address at least three of the Healthy People 2000 priorities and reach at least 40 percent of each state's population. (Baseline data available in 1992)

8.11 Increase to at least 50 percent the proportion of counties that have established culturally and linguistically appropriate community health promotion programs for racial and ethnic minority populations. (Baseline data available in 1992)

Note: This objective will be tracked in counties in which a racial or ethnic group constitutes more than 10 percent of the population.

8.12 Increase to at least 90 percent the proportion of hospitals, health maintenance organizations, and large group practices that provide patient education programs, and to at least 90 percent the proportion of community hospitals that offer community health promotion programs addressing the priority health needs of their communities. (Baseline: 66 percent of 6,821 registered hospitals provided patient education services in 1987; 60 percent of 5,677 community hospitals offered community health promotion programs in 1987)

8.13 Increase to at least 75 percent the proportion of local television network affiliates in the top 20 television markets that have become partners with one or more community organizations around one of the health problems addressed by the Healthy People 2000 objectives. (Baseline data available in 1991)

8.14 Increase to at least 90 percent the proportion of people who are served by a local health department that is effectively carrying out the core functions of public health. (Baseline data available in 1992)

Note: The core functions of public health have been defined as assessment, policy development, and assurance. Local health department refers to any local component of the public health system, defined as an administrative and service unit of local or state government concerned with health and carrying some responsibility for the health of a jurisdiction smaller than a state.

9. Unintentional Injuries
Health Status Objectives

9.1 Reduce deaths caused by unintentional injuries to no more than 29.3 per 100,000 people. (Age-adjusted baseline: 34.5 per 100,000 in 1987)

	Special Population Targets		
	Deaths Caused by		
	Unintentional Injuries		
	(per 100,000)	*1987 Baseline*	*2000 Target*
9.1a	American Indians/Alaska Natives	82.6	66.1
9.1b	Black males	64.9	51.9
9.1c	White males	53.6	42.9

9.2 Reduce nonfatal unintentional injuries so that hospitalizations for this condition are no more than 754 per 100,000 people. (Baseline: 887 per 100,000 in 1988)

9.3 Reduce deaths caused by motor vehicle crashes to no more than 1.9 per 100 million vehicle miles traveled and 16.8 per 100,000 people. (Baseline: 2.4 per 100 million vehicle miles traveled (VMT) and 18.8 per 100,000 people (age adjusted) in 1987)

	Special Population Targets		
	Deaths Caused by Motor		
	Vehicle Crashes (per 100,000)	*1987 Baseline*	*2000 Target*
9.3a	Children aged 14 and younger	6.2	5.5

9.3b	Youth aged 15–24	36.9	33
9.3c	People aged 70 and older	22.6	20
9.3d	American Indians/Alaska Natives	46.8	39.2

Type-Specific Targets

	Deaths Caused by Motor Vehicle Crashes	*1987 Baseline*	*2000 Target*
9.3e	Motorcyclists	40.9/100 million VMT and 1.7/100,000	33/100 million VMT and 1.5/100,000
9.3f	Pedestrians	3.1/100,000	2.7/100,000

9.4 Reduce deaths from falls and fall-related injuries to no more than 2.3 per 100,000 people. (Age-adjusted baseline: 2.7 per 100,000 in 1987)

Special Population Targets

	Deaths from Falls and Fall-Related Injuries (per 100,000)	*1987 Baseline*	*2000 Target*
9.4a	People aged 65–84	18	14.4
9.4b	People aged 85 and older	131.2	105.0
9.4c	Black men aged 30-69	8	5.6

9.5 Reduce drowning deaths to no more than 1.3 per 100,000 people. (Age-adjusted baseline: 2.1 per 100,000 in 1987)

Special Population Targets

	Drowning Deaths (per 100,000)	*1987 Baseline*	*2000 Target*
9.5a	Children aged 4 and younger	4.2	2.3
9.5b	Men aged 15–34	4.5	2.5
9.5c	Black males	6.6	3.6

9.6 Reduce residential fire deaths to no more than 1.2 per 100,000 people. (Age-adjusted baseline: 1.5 per 100,000 in 1987)

Special Population Targets

	Residential Fire Deaths (per 100,000)	*1987 Baseline*	*2000 Target*
9.6a	Children aged 4 and younger	4.4	3.3
9.6b	People aged 65 and older	4.4	3.3
9.6c	Black males	5.7	4.3
9.6d	Black females	3.4	2.6

Type-Specific Target

		1987 Baseline	2000 Target
9.6e	Residential fire deaths caused by smoking	17%	5%

9.7 Reduce hip fractures among people aged 65 and older so that hospitalizations for this condition are no more than 607 per 100,000. (Baseline: 714 per 100,000 in 1988)

Special Population Target

Hip Fractures (per 100,000)		1988 Baseline	2000 Target
9.7a	White women aged 85 and older	2,721	2,177

9.8 Reduce nonfatal poisoning to no more than 88 emergency department treatments per 100,000 people. (Baseline: 103 per 100,000 in 1986)

Special Population Target

Nonfatal Poisoning (per 100,000)		1986 Baseline	2000 Target
9.8a	Among children aged 4 and younger	650	520

9.9 Reduce nonfatal head injuries so that hospitalizations for this condition are no more than 106 per 100,000 people. (Baseline: 125 per 100,000 in 1988)

9.10 Reduce nonfatal spinal cord injuries so that hospitalizations for this condition are no more than 5 per 100,000 people. (Baseline: 5.9 per 100,000 in 1988)

Special Population Target

Nonfatal Spinal Cord Injuries (per 100,000)		1988 Baseline	2000 Target
9.10a	Males	8.9	7.1

9.11 Reduce the incidence of secondary disabilities associated with injuries of the head and spinal cord to no more than 16 and 2.6 per 100,000 people, respectively. (Baseline: 20 per 100,000 for serious head injuries and 3.2 per 100,000 for spinal cord injuries in 1986)

Note: Secondary disabilities are defined as those medical conditions secondary to traumatic head or spinal cord injury that impair independent and productive lifestyles.

Risk Reduction Objectives

9.12 Increase use of occupant protection systems, such as safety belts, inflatable safety restraints, and child safety seats, to at least 85 percent of motor vehicle occupants. (Baseline: 42 percent in 1988)

Special Population Target
Use of Occupant Protection

Systems	1988 Baseline	2000 Target
9.12a Children aged 4 and younger	84%	95%

9.13 Increase use of helmets to at least 80 percent of motorcyclists and at least 50 percent of bicyclists. (Baseline: 60 percent of motorcyclists in 1988 and an estimated 8 percent of bicyclists in 1984)

Services and Protection Objectives

9.14 Extend to 50 states laws requiring safety belt and motorcycle helmet use for all ages. (Baseline: 33 states and the District of Columbia in 1989 for automobiles; 22 states, the District of Columbia, and Puerto Rico for motorcycles)

9.15 Enact in 50 states laws requiring that new handguns be designed to minimize the likelihood of discharge by children. (Baseline: 0 states in 1989)

9.16 Extend to 2,000 local jurisdictions the number whose codes address the installation of fire suppression sprinkler systems in those residences at highest risk for fires. (Baseline data available in 1991)

9.17 Increase the presence of functional smoke detectors to at least one on each habitable floor of all inhabited residential dwellings. (Baseline: 81 percent of residential dwellings in 1989)

9.18 Provide academic instruction on injury prevention and control, preferably as part of quality school health education, in at least 50 percent of public school systems (grades K through 12). (Baseline data available in 1991)

9.19* Extend requirement of the use of effective head, face, eye, and mouth protection to all organizations, agencies, and institutions sponsoring sporting and recreation events that pose risks of injury. (Baseline: Only National Collegiate Athletic Association football, hockey, and lacrosse; high school football; amateur boxing; and amateur ice hockey in 1988)

9.20 Increase to at least 30 the number of states that have design standards for signs, signals, marking, lighting, and other characteristics of the roadway environment to improve the visual stimuli and protect the safety of older drivers and pedestrians. (Baseline data available in 1992)

9.21 Increase to at least 50 percent the proportion of primary care providers who routinely provide age-appropriate counseling on safety precautions to prevent unintentional injury. (Baseline data available in 1992)

9.22 Extend to 50 states emergency medical services and trauma systems linking prehospital and rehabilitation services in order to prevent trauma deaths and long-term disability. (Baseline: 2 states in 1987)

10. Occupational Safety and Health
Health Status Objectives

10.1 Reduce deaths from work-related injuries to no more than 4 per 100,000 full-time workers. (Baseline: Average of 6 per 100,000 during 1983–87)

Special Population Targets

Work-Related Deaths (per 100,000)	1983–87 Average	2000 Target
10.1a Mine workers	30.3	21
10.1b Construction workers	25.0	17
10.1c Transportation workers	15.2	10
10.1d Farm workers	14.0	9.5

10.2 Reduce work-related injuries resulting in medical treatment, lost time from work, or restricted work activity to no more than 6 cases per 100 full-time workers. (Baseline: 7.7 per 100 in 1987)

Special Population Targets

Work-Related Injuries (per 100)	1983–87 Average	2000 Target
10.2a Construction workers	14.9	10
10.2b Nursing and personal care workers	12.7	9
10.2c Farm workers	12.4	8
10.2d Transportation workers	8.3	6
10.2e Mine workers	8.3	6

10.3 Reduce cumulative trauma disorders to an incidence of no more than 60 cases per 100,000 full-time workers. (Baseline: 100 per 100,000 in 1987)

Special Population Targets

Cumulative Trauma Disorders (per 100,000)	1987 Baseline	2000 Target
10.3a Manufacturing industry workers	355	150
10.3b Meat product workers	3,920	2,000

10.4 Reduce occupational skin disorders or diseases to an incidence of no more than 55 per 100,000 full-time workers. (Baseline: Average of 64 per 100,000 during 1983–87)

10.5 Reduce hepatitis B infections among occupationally exposed workers to an incidence of no more than 1,250 cases. (Baseline: An estimated 6,200 cases in 1987)

Risk Reduction Objectives

10.6   Increase to at least 75 percent the proportion of worksites with 50 or more employees that mandate employee use of occupant protection systems, such as seatbelts, during all work-related motor vehicle travel. (Baseline data available in 1991)

10.7   Reduce to no more than 15 percent the proportion of workers exposed to average daily noise levels that exceed 85 dB A. (Baseline data available in 1992)

10.8   Eliminate exposures which result in workers having blood lead concentrations greater than 25 µg/dL of whole blood. (Baseline: 4,804 workers with blood lead levels above 25 µg/dL in 7 states in 1988)

10.9* Increase hepatitis B immunization levels to 90 percent among occupationally exposed workers. (Baseline data available in 1991)

Services and Protection Objectives

10.10 Implement occupational safety and health plans in 50 states for the identification, management, and prevention of leading work-related diseases and injuries within the state. (Baseline: 10 states in 1989)

10.11 Establish in 50 states exposure standards adequate to prevent the major occupational lung diseases to which their worker populations are exposed (byssinosis, asbestosis, coal workers' pneumoconiosis, and silicosis). (Baseline data available in 1991)

10.12 Increase to at least 70 percent the proportion of worksites with 50 or more employees that have implemented programs on worker health and safety. (Baseline data available in 1991)

10.13 Increase to at least 50 percent the proportion of worksites with 50 or more employees that offer back injury prevention and rehabilitation programs. (Baseline: 28.6 percent offered back care activities in 1985)

10.14 Establish in 50 states either public health or labor department programs that provide consultation and assistance to small businesses to implement safety and health programs for their employees. (Baseline data available in 1991)

10.15 Increase to at least 75 percent the proportion of primary care providers who routinely elicit occupational health exposures as a part of patient history and provide relevant counseling. (Baseline data available in 1992)

11. Environmental Health
Health Status Objectives

11.1   Reduce asthma morbidity, as measured by a reduction in asthma hospitalizations to no more than 160 per 100,000 people. (Baseline: 188 per 100,000 in 1987)

Special Population Targets
Asthma Hospitalizations

(per 100,000)	*1987 Baseline*	*2000 Target*
11.1a Blacks and other nonwhites	334	265
11.1b Children	284†	225

†Children aged 14 and younger.

11.2* Reduce the prevalence of serious mental retardation among school-aged children to no more than 2 per 1,000 children. (Baseline: 2.7 per 1,000 children aged 10 in 1985-88)

Note: Community water systems are public or investor-owned water systems that serve large or small communities, subdivisions, or trailer parks with at least 15 service connections or 25 year-round residents.

11.3 Reduce outbreaks of waterborne disease from infectious agents and chemical poisoning to no more than 11 per year. (Baseline: Average of 31 outbreaks per year during 1981–88)

Special Population Target

Average Annual Number of *Waterborne Disease Outbreaks*	*1981–88* *Baseline*	*2000 Target*
11.3a People served by community water systems	13	6

11.4 Reduce the prevalence of blood lead levels exceeding 15 μg/dL and 25 μg/dL among children aged 6 months through 5 years to no more than 500,000 and 0, respectively. (Baseline: An estimated 3 million children had levels exceeding 15 μg/dL, and 234,000 had levels exceeding 25 μg/dL, in 1984)

Special Population Target

Prevalence of Blood Lead *Levels Exceeding 15 μg/dL* *and 25 μg/dL*	*1984 Baseline*	*2000 Target*
11.4a Inner-city low-income black children (annual family income <$6,000 in 1984 dollars)	234,900 and 36,700	75,000 and 0

Risk Reduction Objectives

11.5 Reduce human exposure to criteria air pollution, as measured by an increase to at least 85 percent in the proportion of people who live in counties that have not exceeded any Environmental Protection Agency standard for air quality in the previous 12 months. (Baseline: 49.7 percent in 1988)

Proportion Living in Counties That Have Not Exceeded Criteria Air Pollution Standards in 1988 for:

Ozone	53.6%
Carbon monoxide	87.8%
Nitrogen dioxide	96.6%
Sulfur dioxide	99.3%
Particulates	89.4%
Lead	99.3%
Total (any of above pollutants)	49.7%

Note: An individual living in a county that exceeds an air quality standard may not actually be exposed to unhealthy air. Of all criteria air pollutants, ozone is the most likely to have fairly uniform concentrations throughout an area. Exposure is to criteria air pollutants in ambient air. Due to weather fluctuations, multiyear averages may be the most appropriate way to monitor progress toward this objective.

11.6 Increase to at least 40 percent the proportion of homes in which homeowners/occupants have tested for radon concentrations and that have either been found to pose minimal risk or have been modified to reduce risk to health. (Baseline: Less than 5 percent of homes had been tested in 1989)

Special Population Targets

Testing and Modification as Necessary	*Baseline*	*2000 Target*
11.6a Homes with smokers and former smokers	—	50%
11.6b Homes with children	—	50%

11.7 Reduce human exposure to toxic agents by confining total pounds of toxic agents released into the air, water, and soil each year to no more than:

0.24 billion pounds of those toxic agents included on the Department of Health and Human Services list of carcinogens. (Baseline: 0.32 billion pounds in 1988)

2.6 billion pounds of those toxic agents included on the Agency for Toxic Substances and Disease Registry list of the most toxic chemicals. (Baseline: 2.62 billion pounds in 1988)

11.8 Reduce human exposure to solid-waste-related water, air, and soil contamination, as measured by a reduction in average pounds of municipal solid waste produced per person each day to no more than 3.6 pounds. (Baseline: 4.0 pounds per person each day in 1988)

11.9 Increase to at least 85 percent the proportion of people who receive a supply of drinking water that meets the safe drinking water standards established by the Environmental Protection Agency. (Baseline: 74 percent of 58,099 community water systems serving approximately 80 percent of the population in 1988)

Note: Safe drinking water standards are measured using Maximum Contaminant Level (MCL) standards set by the Environmental Protection Agency which define acceptable levels of contaminants. See Objective 11.3 for definition of community water systems.

11.10 Reduce potential risks to human health from surface water, as measured by a decrease to no more than 15 percent in the proportion of assessed rivers, lakes, and estuaries that do not support beneficial uses, such as fishing and swimming. (Baseline: An estimated 25 percent of assessed rivers, lakes, and estuaries did not support designated beneficial uses in 1988)

Note: Designated beneficial uses, such as aquatic life support, contact recreation (swimming), and water supply, are designated by each state and approved by the Environmental Protection Agency. Support of beneficial use is a proxy measure of risk to human health, as many pollutants causing impaired water uses do not have human health effects (e.g., siltation, impaired fish habitat).

Services and Protection Objectives

11.11 Perform testing for lead-based paint in at least 50 percent of homes built before 1950. (Baseline data available in 1991)

11.12 Expand to at least 35 the number of states in which at least 75 percent of local jurisdictions have adopted construction standards and techniques that minimize elevated indoor radon levels in those new building areas locally determined to have elevated radon levels. (Baseline: 1 state in 1989)

Note: Since construction codes are frequently adopted by local jurisdictions rather than states, progress toward this objective also may be tracked using the proportion of cities and counties that have adopted such construction standards.

11.13 Increase to at least 30 the number of states requiring that prospective buyers be informed of the presence of lead-based paint and radon concentrations in all buildings offered for sale. (Baseline: 2 states required disclosure of lead-based paint in 1989; 1 state required disclosure of radon concentrations in 1989; 2 additional states required disclosure that radon has been found in the state and that testing is desirable in 1989)

11.14 Eliminate significant health risks from National Priority List hazardous waste sites, as measured by performance of cleanup at these sites sufficient to eliminate immediate and significant health threats as specified in health assessments completed at all sites. (Baseline: 1,082 sites were on the list in March of 1990; of these, health assessments have been conducted for approximately 1,000)

Note: The Comprehensive Environmental Response, Compensation, and Liability Act of 1980 required the Environmental Protection Agency to develop criteria for determining priorities among hazardous waste sites and to develop and maintain a list of these priority sites. The resulting list is called the National Priorities List (NPL).

11.15 Establish programs for recyclable materials and household hazardous waste in at least 75 percent of counties. (Baseline: Approximately 850 programs in 41 states collected household toxic waste in 1987; extent of recycling collection unknown)

11.16 Establish and monitor in at least 35 states plans to define and track sentinel environmental diseases. (Baseline: 0 states in 1990)

Note: Sentinel environmental diseases include lead poisoning, other heavy-metal poisoning (e.g., cadmium, arsenic, and mercury), pesticide poisoning, carbon monoxide poisoning, heatstroke, hypothermia, acute chemical poisoning, methoemoglobinemia, and respiratory diseases triggered by environmental factors (e.g., asthma).

12 Food and Drug Safety
Health Status Objectives

12.1 Reduce infections caused by key foodborne pathogens to incidences of no more than:

Disease (per 100,000)	1987 Baseline	2000 Target
Salmonella species	18	16
Campylobacter jejuni	50	25
Escherichia coli 0157:H7	8	4
Listeria monocytogenes	0.7	0.5

12.2 Reduce outbreaks of infections due to *Salmonella enteritidis* to fewer than 25 outbreaks yearly. (Baseline: 77 outbreaks in 1989)

Risk Reduction Objective

12.3 Increase to at least 75 percent the proportion of households in which principal food preparers routinely refrain from leaving perishable food out of the refrigerator for over 2 hours and wash cutting boards and utensils with soap after contact with raw meat and poultry. (Baseline: For refrigeration of perishable foods, 70 percent; for washing cutting boards with soap, 66 percent; and for washing utensils with soap, 55 percent in 1988)

Services and Protection Objectives

12.4 Extend to at least 70 percent the proportion of states and territories that have implemented model food codes for institutional food operations and to at least 70 percent the proportion that have adopted the new uniform food protection code (Unicode) that sets recommended standards for regulation of all food operations.

(Baseline: For institutional food operations currently using FDA's recommended model codes, 20 percent; for the new Unicode to be released in 1991, 0 percent in 1990)

12.5 Increase to at least 75 percent the proportion of pharmacies and other dispensers of prescription medications that use linked systems to provide alerts to potential adverse drug reactions among medications dispensed by different sources to individual patients. (Baseline data available in 1993)

12.6 Increase to at least 75 percent the proportion of primary care providers who routinely review with their patients aged 65 and older all prescribed and over-the-counter medicines taken by their patients each time a new medication is prescribed. (Baseline data available in 1992)

13. Oral Health
Health Status Objectives

13.1 Reduce dental caries (cavities) so that the proportion of children with one or more caries (in permanent or primary teeth) is no more than 35 percent among children aged 6 through 8 and no more than 60 percent among adolescents aged 15. (Baseline: 53 percent of children aged 6 through 8 in 1986–87; 78 percent of adolescents aged 15 in 1986–87)

Special Population Targets

Dental Caries Prevalence	1986–87 Baseline	2000 Target
13.1a Children aged 6–8 whose parents have less than high school education	70%	45%
13.1b American Indian/Alaska Native children aged 6–8	92%† 52%‡	45%
13.1c Black children aged 6–8	61%	40%
13.1d American Indian/Alaska Native adolescents aged 15	93%	70%

†*In primary teeth in 1983–84.*
‡*In permanent teeth in 1983–84.*

13.2 Reduce untreated dental caries so that the proportion of children with untreated caries (in permanent or primary teeth) is no more than 20 percent among children aged 6 through 8 and no more than 15 percent among adolescents aged 15. (Baseline: 27 percent of children aged 6 through 8 in 1986; 23 percent of adolescents aged 15 in 1986–87)

Special Population Targets

Untreated Dental Caries Among Children	1986–87 Baseline	2000 Target
13.2a Children aged 6–8 whose parents have less than high school education	43%	30%
13.2b American Indian/Alaska Native children aged 6–8	64%†	35%
13.2c Black children aged 6–8	38%	25%
13.2d Hispanic children aged 6–8	36%‡	25%

Among Adolescents

13.2e Adolescents aged 15 whose parents have less than high school education	41%	25%
13.2f American Indian/Alaska Native adolescents aged 15	84%†	40%
13.2g Black adolescents aged 15	38%	20%
13.2h Hispanic adolescents aged 15	31–47%‡	25%

†1983–84 baseline.
‡1982–84 baseline.

13.3 Increase to at least 45 percent the proportion of people aged 35 through 44 who have never lost a permanent tooth due to dental caries or periodontal diseases. (Baseline: 31 percent of employed adults had never lost a permanent tooth for any reason in 1985–86)

Note: Never lost a permanent tooth is having 28 natural teeth exclusive of third molars.

13.4 Reduce to no more than 20 percent the proportion of people aged 65 and older who have lost all of their natural teeth. (Baseline: 36 percent in 1986)

Special Population Target

Complete Tooth Loss Prevalence	1986 Baseline	2000 Target
13.4a Low-income people (annual family income <$15,000)	46%	35%

13.5 Reduce the prevalence of gingivitis among people aged 35 through 44 to no more than 30 percent. (Baseline: 42 percent in 1985–86)

Special Population Targets

Gingivitis Prevalence	1985 Baseline	2000 Target
13.5a Low-income people (annual family income <$12,500)	50%	35%
13.5b American Indians/Alaska Natives	95%†	50%
13.5c Hispanics		50%
Mexican Americans	74%‡	
Cubans	79%‡	
Puerto Ricans	82%‡	

†1983–84 baseline.
‡1982–84 baseline.

13.6   Reduce destructive periodontal diseases to a prevalence of no more than 15 percent among people aged 35 through 44. (Baseline: 24 percent in 1985–86)

Note: Destructive periodontal disease is one or more sites with 4 millimeters or greater loss of tooth attachment.

13.7   Reduce deaths due to cancer of the oral cavity and pharynx to no more than 10.5 per 100,000 men aged 45 through 74 and 4.1 per 100,000 women aged 45 through 74. (Baseline: 12.1 per 100,000 men and 4.1 per 100,000 women in 1987)

Risk Reduction Objectives

13.8   Increase to at least 50 percent the proportion of children who have received protective sealants on the occlusal (chewing) surfaces of permanent molar teeth. (Baseline: 11 percent of children aged 8 and 8 percent of adolescents aged 14 in 1986–87)

Note: Progress toward this objective will be monitored based on prevalence of sealants in children at age 8 and at age 14, when the majority of first and second molars, respectively, are erupted.

13.9   Increase to at least 75 percent the proportion of people served by community water systems providing optimal levels of fluoride. (Baseline: 62 percent in 1989)

Note: Optimal levels of fluoride are determined by the mean maximum daily air temperature over a 5-year period and range between 0.7 and 1.2 parts of fluoride per one million parts of water (ppm).

13.10 Increase use of professionally or self-administered topical or systemic (dietary) fluorides to at least 85 percent of people not receiving optimally fluoridated public water. (Baseline: An estimated 50 percent in 1989)

13.11* Increase to at least 75 percent the proportion of parents and caregivers who use feeding practices that prevent baby bottle tooth decay. (Baseline data available in 1991)

Special Population Targets

Appropriate Feeding Practices	Baseline	2000 Target
13.11a Parents and caregivers with less than high school education	—	65%
13.11b American Indian/Alaska Native parents and caregivers	—	65%

Services and Protection Objectives

13.12 Increase to at least 90 percent the proportion of all children entering school programs for the first time who have received an oral health screening, referral, and follow-up for necessary diagnostic, preventive, and treatment services. (Baseline: 66 percent of children aged 5 visited a dentist during the previous year in 1986)

Note: School programs include Head Start, prekindergarten, kindergarten, and 1st grade.

13.13 Extend to all long-term institutional facilities the requirement that oral examinations and services be provided no later than 90 days after entry into these facilities. (Baseline: Nursing facilities receiving Medicaid or Medicare reimbursement will be required to provide for oral examinations within 90 days of patient entry beginning in 1990; baseline data unavailable for other institutions)

Note: Long-term institutional facilities include nursing homes, prisons, juvenile homes, and detention facilities.

13.14 Increase to at least 70 percent the proportion of people aged 35 and older using the oral health care system during each year. (Baseline: 54 percent in 1986)

Special Population Targets

Proportion Using Oral Health Care System During Each Year	1986 Baseline	2000 Target
13.14a Edentulous people	11%	50%
13.14b People aged 65 and older	42%	60%

13.15 Increase to at least 40 the number of states that have an effective system for recording and referring infants with cleft lips and/or palates to craniofacial anomaly teams. (Baseline: In 1988, approximately 25 states had a central recording mechanism for cleft lip and/or palate and approximately 25 states had an organized referral system to craniofacial anomaly teams)

13.16* Extend requirement of the use of effective head, face, eye, and mouth protection to all organizations, agencies, and institutions sponsoring sporting and recreation events that pose risks of injury. (Baseline: Only National Collegiate Athletic Association football, hockey, and lacrosse; high school football; amateur boxing; and amateur ice hockey in 1988)

14. Maternal and Infant Health
Health Status Objectives

14.1 Reduce the infant mortality rate to no more than 7 per 1,000 live births. (Baseline: 10.1 per 1,000 live births in 1987)

Special Population Targets

Infant Mortality (per 1,000 live births)	1987 Baseline	2000 Target
14.1a Blacks	17.9	11
14.1b American Indians/Alaska Natives	12.5†	8.5
14.1c Puerto Ricans	12.9†	8

Type-Specific Targets

Neonatal and Postneonatal Mortality (per 1,000 live births)	1987 Baseline	2000 Target
14.1d Neonatal mortality	6.5	4.5
14.1e Neonatal mortality among blacks	11.7	7
14.1f Neonatal mortality among Puerto Ricans	8.6†	5.2
14.1g Postneonatal mortality	3.6	2.5
14.1h Postneonatal mortality among blacks	6.1	4
14.1i Postneonatal mortality among American Indians/ Alaska Natives	6.5†	4
14.1j Postneonatal mortality among Puerto Ricans	4.3†	2.8

†1984 baseline.

Note: Infant mortality is deaths of infants under 1 year; neonatal mortality is deaths of infants under 28 days; and postneonatal mortality is deaths of infants aged 28 days up to 1 year.

14.2 Reduce the fetal death rate (20 or more weeks of gestation) to no more than 5 per 1,000 live births plus fetal deaths. (Baseline: 7.6 per 1,000 live births plus fetal deaths in 1987)

	Special Population Target	
Fetal Deaths	*1987 Baseline*	*2000 Target*
14.2a Blacks	12.8†	7.5†

†Per 1,000 live births plus fetal deaths.

14.3 Reduce the maternal mortality rate to no more than 3.3 per 100,000 live births. (Baseline: 6.6 per 100,000 in 1987)

	Special Population Target	
Maternal Mortality	*1987 Baseline*	*2000 Target*
14.3a Blacks	14.2†	5†

†Per 1,000 live births.

Note: The objective uses the maternal mortality rate as defined by the National Center for Health Statistics. However, if other sources of maternal mortality data are used, a 50 percent reduction in maternal mortality is the intended target.

14.4 Reduce the incidence of fetal alcohol syndrome to no more than 0.12 per 1,000 live births. (Baseline: 0.22 per 1,000 live births in 1987)

	Special Population Targets	
Fetal Alcohol Syndrome (per 1,000 live births)	*1987 Baseline*	*2000 Target*
14.4a American Indians/Alaska Natives	4	2
14.4b Blacks	0.8	0.4

Risk Reduction Objectives

14.5 Reduce low birth weight to an incidence of no more than 5 percent of live births and very low birth weight to no more than 1 percent of live births. (Baseline: 6.9 and 1.2 percent, respectively, in 1987)

	Special Population Targets	
Low Birth Weight	*1987 Baseline*	*2000 Target*
14.5a Blacks	12.7%	9%
Very Low Birth Weight	*1987 Baseline*	*2000 Target*
14.5b Blacks	2.7%	2%

Note: Low birth weight is weight at birth of less than 2,500 grams; very low birth weight is weight at birth of less than 1,500 grams.

14.6 Increase to at least 85 percent the proportion of mothers who achieve the minimum recommended weight gain during their pregnancies. (Baseline: 67 percent of married women in 1980)

Note: Recommended weight gain is pregnancy weight gain recommended in the 1990 National Academy of Science's report, Nutrition During Pregnancy.

14.7 Reduce severe complications of pregnancy to no more than 15 per 100 deliveries. (Baseline: 22 hospitalizations (prior to delivery) per 100 deliveries in 1987)

Note: Severe complications of pregnancy will be measured using hospitalizations due to pregnancy-related complications.

14.8 Reduce the cesarean delivery rate to no more than 15 per 100 deliveries. (Baseline: 24.4 per 100 deliveries in 1987)

Type-Specific Targets

Cesarean Delivery (per 100 deliveries)	1987 Baseline	2000 Target
14.8a Primary (first time) cesarean delivery	17.4	12
14.8b Repeat cesarean deliveries	91.2†	65†

†*Among women who had a previous cesarean delivery.*

14.9* Increase to at least 75 percent the proportion of mothers who breastfeed their babies in the early postpartum period and to at least 50 percent the proportion who continue breastfeeding until their babies are 5 to 6 months old. (Baseline: 54 percent at discharge from birth site and 21 percent at 5 to 6 months in 1988)

Special Population Targets

Mothers Breastfeeding Their Babies During Early Postpartum Period	1988 Baseline	2000 Target
14.9a Low-income mothers	32%	75%
14.9b Black mothers	25%	75%
14.9c Hispanic mothers	51%	75%
14.9d American Indian/Alaska Native mothers	46%	75%
At Age 5–6 Months		
14.9e Low-income mothers	9%	50%
14.9f Black mothers	8%	50%
14.9g Hispanic mothers	16%	50%
14.9h American Indian/Alaska Native mothers	28%	50%

14.10 Increase abstinence from tobacco use by pregnant women to at least 90 percent and increase abstinence from alcohol, cocaine, and marijuana by pregnant women by at least 20 percent. (Baseline: 75 percent of pregnant women abstained from tobacco use in 1985)

Note: Data for alcohol, cocaine, and marijuana use by pregnant women will be available from the National Maternal and Infant Health Survey, CDC, in 1991.

Services and Protection Objectives

14.11   Increase to at least 90 percent the proportion of all pregnant women who receive prenatal care in the first trimester of pregnancy. (Baseline: 76 percent of live births in 1987)

	Special Population Targets		
	Proportion of Pregnant Women Receiving Early Prenatal Care	*1987 Baseline*	*2000 Target*
14.11a	Black women	61.1†	90†
14.11b	American Indian/Alaska Native women	60.2†	90†
14.11c	Hispanic women	61.0†	90†
	†Percentage of live births.		

14.12* Increase to at least 60 percent the proportion of primary care providers who provide age-appropriate preconception care and counseling. (Baseline data available in 1992)

14.13   Increase to at least 90 percent the proportion of women enrolled in prenatal care who are offered screening and counseling on prenatal detection of fetal abnormalities. (Baseline data available in 1991)

Note: This objective will be measured by tracking use of maternal serum alpha-fetoprotein screening tests.

14.14   Increase to at least 90 percent the proportion of pregnant women and infants who receive risk-appropriate care. (Baseline data available in 1991)

Note: This objective will be measured by tracking the proportion of very low birth weight infants (less than 1,500 grams) born in facilities covered by a neonatologist 24 hours a day.

14.15   Increase to at least 95 percent the proportion of newborns screened by state-sponsored programs for genetic disorders and other disabling conditions and to 90 percent the proportion of newborns testing positive for disease who receive appropriate treatment. (Baseline: For sickle cell anemia, with 20 states reporting, approximately 33 percent of live births screened (57 percent of black infants); for galactosemia, with 38 states reporting, approximately 70 percent of live births screened)

Note: As measured by the proportion of infants served by programs for sickle cell anemia and galactosemia. Screening programs should be appropriate for state demographic characteristics.

14.16 Increase to at least 90 percent the proportion of babies aged 18 months and younger who receive recommended primary care services at the appropriate intervals. (Baseline data available in 1992)

15. Heart Disease and Stroke
Health Status Objectives

15.1* Reduce coronary heart disease deaths to no more than 100 per 100,000 people. (Age-adjusted baseline: 135 per 100,000 in 1987)

Special Population Target

	Coronary Deaths (per 100,000)	1987 Baseline	2000 Target
15.1a	Blacks	163	115

15.2 Reduce stroke deaths to no more than 20 per 100,000 people. (Age-adjusted baseline: 30.3 per 100,000 in 1987)

Special Population Target

	Stroke Deaths (per 100,000)	1987 Baseline	2000 Target
15.2a	Blacks	51.2	27

15.3 Reduce the increase in end-stage renal disease (requiring maintenance dialysis or transplantation) to attain an incidence of no more than 13 per 100,000. (Baseline: 13.9 per 100,000 in 1987)

Special Population Target

	ESRD Incidence (per 100,000)	1987 Baseline	2000 Target
15.3a	Blacks	32.4	30

Risk Reduction Objectives

15.4 Increase to at least 50 percent the proportion of people with high blood pressure whose blood pressure is under control. (Baseline: 11 percent controlled among people aged 18 through 74 in 1976–80; an estimated 24 percent for people aged 18 and older in 1982–84)

Special Population Target

	High Blood Pressure Control	1976–80 Baseline	1982–84 Baseline	2000 Target
15.4a	Men with high blood pressure	6%	16%	40%

Note: People with high blood pressure have blood pressure equal to or greater than 140 mm Hg systolic and/or 90 mm Hg diastolic and/or take antihypertensive medication. Blood pressure control is defined as maintaining a blood pressure less than 140 mm Hg systolic and 90 mm Hg diastolic. In NHANES II and the Seven States Study, control of hypertension did not include nonpharmacologic treatment. In NHANES III, those controlling their high blood pressure without medication (e.g., through weight loss, low-sodium diets, or restriction of alcohol) will be included.

15.5 Increase to at least 90 percent the proportion of people with high blood pressure who are taking action to help control their blood pressure. (Baseline: 79 percent of aware hypertensives aged 18 and older were taking action to control their blood pressure in 1985)

Special Population Targets

Taking Action to Control Blood Pressure		1985 Baseline	2000 Target
15.5a	White hypertensive men aged 18–34	51%†	80%
15.5b	Black hypertensive men aged 18-34	63%†	80%

†Baseline for aware hypertensive men.

Note: High blood pressure is defined as blood pressure equal to or greater than 140 mm Hg systolic and/or 90 mm Hg diastolic and/or taking antihypertensive medication. Actions to control blood pressure include taking medication, dieting to lose weight, cutting down on salt, and exercising.

15.6 Reduce the mean serum cholesterol level among adults to no more than 200 mg/dL. (Baseline: 213 mg/dL among people aged 20 through 74 in 1976–80, 211 mg/dL for men and 215 mg/dL for women)

15.7 Reduce the prevalence of blood cholesterol levels of 240 mg/dL or greater to no more than 20 percent among adults. (Baseline: 27 percent for people aged 20 through 74 in 1976–80, 29 percent for women and 25 percent for men)

15.8 Increase to at least 60 percent the proportion of adults with high blood cholesterol who are aware of their condition and are taking action to reduce their blood cholesterol to recommended levels. (Baseline: 11 percent of all people aged 18 and older, and thus an estimated 30 percent of people with high blood cholesterol, were aware that their blood cholesterol level was high in 1988)

15.9* Reduce dietary fat intake to an average of 30 percent of calories or less and average saturated fat intake to less than 10 percent of calories among people aged 2 and older. (Baseline: 36 percent of calories from total fat and 13 percent from saturated fat for people aged 20 through 74 in 1976–80; 36 percent and 13 percent for women aged 19 through 50 in 1985)

15.10* Reduce overweight to a prevalence of no more than 20 percent among people aged 20 and older and no more than 15 percent among adolescents aged 12 through 19. (Baseline: 26 percent for people aged 20 through 74 in 1976–80, 24 percent for men and 27 percent for women; 15 percent for adolescents aged 12 through 19 in 1976–80)

Special Population Targets

Overweight Prevalence	1976–80 *Baseline†*	*2000 Target*
15.10a Low-income women aged 20 and older	37%	25%
15.10b Black women aged 20 and older	44%	30%
15.10c Hispanic women aged 20 and older		25%
Mexican American women	39%‡	
Cuban women	34%‡	
Puerto Rican women	37%‡	
15.10d American Indians/Alaska Natives	29–75%§	30%
15.10e People with disabilities	36%+	25%
15.10f Women with high blood pressure	50%	41%
15.10g Men with high blood pressure	39%	35%

†1976–80 baseline for people aged 20–74.
‡1982–84 baseline for Hispanics aged 20–74.
§1984–88 estimates for different tribes.
+1985 baseline for people aged 20–74 who report any limitation in activity due to chronic conditions.

Note: For people aged 20 and older, overweight is defined as body mass index (BMI) equal to or greater than 27.8 for men and 27.3 for women. For adolescents, overweight is defined as BMI equal to or greater than 23.0 for males aged 12 through 14, 24.3 for males aged 15 through 17, 25.8 for males aged 18 through 19, 23.4 for females aged 12 through 14, 24.8 for females aged 15 through 17, and 25.7 for females aged 18 through 19. The values for adolescents are the age- and gender-specific 85th percentile values of the 1976–80 National

Health and Nutrition Examination Survey (NHANES II), corrected for sample variation. BMI is calculated by dividing weight in kilograms by the square of height in meters. The cut points used to define overweight approximate the 120 percent of desirable body weight definition used in the 1990 objectives.

15.11* Increase to at least 30 percent the proportion of people aged 6 and older who engage regularly, preferably daily, in light to moderate physical activity for at least 30 minutes per day. (Baseline: 22 percent of people aged 18 and older were active for at least 30 minutes 5 or more times per week and 12 percent were active 7 or more times per week in 1985)

Note: Light to moderate physical activity requires sustained, rhythmic muscular movements, is at least equivalent to sustained walking, and is performed at less than 60 percent of maximum heart rate for age. Maximum heart rate equals roughly 220 beats per minute minus age. Examples may include walking, swimming, cycling, dancing, gardening and yardwork, various domestic and occupational activities, and games and other childhood pursuits.

15.12* Reduce cigarette smoking to a prevalence of no more than 15 percent among people aged 20 and older. (Baseline: 29 percent in 1987, 32 percent for men and 27 percent for women)

Special Population Targets		
Cigarette Smoking Prevalence	1987 Baseline	2000 Target
15.12a People with a high school education or less aged 20 and older	34%	20%
15.12b Blue-collar workers aged 20 and older	36%	20%
15.12c Military personnel	42%†	20%
15.12d Blacks aged 20 and older	34%	18%
15.12 Hispanics aged 20 and older	33%‡	18%
15.12f American Indians/Alaska Natives	42–70%§	20%
15.12g Southeast Asian men	55%+	20%
15.12h Women of reproductive age	29%††	12%
15.12i Pregnant women	25%‡‡	10%
15.12j Women who use oral contraceptives	36%§§	10%

†1988 baseline.
‡1982–84 baseline for Hispanics aged 20–74.
§1979–87 estimates for different tribes.
+1984–88 baseline.
††Baseline for women aged 18–44.

‡‡*1985 baseline.*
§§*1983 baseline.*

Note: A cigarette smoker is a person who has smoked at least 100 cigarettes and currently smokes cigarettes.

Services and Protection Objectives

15.13 Increase to at least 90 percent the proportion of adults who have had their blood pressure measured within the preceding 2 years and can state whether their blood pressure was normal or high. (Baseline: 61 percent of people aged 18 and older had their blood pressure measured within the preceding 2 years and were given the systolic and diastolic values in 1985)

Note: A blood pressure measurement within the preceding 2 years refers to a measurement by a health professional or other trained observer.

15.14 Increase to at least 75 percent the proportion of adults who have had their blood cholesterol checked within the preceding 5 years. (Baseline: 59 percent of people aged 18 and older had "ever" had their cholesterol checked in 1988; 52 percent were checked "within the preceding 2 years" in 1988)

15.15 Increase to at least 75 percent the proportion of primary care providers who initiate diet and, if necessary, drug therapy at levels of blood cholesterol consistent with current management guidelines for patients with high blood cholesterol. (Baseline data available in 1991)

Note: Current treatment recommendations are outlined in detail in the Report of the Expert Panel on the Detection, Evaluation, and Treatment of High Blood Cholesterol in Adults, released by the National Cholesterol Education Program in 1987. Guidelines appropriate for children are currently being established. Treatment recommendations are likely to be refined over time. Thus, for the year 2000, "current" means whatever recommendations are then in effect.

15.16 Increase to at least 50 percent the proportion of worksites with 50 or more employees that offer high blood pressure and/or cholesterol education and control activities to their employees. (Baseline: 16.5 percent offered high blood pressure activities and 16.8 percent offered nutrition education activities in 1985)

15.17 Increase to at least 90 percent the proportion of clinical laboratories that meet the recommended accuracy standard for cholesterol measurement. (Baseline: 53 percent in 1985)

16. Cancer
Health Status Objectives

16.1* Reverse the rise in cancer deaths to achieve a rate of no more than 130 per 100,000 people. (Age-adjusted baseline: 133 per 100,000 in 1987)

Note: In its publications, the National Cancer Institute age-adjusts cancer death rates to the 1970 U.S. population. Using the 1970 standard, the equivalent baseline and target values for this objective would be 171 and 175 per 100,000, respectively.

16.2* Slow the rise in lung cancer deaths to achieve a rate of no more than 42 per 100,000 people. (Age-adjusted baseline: 37.9 per 100,000 in 1987)

Note: In its publications, the National Cancer Institute age-adjusts cancer death rates to the 1970 U.S. population. Using the 1970 standard, the equivalent baseline and target values for this objective would be 47.9 and 53 per 100,000, respectively.

16.3 Reduce breast cancer deaths to no more than 20.6 per 100,000 women. (Age-adjusted baseline: 22.9 per 100,000 in 1987)

Note: In its publications, the National Cancer Institute age-adjusts cancer death rates to the 1970 U.S. population. Using the 1970 standard, the equivalent baseline and target values for this objective would be 27.2 and 25.2 per 100,000, respectively.

16.4 Reduce deaths from cancer of the uterine cervix to no more than 1.3 per 100,000 women. (Age adjusted baseline: 2.8 per 100,000 in 1987)

Note: In its publications, the National Cancer Institute age-adjusts cancer death rates to the 1970 U.S. population. Using the 1970 standard, the equivalent baseline and target values for this objective would be 3.2 and 1.5 per 100,000, respectively.

16.5 Reduce colorectal cancer deaths to no more than 13.2 per 100,000 people. (Age-adjusted baseline: 14.4 per 100,000 in 1987)

Note: In its publications, the National Cancer Institute age-adjusts cancer death rates to the 1970 U.S. population. Using the 1970 standard, the equivalent baseline and target values for this objective would be 20.1 and 18.7 per 100,000, respectively.

Risk Reduction Objectives

16.6* Reduce cigarette smoking to a prevalence of no more than 15 percent among people aged 20 and older. (Baseline: 29 percent in 1987, 32 percent for men and 27 percent for women)

Special Population Targets

Cigarette Smoking Prevalence	1987 Baseline	2000 Target
16.6a People with a high school education or less aged 20 and older	34%	20%
16.6b Blue-collar workers aged 20 and older	36%	20%
16.6c Military personnel	42%†	20%

16.6d	Blacks aged 20 and older	34%	18%
16.6e	Hispanics aged 20 and older	33%†	18%
16.6f	American Indians/Alaska Natives	42–70%§	20%
16.6g	Southeast Asian men	55%+	20%
16.6h	Women of reproductive age	29%††	12%
16.6i	Pregnant women	25%††	10%
16.6j	Women who use oral contraceptives	36%§§	10%

†1988 baseline.
†1982-84 baseline for Hispanics aged 20–74.
§1979–87 estimates for different tribes.
+1984–88 baseline.
††Baseline for women aged 18–44.
†††1985 baseline.
§§1983 baseline.

Note: A cigarette smoker is a person who has smoked at least 100 cigarettes and currently smokes cigarettes.

16.7* Reduce dietary fat intake to an average of 30 percent of calories or less and average saturated fat intake to less than 10 percent of calories among people aged 2 and older. (Baseline: 36 percent of calories from total fat and 13 percent from saturated fat for people aged 20 through 74 in 1976–80; 36 percent and 13 percent for women aged 19 through 50 in 1985)

Note: The inclusion of a saturated fat target in this objective should not be interpreted as evidence that reducing only saturated fat will reduce cancer risk. Epidemiologic and experimental animal studies suggest that the amount of fat consumed rather than the specific type of fat can influence the risk of some cancers.

16.8* Increase complex carbohydrate and fiber-containing foods in the diets of adults to 5 or more daily servings for vegetables (including legumes) and fruits, and to 6 or more daily servings for grain products. (Baseline: 2½ servings of vegetables and fruits and 3 servings of grain products for women aged 19 through 50 in 1985)

16.9 Increase to at least 60 percent the proportion of people of all ages who limit sun exposure, use sunscreens and protective clothing when exposed to sunlight, and avoid artificial sources of ultraviolet light (e.g., sunlamps, tanning booths). (Baseline data available in 1992)

Services and Protection Objectives

16.10 Increase to at least 75 percent the proportion of primary care providers who routinely counsel patients about tobacco use cessation, diet modification, and cancer-screening recommendations. (Baseline: About 52 percent of internists reported counseling more than 75 percent of their smoking patients about smoking cessation in 1986)

16.11 Increase to at least 80 percent the proportion of women aged 40 and older who have ever received a clinical breast examination and a mammogram, and to at least 60 percent those aged 50 and older who have received them within the preceding 1 to 2 years. (Baseline: 36 percent of women aged 40 and older "ever" in 1987; 25 percent of women aged 50 and older "within the preceding 2 years" in 1987)

Special Population Targets

	Clinical Breast Exam & Mammogram Ever Received	1987 Baseline	2000 Target
16.11a	Hispanic women aged 40 and older	20%	80%
16.11b	Low-income women aged 40 and older (annual family income <$10,000)	22%	80%
16.11c	Women aged 40 and older with less than high school education	23%	80%
16.11d	Women aged 70 and older	25%	80%
16.11e	Black women aged 40 and older	28%	80%
	Received Within Preceding 2 Years		
16.11f	Hispanic women aged 50 and older	18%	60%
16.11g	Low-income women aged 50 and older (annual family income <$10,000)	15%	60%
16.11h	Women aged 50 and older with less than high school education	16%	60%
16.11i	Women aged 70 and older	18%	60%
16.11j	Black women aged 50 and older	19%	60%

16.12 Increase to at least 95 percent the proportion of women aged 18 and older with uterine cervix who have ever received a Pap test, and to at least 85 percent those who received a Pap test within the preceding 1 to 3 years. (Baseline: 88 percent "ever" and 75 percent "within the preceding 3 years" in 1987)

Special Population Targets

Pap Test Ever Received		1987 Baseline	2000 Target
16.12a	Hispanic women aged 18 and older	75%	95%
16.12b	Women aged 70 and older	76%	95%
16.12c	Women aged 18 and older with less than high school education	79%	95%
16.12d	Low-income women aged 18 and older (annual family income <$10,000)	80%	95%

Received Within Preceding 3 Years			
16.12e	Hispanic women aged 18 and older	66%	80%
16.12f	Women aged 70 and older	44%	70%
16.12g	Women aged 18 and older with less than high school education	58%	75%
16.12h	Low-income women aged 18 and older (annual family income <$10,000)	64%	80%

16.13 Increase to at least 50 percent the proportion of people aged 50 and older who have received fecal occult blood testing within the preceding 1 to 2 years, and to at least 40 percent those who have ever received proctosigmoidoscopy. (Baseline: 27 percent received fecal occult blood testing during the preceding 2 years in 1987; 25 percent had ever received proctosigmoidoscopy in 1987)

16.14 Increase to at least 40 percent the proportion of people aged 50 and older visiting a primary care provider in the preceding year who have received oral, skin, and digital rectal examinations during one such visit. (Baseline: An estimated 27 percent received a digital rectal exam during a physician visit within the preceding year in 1987)

16.15 Ensure that Pap tests meet quality standards by monitoring and certifying all cytology laboratories. (Baseline data available in 1991)

16.16 Ensure that mammograms meet quality standards by monitoring and certifying at least 80 percent of mammography facilities. (Baseline: An estimated 18 to 21 percent certified by the American College of Radiology as of June 1990)

17. Diabetes and Chronic Disabling Conditions
Health Status Objectives

Chronic Disabling Conditions

17.1* Increase years of healthy life to at least 65 years. (Baseline: An estimated 62 years in 1980)

Special Population Targets

	Years of Healthy Life	1980 Baseline	2000 Target
17.1a	Blacks	56	60
17.1b	Hispanics	62	65
17.1c	People aged 65 and older	12†	14†

†Years of healthy life remaining at age 65.

Note: Years of healthy life (also referred to as quality-adjusted life years) is a summary measure of health that combines mortality (quantity of life) and morbidity and disability (quality of life) into a single measure. For people aged 65 and older, active life expectancy, a related summary measure, also will be tracked.

17.2 Reduce to no more than 8 percent the proportion of people who experience a limitation in major activity due to chronic conditions. (Baseline: 9.4 percent in 1988)

Special Population Targets

	Prevalence of Disability	1988 Baseline	2000 Target
17.2a	Low-income people (annual family income <$10,000 in 1988)	18.9%	15%
17.2b	American Indians/Alaska Natives	13.4%†	11%
17.2c	Blacks	11.2%	9%

†1983–85 baseline.

Note: Major activity refers to the usual activity for one's age-gender group whether it is working, keeping house, going to school, or living independently. Chronic conditions are defined as conditions that either (1) were first noticed 3 or more months ago or (2) belong to a group of conditions such as heart disease and diabetes, which are considered chronic regardless of when they began.

17.3 Reduce to no more than 90 per 1,000 people the proportion of all people aged 65 and older who have difficulty in performing two or more personal care activities, thereby preserving independence. (Baseline: 111 per 1,000 in 1984–85)

Special Population Targets

	Difficulty Performing Self-Care Activities (per 1,000)	1984–85 Baseline	2000 Target
17.3a	People aged 85 and older	371	325

Note: Personal care activities are bathing, dressing, using the toilet, getting in and out of bed or chair, and eating.

17.4 Reduce to no more than 10 percent the proportion of people with asthma who experience activity limitation. (Baseline: Average of 19.4 percent during 1986–88)

Note: Activity limitation refers to any self-reported limitation in activity attributed to asthma.

17.5 Reduce activity limitation due to chronic back conditions to a prevalence of no more than 19 per 1,000 people. (Baseline: Average of 21.9 per 1,000 during 1986–88)

Note: Chronic back conditions include intervertebral disk disorders, curvature of the back or spine, and other self-reported chronic back impairments such as permanent stiffness or deformity of the back or repeated trouble with the back. Activity limitation refers to any self-reported limitation in activity attributed to a chronic back condition.

17.6 Reduce significant hearing impairment to a prevalence of no more than 82 per 1,000 people. (Baseline: Average of 88.9 per 1,000 during 1986–88)

	Special Population Target	
Hearing Impairment	1986–88	
(per 1,000)	Baseline	2000 Target
17.6a People aged 45 and older	203	180

Note: Hearing impairment covers the range of hearing deficits from mild loss in one ear to profound loss in both ears. Generally, inability to hear sounds at levels softer (less intense) than 20 decibels (dB) constitutes abnormal hearing. Significant hearing impairment is defined as having hearing thresholds for speech poorer than 25 dB. However, for this objective, self-reported hearing impairment (i.e., deafness in one or both ears or any trouble hearing in one or both ears) will be used as a proxy measure for significant hearing impairment.

17.7 Reduce significant visual impairment to a prevalence of no more than 30 per 1,000 people. (Baseline: Average of 34.5 per 1,000 during 1986–88)

	Special Population Target	
	1986–88	
Visual Impairment (per 1,000)	Baseline	2000 Target
17.7a People aged 65 and older	87.7	70

Note: Significant visual impairment is generally defined as a permanent reduction in visual acuity and/or field of vision which is not correctable with eyeglasses or contact lenses. Severe visual impairment is defined as inability to read ordinary newsprint even with corrective lenses. For this objective, self-reported blindness in one or both eyes and other self-reported visual impairments (i.e., any trouble seeing with one or both eyes even when wearing glasses or color blindness) will be used as a proxy measure for significant visual impairment.

17.8* Reduce the prevalence of serious mental retardation in school-aged children to no more than 2 per 1,000 children. (Baseline: 2.7 per 1,000 children aged 10 in 1985–88)

Note: Serious mental retardation is defined as an intelligence quotient (IQ) less than 50. This includes individuals defined by the American Association of Mental Retardation as profoundly retarded (IQ of 20 or less), severely retarded (IQ of 21–35), and moderately retarded (IQ of 36–50).

Diabetes

17.9 Reduce diabetes-related deaths to no more than 34 per 100,000 people. (Age-adjusted baseline: 38 per 100,000 in 1986)

Special Population Targets		
Diabetes-Related Deaths		
(per 100,000)	*1986 Baseline*	*2000 Target*
17.9a Blacks	65	58
17.9b American Indians/Alaska Natives	54	48

Note: Diabetes-related deaths refer to deaths from diabetes as an underlying or contributing cause.

17.10 Reduce the most severe complications of diabetes as follows:

Complications Among People with Diabetes	*1988 Baseline*	*2000 Target*
End-stage renal disease	1.5/1,000†	1.4/1,000
Blindness	2.2/1,000	1.4/1,000
Lower-extrmity amputation	8.1/1,000†	4.9/1,000
Perinatal mortality‡	5%	2%
Major congenital malformations‡	8%	4%

†1987 baseline.
‡Among infants of women with established diabetes.

Special Population Targets for ESRD		
ESRD Due to Diabetes	*1983–86*	
(per 1,000)	*Baseline*	*2000 Target*
17.10a Blacks with diabetes	2.2	2
17.10b American Indians/Alaska Natives with diabetes	2.1	1.9

Special Population Target for Amputations

	Lower Extremity Amputations Due to Diabetes (per 1,000)	1984–87 Baseline	2000 Target
17.10c	Blacks with diabetes	10.2	6.1

Note: End-stage renal disease (ESRD) is defined as requiring maintenance dialysis or transplantation and is limited to ESRD due to diabetes. Blindness refers to blindness due to diabetic eye disease.

17.11 Reduce diabetes to an incidence of no more than 2.5 per 1,000 people and a prevalence of no more than 25 per 1,000 people. (Baseline: 2.9 per 1,000 in 1987; 28 per 1,000 in 1987)

Special Population Targets

	Prevalence of Diabetes (per 1,000)	1982–84 Baseline†	2000 Target
17.11a	American Indians/Alaska Natives	69‡	62
17.11b	Puerto Ricans	55	49
17.11c	Mexican Americans	54	49
17.11d	Cuban Americans	36	32
17.11e	Blacks	36§	32

†1982–84 baseline for people aged 20–74.
‡1987 baseline for American Indians/Alaska Natives aged 15 and older.
§1987 baseline for blacks of all ages.

Risk Reduction Objectives

17.12* Reduce overweight to a prevalence of no more than 20 percent among people aged 20 and older and no more than 15 percent among adolescents aged 12 through 19. (Baseline: 26 percent for people aged 20 through 74 in 1976–80, 24 percent for men and 27 percent for women; 15 percent for adolescents aged 12 through 19 in 1976–80)

Special Population Targets

	Overweight Prevalence	1976–80 Baseline†	2000 Target
17.12a	Low-income women aged 20 and older	37%	25%
17.12b	Black women aged 20 and older	44%	30%
17.12c	Hispanic women aged 20 and older		25%
	Mexican American women	39%‡	
	Cuban women	34%‡	
	Puerto Rican women	37%‡	

17.12d American Indians/Alaska Natives	29–75%§	30%
17.12e People with disabilities	36%+	25%
17.12f Women with high blood pressure	50%	41%
17.12g Men with high blood pressure	39%	35%

†1976–80 baseline for people aged 20–74.

‡1982–84 baseline for Hispanics aged 20–74.

§1984–88 estimates for different tribes.

+1985 baseline for people aged 20–74 who report any limitation in activity due to chronic conditions.

Note: For people aged 20 and older, overweight is defined as body mass index (BMI) equal to or greater than 27.8 for men and 27.3 for women. For adolescents, overweight is defined as BMI equal to or greater than 23.0 for males aged 12 through 14, 24.3 for males aged 15 through 17, 25.8 for males aged 18 through 19, 23.4 for females aged 12 through 14, 24.8 for females aged 15 through 17, and 25.7 for females aged 18 through 19. The values for adolescents are the age- and gender-specific 85th percentile values of the 1976–80 National Health and Nutrition Examination Survey (NHANES II), corrected for sample variation. BMI is calculated by dividing weight in kilograms by the square of height in meters. The cut points used to define overweight approximate the 120 percent of desirable body weight definition used in the 1990 objectives.

17.13* Increase to at least 30 percent the proportion of people aged 6 and older who engage regularly, preferably daily, in light to moderate physical activity for at least 30 minutes per day. (Baseline: 22 percent of people aged 18 and older were active for at least 30 minutes 5 or more times per week and 12 percent were active 7 or more times per week in 1985)

Note: Light to moderate physical activity requires sustained, rhythmic muscular movements, is at least equivalent to sustained walking, and is performed at less than 60 percent of maximum heart rate for age. Maximum heart rate equals roughly 220 beats per minute minus age. Examples may include walking, swimming, cycling, dancing, gardening and yardwork, various domestic and occupational activities, and games and other childhood pursuits.

Services and Protection Objectives

17.14 Increase to at least 40 percent the proportion of people with chronic and disabling conditions who receive formal patient education including information about community and self-help resources as an integral part of the management of their condition. (Baseline data available in 1991)

Type-Specific Targets

Patient Education	1983–84 Baseline	2000 Target
17.14a People with diabetes	32% (classes) 68% (counseling)	75%
17.14b People with asthma	—	50%

17.15 Increase to at least 80 percent the proportion of providers of primary care for children who routinely refer or screen infants and children for impairments of vision, hearing, speech and language, and assess other developmental milestones as part of well-child care. (Baseline data available in 1992)

17.16 Reduce the average age at which children with significant hearing impairment are identified to no more than 12 months. (Baseline: Estimated as 24 to 30 months in 1988)

17.17 Increase to at least 60 percent the proportion of providers of primary care for older adults who routinely evaluate people aged 65 and older for urinary incontinence and impairments of vision, hearing, cognition, and functional status. (Baseline data available in 1992)

17.18 Increase to at least 90 percent the proportion of perimenopausal women who have been counseled about the benefits and risks of estrogen replacement therapy (combined with progestin, when appropriate) for prevention of osteoporosis. (Baseline data available in 1991)

17.19 Increase to at least 75 percent the proportion of worksites with 50 or more employees that have a voluntarily established policy or program for the hiring of people with disabilities. (Baseline: 37 percent of medium and large companies in 1986)

Note: Voluntarily established policies and programs for the hiring of people with disabilities are encouraged for worksites of all sizes. This objective is limited to worksites with 50 or more employees for tracking purposes.

17.20 Increase to 50 the number of states that have service systems for children with or at risk of chronic and disabling conditions, as required by Public Law 101–239. (Baseline data available in 1991)

Note: Children with or at risk of chronic and disabling conditions, often referred to as children with special health care needs, include children with psychosocial as well as physical problems. This population encompasses children with a wide variety of actual or potential disabling conditions, including children with or at risk for cerebral palsy, mental retardation, sensory deprivation, developmental disabilities, spina bifida, hemophilia, other genetic disorders, and health-

related educational and behavioral problems. Service systems for such children are organized networks of comprehensive, community-based, coordinated, and family-centered services.

18. HIV Infection
Health Status Objectives

18.1 Confine annual incidence of diagnosed AIDS cases to no more than 98,000 cases. (Baseline: An estimated 44,000 to 50,000 diagnosed cases in 1989)

Special Population Targets

	Diagnosed AIDS Cases	1989 Baseline	2000 Target
18.1a		26,000–	
	Gay and bisexual men	28,000	48,000
18.1b		14,000–	
	Blacks	15,000	37,000
18.1c	Hispanics	7,000–8,000	18,000

Note: Targets for this objective are equal to upper bound estimates of the incidence of diagnosed AIDS cases projected for 1993.

18.2 Confine the prevalence of HIV infection to no more than 800 per 100,000 people. (Baseline: An estimated 400 per 100,000 in 1989)

Special Population Targets

Estimated Prevalence of HIV Infection (per 100,000)		1989 Baseline	2000 Target
18.2a		2,000–	
	Homosexual men	42,000†	20,000
18.2b		30,000–	
	Intravenous drug abusers	40,000‡	40,000
18.2c	Women giving birth to live-born infants	150	100

†*Per 100,000 homosexual men aged 15 through 24 based on men tested in selected sexually transmitted disease clinics in unlinked surveys; most studies find HIV prevalence of between 2,000 and 21,000 per 100,000.*

‡*Per 100,000 intravenous drug abusers aged 15 through 24 in the New York city vicinity: in areas other than major metropolitan centers, infection rates in people entering selected drug treatment programs tested in unlinked surveys are often under 500 per 100,000.*

Risk Reduction Objectives

18.3* Reduce the proportion of adolescents who have engaged in sexual intercourse to no more than 15 percent by age 15 and no more than 40 percent by age 17. (Baseline: 27 percent of girls and

33 percent of boys by age 15; 50 percent of girls and 66 percent of boys by age 17; reported in 1988)

18.4* Increase to at least 50 percent the proportion of sexually active, unmarried people who used a condom at last sexual intercourse. (Baseline: 19 percent of sexually active, unmarried women aged 15 through 44 reported that their partners used a condom at last sexual intercourse in 1988)

	Special Population Targets		
	Use of Condoms	*1988 Baseline*	*2000 Target*
18.4a	Sexually active young women aged 15–19 (by their partners)	25%	60%
18.4b	Sexually active young men aged 15–19	57%	75%
18.4c	Intravenous drug abusers	—	60%

Note: Strategies to achieve this objective must be undertaken sensitively to avoid indirectly encouraging or condoning sexual activity among teens who are not yet sexually active.

18.5 Increase to at least 50 percent the estimated proportion of all intravenous drug abusers who are in drug abuse treatment programs. (Baseline: An estimated 11 percent of opiate abusers were in treatment in 1989)

18.6 Increase to at least 50 percent the estimated proportion of intravenous drug abusers not in treatment who use only uncontaminated drug paraphernalia ("works"). (Baseline: 25 to 35 percent of opiate abusers in 1989)

18.7 Reduce to no more than 1 per 250,000 units of blood and blood components the risk of transfusion-transmitted HIV infection. (Baseline: 1 per 40,000 to 150,000 units in 1989)

Services and Protection Objectives

18.8 Increase to at least 80 percent the proportion of HIV-infected people who have been tested for HIV infection. (Baseline: An estimated 15 percent of approximately 1,000,000 HIV-infected people had been tested at publicly funded clinics, in 1989)

18.9* Increase to at least 75 percent the proportion of primary care and mental health care providers who provide age-appropriate counseling on the prevention of HIV and other sexually transmitted diseases. (Baseline: 10 percent of physicians reported that they regularly assessed the sexual behaviors of their patients in 1987)

	Special Population Target		
	Counseling on HIV and STD Prevention	*1987 Baseline*	*2000 Target*
18.9a	Providers practicing in high-incidence areas	—	90%

Note: Primary care providers include physicians, nurses, nurse prac-titioners, and physician assistants. Areas of high AIDS and sexually transmitted disease incidence are cities and states with incidence rates of AIDS cases, HIV seroprevalence, gonorrhea, or syphilis that are at least 25 percent above the national average.

18.10 Increase to at least 95 percent the proportion of schools that have age-appropriate HIV education curricula for students in 4th through 12th grade, preferably as part of quality school health education. (Baseline: 66 percent of school districts re-quired HIV education but only 5 percent required HIV educa-tion in each year for 7th through 12th grade in 1989)

Note: Strategies to achieve this objective must be undertaken sensi-tively to avoid indirectly encouraging or condoning sexual activity among teens who are not yet sexually active.

18.11 Provide HIV education for students and staff in at least 90 percent of colleges and universities. (Baseline data available in 1995)

18.12 Increase to at least 90 percent the proportion of cities with populations over 100,000 that have outreach programs to con-tact drug abusers (particularly intravenous drug abusers) to deliver HIV risk reduction messages. (Baseline data available in 1995)

Note: HIV risk reduction messages include messages about reducing or eliminating drug use, entering drug treatment, disinfection of injection equipment if still injecting drugs, and safer sex practices.

18.13* Increase to at least 50 percent the proportion of family planning clinics, maternal and child health clinics, sexually transmitted disease clinics, tuberculosis clinics, drug treatment centers, and primary care clinics that screen, diagnose, treat, counsel, and provide (or refer for) partner notification services for HIV infec-tion and bacterial sexually transmitted diseases (gonorrhea, syphilis, and chlamydia). (Baseline: 40 percent of family plan-ning clinics for bacterial sexually transmitted diseases in 1989)

18.14 Extend to all facilities where workers are at risk for occupa-tional transmission of HIV regulations to protect workers from exposure to bloodborne infections, including HIV infection. (Baseline data available in 1992)

Note: The Occupational Safety and Health Administration (OSHA) is expected to issue regulations requiring worker protection from expo-sure to bloodborne infections, including HIV, during 1991. Imple-mentation of the OSHA regulations would satisfy this objective.

19. Sexually Transmitted Diseases
Health Status Objectives

19.1 Reduce gonorrhea to an incidence of no more than 225 cases per 100,000 people. (Baseline: 300 per 100,000 in 1989)

Special Population Targets

Gonorrhea Incidence (per 100,000)	1989 Baseline	2000 Target
19.1a Blacks	1,990	1,300
19.1b Adolescents aged 15–19	1,123	750
19.1c Women aged 15–44	501	290

19.2 Reduce *Chlamydia trachomatis* infections, as measured by a decrease in the incidence of nongonococcal urethritis to no more than 170 cases per 100,000 people. (Baseline: 215 per 100,000 in 1988)

19.3 Reduce primary and secondary syphilis to an incidence of no more than 10 cases per 100,000 people. (Baseline: 18.1 per 100,000 in 1989)

Special Population Target

Gonorrhea Incidence (per 100,000)	1989 Baseline	2000 Target
19.3a Blacks	118	65

19.4 Reduce congenital syphilis to an incidence of no more than 50 cases per 100,000 live births. (Baseline: 100 per 100,000 live births in 1989)

19.5 Reduce genital herpes and genital warts, as measured by a reduction to 142,000 and 385,000, respectively, in the annual number of first-time consultations with a physician for the conditions. (Baseline: 167,000 and 451,000 in 1988)

19.6 Reduce the incidence of pelvic inflammatory disease, as measured by a reduction in hospitalizations for pelvic inflammatory disease to no more than 250 per 100,000 women aged 15 through 44. (Baseline: 311 per 100,000 in 1988)

19.7 Reduce the rate of repeat gonorrhea infection to no more than 15 percent within the previous year. (Baseline: 20 percent in 1988)

Note: As measured by a reduction in the proportion of gonorrhea patients who, within the previous year, were treated for a separate case of gonorrhea.

Risk Reduction Objectives

19.8* Reduce the proportion of adolescents who have engaged in sexual intercourse to no more than 15 percent by age 15 and no more than 40 percent by age 17. (Baseline: 27 percent of girls and

33 percent of boys by age 15; 50 percent of girls and 66 percent of boys by age 17; reported in 1988)

19.9* Increase to at least 50 percent the proportion of sexually active, unmarried people who used a condom at last sexual intercourse. (Baseline: 19 percent of sexually active, unmarried women aged 15 through 44 reported that their partners used a condom at last sexual intercourse in 1988)

Special Population Targets

Use of Condoms	1988 Baseline	2000 Target
19.9a Sexually active young women aged 15–19 (by their partners)	25%	60%
19.9b Sexually active young men aged 15–19	57%	75%
19.9c Intravenous drug abusers	—	60%

Note: Strategies to achieve this objective must be undertaken sensitively to avoid indirectly encouraging or condoning sexual activity among teens who are not yet sexually active.

Services and Protection Objectives

19.10* Increase to at least 50 percent the proportion of family planning clinics, maternal and child health clinics, sexually transmitted disease clinics, tuberculosis clinics, drug treatment centers, and primary care clinics that screen, diagnose, treat, counsel, and provide (or refer for) partner notification services for HIV infection and bacterial sexually transmitted diseases (gonorrhea, syphilis, and chlamydia). (Baseline: 40 percent of family planning clinics for bacterial sexually transmitted diseases in 1989)

19.11 Include instruction in sexually transmitted disease transmission prevention in the curricula of all middle and secondary schools, preferably as part of quality school health education. (Baseline: 95 percent of schools reported offering at least one class on sexually transmitted diseases as part of their standard curricula in 1988)

Note: Strategies to achieve this objective must be undertaken sensitively to avoid indirectly encouraging or condoning sexual activity among teens who are not yet sexually active.

19.12 Increase to at least 90 percent the proportion of primary care providers treating patients with sexually transmitted diseases who correctly manage cases, as measured by their use of appropriate types and amounts of therapy. (Baseline: 70 percent in 1988)

19.13* Increase to at least 75 percent the proportion of primary care and mental health care providers who provide age-appropriate

counseling on the prevention of HIV and other sexually transmitted diseases. (Baseline: 10 percent of physicians reported
that they regularly assessed the sexual behaviors of their patients in 1987)

Special Population Target

Counseling on HIV and STD Prevention	1987 Baseline	2000 Target
19.13a Providers practicing in high-incidence areas	—	90%

*Note: Primary care providers include physicians, nurses, nurse prac-
titioners, and physician assistants. Areas of high AIDS and sexually
transmitted disease incidence are cities and states with incidence rates
of AIDS cases, HIV seroprevalence, gonorrhea, or syphilis that are at
least 25 percent above the national average.*

19.14 Increase to at least 50 percent the proportion of all patients with
bacterial sexually transmitted diseases (gonorrhea, syphilis, and
chlamydia) who are offered provider referral services. (Baseline:
20 percent of those treated in sexually transmitted disease clinics
in 1988)

*Note: Provider referral (previously called contact tracing) is the process
whereby health department personnel directly notify the sexual partners of infected individuals of their exposure to an infected individual.*

20. Immunization and Infectious Diseases
Health Status Objectives

20.1 Reduce indigenous cases of vaccine-preventable diseases as
follows:

Disease	1988 Baseline	2000 Target
Diphtheria among people aged 25 and younger	1	0
Tetanus among people aged 25 and younger	3	0
Polio (wild-type virus)	0	0
Measles	3,058	0
Rubella	225	0
Congenital rubella syndrome	6	0
Mumps	4,866	500
Pertussis	3,450	1,000

20.2 Reduce epidemic-related pneumonia and influenza deaths
among people aged 65 and older to no more than 7.3 per 100,000.
(Baseline: Average of 9.1 per 100,000 during 1980 through 1987)

Note: Epidemic-related pneumonia and influenza deaths are those that occur above and beyond the normal yearly fluctuations of mortality. Because of the extreme variability in epidemic-related deaths from year to year, the target is a 3-year average.

20.3* Reduce viral hepatitis as follows:

(Per 100,000)	1987 Baseline	2000 Target
Hepatitis B (HBV)	63.5	40
Hepatitis A	31	23
Hepatitis C	18.3	13.7

Special Population Targets for HBV

	HBV Cases	1987 Estimated Baseline	2000 Target
20.3a	Intravenous drug abusers	30,000	22,500
20.3b	Heterosexually active people	33,000	22,000
20.3c	Homosexual men	25,300	8,500
20.3d	Children of Asians/Pacific Islanders	8,900	1,800
20.3e	Occupationally exposed workers	6,200	1,250
20.3f	Infants	3,500	550 new carriers
20.3g	Alaska Natives	15	1

20.4 Reduce tuberculosis to an incidence of no more than 3.5 cases per 100,000 people. (Baseline: 9.1 per 100,000 in 1988)

Special Population Targets

Tuberculosis Cases (per 100,000)		1988 Baseline	2000 Target
20.4a	Asians/Pacific Islanders	36.3	15
20.4b	Blacks	28.3	10
20.4c	Hispanics	18.3	5
20.4d	American Indians/Alaska Natives	18.1	5

20.5 Reduce by at least 10 percent the incidence of surgical wound infections and nosocomial infections in intensive care patients. (Baseline data available in late 1990)

20.6 Reduce selected illness among international travelers as follows:

Incidence	1987 Baseline	2000 Target
Typhoid fever	280	140
Hepatitis A	1,280	640
Malaria	2,000	1,000

20.7 Reduce bacterial meningitis to no more than 4.7 cases per 100,000 people. (Baseline: 6.3 per 100,000 in 1986)

Special Population Target
Bacterial Meningitis Cases

(per 100,000)	*1986 Baseline*	*2000 Target*
20.7a Alaska Natives	33	8

20.8 Reduce infectious diarrhea by at least 25 percent among children in licensed child care centers and children in programs that provide an individualized education program (IEP) or individualized health plan (IHP). (Baseline data available in 1992)

20.9 Reduce acute middle-ear infections among children aged 4 and younger, as measured by days of restricted activity or school absenteeism, to no more than 105 days per 100 children. (Baseline: 131 days per 100 children in 1987)

20.10 Reduce pneumonia-related days of restricted activity as follows:

	1987 Baseline	*2000 Target*
People aged 65 and older (per 100 people)	48 days	38 days
Children aged 4 and younger (per 100 children)	27 days	24 days

Risk Reduction Objectives

20.11 Increase immunization levels as follows:

Basic immunization series among children under age 2: at least 90 percent. (Baseline: 70–80 percent estimated in 1989)

Basic immunization series among children in licensed child care facilities and kindergarten through postsecondary education institutions: at least 95 percent. (Baseline: For licensed child care, 94 percent; 97 percent for children entering school for the 1987–1988 school year; and for postsecondary institutions, baseline data available in 1992)

Pneumococcal pneumonia and influenza immunization among institutionalized chronically ill or older people: at least 80 percent. (Baseline data available in 1992)

Pneumococcal pneumonia and influenza immunization among noninstitutionalized, high-risk populations, as defined by the Immunization Practices Advisory Committee: at least 60 percent. (Baseline: 10 percent estimated for pneumococcal vaccine and 20 percent for influenza vaccine in 1985)

Hepatitis B immunization among high-risk populations, including infants of surface antigen-positive mothers to at least 90 percent; occupationally exposed workers to at least 90 percent; IV-drug users in drug treatment programs to at least 50 percent;

and homosexual men to at least 50 percent. (Baseline data available in 1992)

20.12 Reduce postexposure rabies treatments to no more than 9,000 per year. (Baseline: 18,000 estimated treatments in 1987)

Services and Protection Objectives

20.13 Expand immunization laws for schools, preschools, and day care settings to all states for all antigens. (Baseline: 9 states and the District of Columbia in 1990)

20.14 Increase to at least 90 percent the proportion of primary care providers who provide information and counseling about immunizations and offer immunizations as appropriate for their patients. (Baseline data available in 1992)

20.15 Improve the financing and delivery of immunizations for children and adults so that virtually no American has a financial barrier to receiving recommended immunizations. (Baseline: Financial coverage for immunizations was included in 45 percent of employment-based insurance plans with conventional insurance plans; 62 percent with preferred provider organization plans; and 98 percent with health maintenance organization plans in 1989; Medicaid covered basic immunizations for eligible children and Medicare covered pneumococcal immunization for eligible older adults in 1990)

20.16 Increase to at least 90 percent the proportion of public health departments that provide adult immunization for influenza, pneumococcal disease, hepatitis B, tetanus, and diphtheria. (Baseline data available in 1991)

20.17 Increase to at least 90 percent the proportion of local health departments that have ongoing programs for actively identifying cases of tuberculosis and latent infection in populations at high risk for tuberculosis. (Baseline data available in 1991)

Note: Local health department refers to any local component of the public health system, defined as an administrative and service unit of local or state government concerned with health and carrying some responsibility for the health of a jurisdiction smaller than a state.

20.18 Increase to at least 85 percent the proportion of people found to have tuberculosis infection who completed courses of preventive therapy. (Baseline: 89 health departments reported that 66.3 percent of 95,201 persons placed on preventive therapy completed their treatment in 1987)

20.19 Increase to at least 85 percent the proportion of tertiary care hospital laboratories and to at least 50 percent the proportion of secondary care hospital and health maintenance organization laboratories possessing technologies for rapid viral diagnosis of influenza. (Baseline data available in 1992)

21. Clinical Preventive Services
Health Status Objective

21.1* Increase years of healthy life to at least 65 years. (Baseline: An estimated 62 years in 1980)

Special Population Targets

Years of Healthy Life		1980 Baseline	2000 Target
21.1a	Blacks	56	60
21.1b	Hispanics	62	65
21.1c	People aged 65 and older	12†	14†

†*Years of health life remaining at age 65.*

Note: Years of healthy life (also referred to as quality-adjusted life years) is a summary measure of health that combines mortality (quantity of life) and morbidity and disability (quality of life) into a single measure. For people aged 65 and older, active life expectancy, a related summary measure, also will be tracked.

Risk Reduction Objective

Special Population Targets

Receipt of Recommended Services		Baseline	2000 Target
21.2a	Infants up to 24 months	—	90%
21.2b	Children aged 2–12	—	80%
21.2c	Adolescents aged 13–18	—	50%
21.2d	Adults aged 19 –39	—	40%
21.2e	Adults aged 40–64	—	40%
21.2f	Adults aged 65 and older	—	40%
21.2g	Low-income people	—	50%
21.2h	Blacks	—	50%
21.2i	Hispanics	—	50%
21.2j	Asians/Pacific Islanders	—	50%
21.2k	American Indians/Alaska Natives	—	70%
21.2l	People with disabilities	—	80%

Services and Protection Objectives

21.3 Increase to at least 95 percent the proportion of people who have a specific source of ongoing primary care for coordination of their preventive and episodic health care. (Baseline: Less than 82 percent in 1986, as 18 percent reported having no physician, clinic, or hospital as a regular source of care)

Special Population Targets

Percentage with Source of Care		1986 Baseline	2000 Target
21.3a	Hispanics	70%	95%
21.3b	Blacks	80%	95%
21.3c	Low-income people	80%	95%

21.4 Improve financing and delivery of clinical preventive services so that virtually no American has a financial barrier to receiving, at a minimum, the screening, counseling, and immunization services recommended by the U.S. Preventive Services Task Force. (Baseline data available in 1992)

21.5 Assure that at least 90 percent of people for whom primary care services are provided directly by publicly funded programs are offered, as a minimum, the screening, counseling, and immunization services recommended by the U.S. Preventive Services Task Force. (Baseline data available in 1992)

Note: Publicly funded programs that provide primary care services directly include federally funded programs such as the Maternal and Child Health Program, Community and Migrant Health Centers, and the Indian Health Service as well as primary care service settings funded by state and local governments. This objective does not include services covered indirectly through the Medicare and Medicaid programs.

21.6 Increase to at least 50 percent the proportion of primary care providers who provide their patients with the screening, counseling, and immunization services recommended by the U.S. Preventive Services Task Force. (Baseline data available in 1992)

21.7 Increase to at least 90 percent the proportion of people who are served by a local health department that assesses and assures access to essential clinical preventive services. (Baseline data available in 1992)

Note: Local health department refers to any local component of the public health system, defined as an administrative and service unit of local or state government concerned with health and carrying some responsibility for the health of a jurisdiction smaller than a state.

21.8 Increase the proportion of all degrees in the health professions and allied and associated health profession fields awarded to members of underrepresented racial and ethnic minority groups as follows:

Degrees Awarded To:	1985–86 Baseline	2000 Target
Blacks	5%	8%
Hispanics	3%	6.4%
American Indians/Alaska Natives	0.3%	0.6%

Note: Underrepresented minorities are those groups consistently below parity in most health profession schools—blacks, Hispanics, and American Indians and Alaska Natives.

22. Surveillance and Data Systems Objectives

22.1 Develop a set of health status indicators appropriate for federal, state, and local health agencies and establish use of the set in at least 40 states. (Baseline: No such set exists in 1990)

22.2 Identify, and create where necessary, national data sources to measure progress toward each of the year 2000 national health objectives. (Baseline: 77 percent of the objectives have baseline data in 1990)

Type-Specific Target

1989 Baseline   2000 Target

22.2a   State level data for at least two-thirds of the objectives   23 states†   35 states

†*Measured using the 1989 Draft Year 2000 National Health Objectives.*

22.3 Develop and disseminate among federal, state, and local agencies procedures for collecting comparable data for each of the year 2000 national health objectives and incorporate these into Public Health Service data collection systems. (Baseline: Although such surveys as the National Health Interview Survey may serve as a model, widely accepted procedures do not exist in 1990)

22.4 Develop and implement a national process to identify significant gaps in the nation's disease prevention and health promotion data, including data for racial and ethnic minorities, people with low incomes, and people with disabilities, and establish mechanisms to meet these needs. (Baseline: No such process exists in 1990)

Note: Disease prevention and health promotion data include disease status, risk factors, and services receipt data. Public health problems include such issue areas as HIV infection, domestic violence, mental health, environmental health, occupational health, and disabling conditions.

22.5 Implement in all states periodic analysis and publication of data needed to measure progress toward objectives for at least 10 of the priority areas of the national health objectives. (Baseline: 20 states reported they disseminate the analyses they use to assess state progress toward the health objectives to the public and to the health professionals in 1989)

Type-Specific Target

1989 Baseline   2000 Target

22.5a   Periodic analysis and publication of state progress toward the national objectives for each racial or ethnic group that makes up at least 10 percent of the state population   —   25 states

Note: Periodic is at least once every 3 years. Objectives include, at a minimum, one from each objectives category: health status, risk reduction, and services and protection.

22.6 Expand in all states systems for the transfer of health information related to the national health objectives among federal, state, and local agencies. (Baseline: 30 states reported that they have some capability for transfer of health data, tables, graphs, and maps to federal, state, and local agencies that collect and analyze data in 1989)

Note: Information related to the national health objectives includes state and national level baseline data, disease prevention/health promotion evaluation results, and data generated to measure progress.

22.7 Achieve timely release of national surveillance and survey data needed by health professionals and agencies to measure progress toward the national health objectives. (Baseline data available in 1993)

Note: Timely release (publication of provisional or final data or public use data tapes) should be based on the use of the data, but is at least within one year of the end of data collection.

Age-Related Objectives

Reduce the death rate for adolescents and young adults by 15 percent to no more than 85 per 100,000 people aged 15 through 24. (Baseline: 99.4 per 100,000 in 1987)

Reduce the death rate for adults by 20 percent to no more than 340 per 100,000 people aged 25 through 64. (Baseline: 423 per 100,000 in 1987)

Suggestions for Further Reading

Ames, E. E., L. A. Trucano, J. C. Wan, and M. H. Harris. 1992. *Designing School Health Curricula: Planning for Good Health.* Dubuque, IA: W. C. Brown.

Fodor, J. and G. Dalis. 1974. *Health Instruction: Theory Application.* Philadelphia: Lea and Febiger.

Green, L. W., and M. W. Kreuter. 1991. *Health Promotion and Planning an Educational and Environmental Approach.* Mountain View, CA: Mayfield.

Greenberg, J. S. 1988. *Health Education: Learner-Centered Instructional Strategies.* Dubuque, IA: W. C. Brown.

Greenberg, J. S., and C. E. Bruess. 1981. *Sex Education: Theory and Practice.* Belmont, CA: Wadsworth.

Hoff, R. 1988. *I Can See You Naked.* New York: Andrews and McMeel.

Means, R. K. 1962. *A History of Health Education in the U.S.* Philadelphia: Lea and Febiger.

Meeks, L., and P. Heit. 1992. *Health Education Strategies.* Meeks/Heit Publishing. Blacklick, OH.

National Task Force on the Preparation and Practice of Health Educators, Inc. 1983. *A Guide for the Development of Competency-Based Curricula for Entry Level Health Educators.* New York.

National Task Force on the Preparation and Practice of Health Educators, Inc. 1985. *A Framework for the Development of Competency-Based Curricula for Entry Level Health Educators.* New York.

Report of the Secretary's Task Force on Black and Minority Health. 1985. Washington, DC: U.S. Department of Health and Human Services.

U.S. Department of Health and Human Services. 1980. Promoting Health/Preventing Disease: Objectives for the Nation. U.S. Public Health Service.

U.S. Department of Health and Human Services. 1981. National Conference for Institutions Preparing Health Educators: Proceedings. Birmingham, AL., DHHS Publication 81-50171.

U.S. Department of Health and Human Services. 1992. Healthy Communities 2000: Model Standards. U.S. Public Health Service.

U.S. Department of Health and Human Services. 1992. *Healthy People 2000: National Health Promotion Objectives Full Report, With Commentary.* Boston: Jones and Bartlett Publishers.

Glossary

Entry Level Health Educator Competencies Addressed In This Chapter

Responsibility VI: Acting as a Resource Person in Health Education

Competency A: Utilize computerized health information retrieval systems effectively.

Competency B: Establish effective consultative relationships with those requesting assistance in solving health-related problems.

Competency C: Interpret and respond to requests for health information.

Competency D: Select effective resource materials for dissemination.

Taken from *A Framework for the Development of Competency-Based Curricula for Entry Level Health Educators,* National Task Force on the Preparation and Practice of Health Educators, Inc., 1985. Reprinted by permission.

Method Selection in Health Education

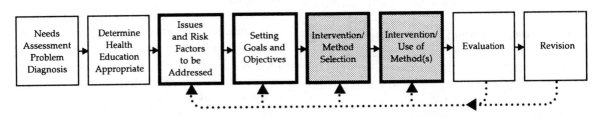

Heavy-bordered boxes indicate subjects addressed in this text; shaded boxes indicate subject(s) of current chapter.

American sign language The native language of most culturally deaf Americans, this is a visually based language that bears little relationship to English, particularly in grammar and syntax.

CD-ROM Compact disk read-only memory.

Certified Health Education Specialist (CHES) An individual who is credentialed as a result of demonstrating competency based on criteria established by the National Commission for Health Education Credentialing, Inc. (NCHEC). (1990 Joint Committee on Health Education Terminology)

Community health education The application of a variety of methods that result in the education and mobilization of community members in actions for resolving health issues and problems that affect the community. These methods include, but are not limited to: group process, mass media, communication, community organization, organization development, strategic planning, skills training, legislation, policy making, and advocacy. (1990 Joint Committee on Health Education Terminology)

Community health educator A practitioner professionally prepared in the field of community/public health education who demonstrates competence in the planning, implementation, and evaluation of a broad range of health-promoting or health enhancing programs for community groups. (1990 Joint Committee on Health Education Terminology)

Comprehensive school health program The development, delivery, and evaluation of a planned curriculum, preschool through 12, with goals, objectives, content sequence, and specific classroom lessons. It includes, but is not limited to, the following major content areas:

> Community health
> Consumer health
> Environmental health
> Family life

> Mental and emotional health
> Injury prevention and safety
> Nutrition
> Personal health
> Prevention and control of disease
> Substance use and abuse

(1990 Joint Committee on Health Education Terminology)

Contact time The time spent with a target group as part of a health education intervention.

Deaf A hearing impairment so severe that an individual is impaired in processing linguistic information through hearing. (Federal Register, 1977)

Demographics Information such as ages, ethnicity, gender, and other characteristics that describe a population and may impact objectives and method selection.

Diffusion The process of making innovations/ methods available and understandable to practicing health educators.

Disability A total or partial behavioral, mental, physical, or sensorial loss of functioning. (Mandell & Fiscus, 1981)

Exceptional A label usually associated with an individual whose performance is atypical and often deviates from what is expected. The performance could be superior or inferior to what is expected. (Mandell & Fiscus, 1981)

Facilitator The leader or teacher of a method or strategy.

Family life Also known as family living, human sexuality, sex education. Scope and depth of information can vary in the extreme, according to the specific situation.

Goal A broad statement of direction used to present the overall intent of a program or course. Unlike an objective, it does not need to be stated in measurable terms.

Handicap Environmental restrictions placed on a person's life as a result of a disability or exceptionality. (Mandell & Fiscus, 1981)

Hard of hearing A hearing impairment, either permanent or fluctuating, which adversely affects an individual's educational performance. (Federal Register, 1977)

Health advising A process of informing and assisting individuals or groups in making decisions and solving problems related to health. (1990 Joint Committee on Health Education Terminology)

Health education (1) A discipline dedicated to the improvement of the health status of individuals and the community. (2) The process of favorably and voluntarily influencing the health behavior of others.

Health education administrator A professional health educator who has the authority and responsibility for the management and coordination of all health education policies, activities, and resources within a particular setting or circumstance. (1990 Joint Committee on Health Education Terminology)

Health education coordinator A professional health educator who is responsible for the management and coordination of all health education policies, activities, and resources within a particular setting or circumstance. (1990 Joint Committee on Health Education Terminology)

Health education field The multi-disciplinary practice concerned with designing, implementing, and evaluating educational programs that enable individuals, families, groups, organizations, and communities to play active roles in achieving, protecting, and sustaining health. (1990 Joint Committee on Health Education Terminology)

Health education process The continuum of learning that enables people, as individuals and as members of social structures, to voluntarily make decisions, modify behaviors, and change social conditions in ways that are health enhancing.

Health education program A planned combination of activities developed with the involvement of specific populations and based on a needs assessment, sound principles of educa-

tion, and periodic evaluation using a clear set of goals and objectives. (1990 Joint Committee on Health Education Terminology)

Health educator A practitioner professionally prepared in the field of health education who demonstrates competence in both theory and practice, and who accepts responsibility to advance the aims of the health education profession. (1990 Joint Committee on Health Education Terminology)

Health information The content of communications based on data derived from systematic and scientific methods as they relate to health issues, policies, programs, services, and other aspects of individual and public health, which can be used for informing various populations and for planning health education activities. (1990 Joint Committee on Health Education Terminology)

Health literacy The capacity of an individual to obtain, interpret, and understand basic health information and services and the competence to use such information and services in ways that are health enhancing. (1990 Joint Committee on Health Education Terminology)

Health promotion and disease prevention The aggregate of all purposeful activities designed to improve personal and public health through a combination of strategies, including the competent implementation of behavioral change strategies, health education, health protection measures, risk factor detection, health enhancement and health maintenance. (1990 Joint Committee on Health Education Terminology)

Healthy lifestyle A set of health-enhancing behaviors shaped by internally consistent values, attitudes, beliefs and external social and cultural forces. (1990 Joint Committee on Health Education Terminology)

Hispanic A classification of national background. A Hispanic person may be from any ethnic group.

Implementation The carrying out of or operationalizing of a plan of action.

Innovation An educational tool or method perceived as being new to potential users.

Intervention The total overall strategy to achieve our objectives.

Lesson/presentation plan The organized plan for a presentation.

Long-range goals The very broad outcome intentions for the unit. These are optimal behaviors the educator hopes to achieve; they need not be easily measurable.

Method One component of the intervention such as an educational game or a health fair. We use the term interchangeably with strategy.

Objective A precise statement of intended outcome; it must be stated in measurable terms.

Official health agency A publicly supported government organization mandated by public law and/or regulation for the protection and improvement of the health of the public.

Post-secondary health education program A planned set of health education policies, procedures, activities, and services that are directed to students, faculty and/or staff of colleges, universities, and other higher education institutions. This includes, but is not limited to:

general health courses for students
employee and student health promotion activities
health services
professional preparation of health educators and other professionals
self-help groups
student life

(1990 Joint Committee on Health Education Terminology)

Postlingual deafness Deafness that occurs after spoken language has been developed.

Prelingual deafness Deafness that occurs before spoken language skills have been developed.

Private health agency A profit or nonprofit organization devoted to providing primary, secondary, and/or tertiary health services which may include health education. (1990 Joint Committee on Health Education Terminology)

School health education One component of the comprehensive school health program which includes the development, delivery, and evaluation of a planned instructional program and other activities for students preschool through grade 12, for parents and for school staff. It is designed to influence positively the health knowledge, attitudes, and skills of individuals. (1990 Joint Committee on Health Education Terminology)

School health educator A practitioner who is professionally prepared in the field of school health education; meets state teaching requirements; and has demonstrated competence in the development, delivery, and evaluation of curricula for students and adults in the school setting that enhance health knowledge, attitudes, and problem-solving skills. (1990 Joint Committee on Health Education Terminology)

School health services That part of the school health program provided by physicians, nurses, dentists, health educators, other allied health personnel, social workers, teachers and others to appraise, protect and promote the health of students and school personnel. These services are designed to ensure access to and appropriate use of primary health care services, prevent and control communicable disease, provide emergency care for injury or sudden illness, promote and provide optimum sanitary conditions in a safe school facility and environment, and provide concurrent learning opportunities which are conducive to the maintenance and promotion of individual and community health. (1990 Joint Committee on Health Education Terminology)

Self-efficacy Belief or expectation by an individual that he or she can carry out the desired behavior.

Sex educator An individual who teaches about human sexuality. Although professional certification can be obtained through AASECT (American Association of Sex Educators, Counselors & Therapists), many individuals may have little or no training.

Simulation The simulation is contrived experience used to expose someone to a certain prescribed set of circumstances based on a model. It has the appearance of some real-life phenomenon.

Strategy One component of the intervention such as an educational game or a health fair. We use the term interchangeably with method.

Target population The population for whom we are targeting our health education intervention.

Two-committee system A system designed to minimize complaint and maximize community involvement when developing materials and programs that might be viewed as controversial.

Unit plan An orderly self-contained collection of activities designed to meet a set of given objectives.

Visually impaired Individuals who have defective or impaired vision. Definitions of impairment or blindness can be either legally or educationally based. (Meyen 1978)

Voluntary health organization A nonprofit association supported by contributions dedicated to conducting research and providing education and/or services related to particular health problems or concerns. (1990 Joint Committee on Health Education Terminology)

REFERENCES

Federal Register (Part IV). Washington DC: Department of Health, Education, and Welfare, August 23, 1977, 42 (163).

Mandell, C. J. and E. Fiscus. E. 1981. *Understanding exceptional people.* St. Paul, MN: West Publishing Co.

Meyen, E. L. (1978). *Exceptional children and youth.* Denver: Love Publishing Co.

Report of the 1990 Joint Committee on Health Education Terminology, *Journal of Health Education,* March–April 1991, Volume 22, No. 2.

Index